Here Is What They Are Saying

"Thank you for making my pregnancy a positive experience. Before seeing you I didn't even know how to move. You taught me how to take care of myself."
—E.E. (pregnant patient with pubic pain)

"My weekly visits to you were a godsend. You keep me out of pain and you prepared me for labor by keeping me calm and showing me how to use my pelvic floor muscles and my abdominal muscles correctly."
—V.D. (pregnant patient with low back pain)

"Before I came in for treatment I was a mess. I didn't think I could make it through the pregnancy without you. I have a high power job and you made the exercises simple and easy to do at work."
—J. M. (pregnant patient with sacroiliac pain)

"At first I didn't like the belts. I am in the fashion world and I need to look good. But the belts helped me to function. Thank you for showing me how to wear them so they were less conspicuous. Thank you for drilling into me that without those belts I wouldn't be able to function. You were right. I am grateful to all of you."
—K.M. (pregnant patient with sacroiliac joint pain)

"I am convinced that my labor and delivery were easy because of your help. I also had an easier time after the baby came because I followed your exercises. I kept hearing your voice in my head: 'Sit straight'; 'Don't slouch'; 'Don't work all day sitting without standing up.' You saved my life. I recommend all women seek prenatal physical therapy."
— J.V. (pregnant patient with vulvodynia)

"I didn't know anything about the pelvic floor muscles and having to massage these muscles was not high on my list. You showed me how to do this massage correctly and I didn't tear in childbirth. I owe you big time."
—K.W. (pregnant patient with pelvic floor muscle spasms)

D0746286

ENDING PAIN IN PREGNANCY

Trade Secrets for an Injury-Free Childbirth,
Relieving Pelvic Girdle Pain, and
Creating Powerful Pelvic Muscles

Isa Herrera
MSPT, CSCS

Published in the United States by Duplex Publishing, New York
1st Edition
10 Digit ISBN: 0692237216
13 Digit EAN: 978-0692237216

Medical Disclaimer:

Consult and seek the advice of your Doctor and/or Physical Therapist before attempting these exercises or self-help tools found in *Ending Pain in Pregnancy*. The medical information in this book is provided for informational purposes only, and is not to be used or relied on for any diagnostic or treatment purposes. This information is intended to be educational only and does not create any patient-physical therapist relationship, and should not be used as a substitute for professional diagnosis and treatment. Serious injury could result from improper performance of these techniques and exercises. If pain occurs with any exercise STOP immediately. Neither Renew Physical Therapy, PC nor Isa Herrera, MSPT, CSCS can be held liable for injury caused by the improper performance of these exercises or self-help tools. The self-help tips found in this book are merely a guide; this book is not intended as a prescription for Physical Therapy. To prevent injury seek the advice of your doctor or physical therapist before attempting any exercise, self-help tip or implementation of any of the information in this book.

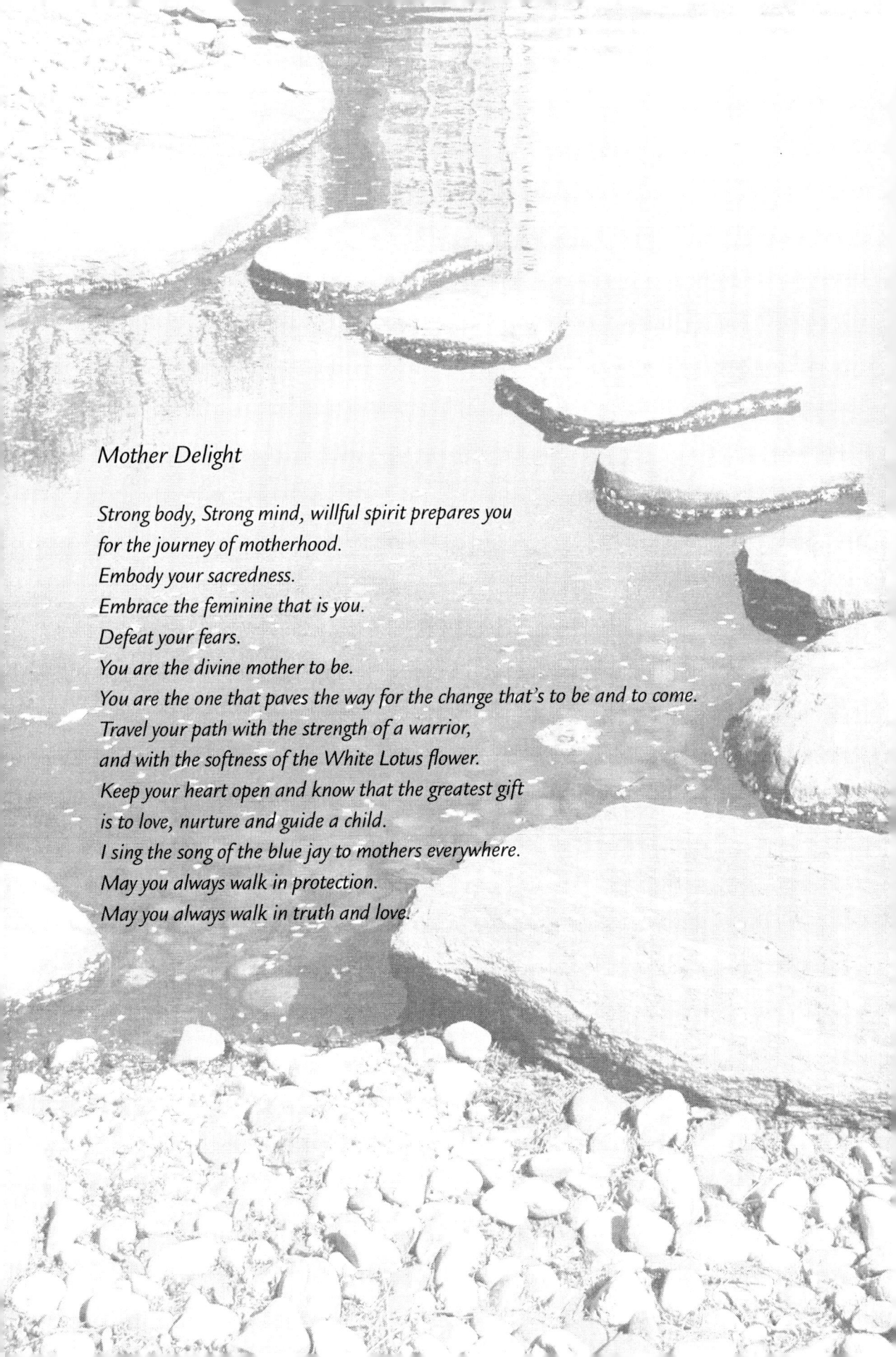

Mother Delight

Strong body, Strong mind, willful spirit prepares you
for the journey of motherhood.
Embody your sacredness.
Embrace the feminine that is you.
Defeat your fears.
You are the divine mother to be.
You are the one that paves the way for the change that's to be and to come.
Travel your path with the strength of a warrior,
and with the softness of the White Lotus flower.
Keep your heart open and know that the greatest gift
is to love, nurture and guide a child.
I sing the song of the blue jay to mothers everywhere.
May you always walk in protection.
May you always walk in truth and love.

Special Thanks

David Ondrick
Digital Production, Project Management and Editing
Thank you for your tech support, ideas and doing whatever is needed to get the
job done. You do it with grace. You listen to me and have always supported me
through all three books. Without you I don't think I could do all the work.
You have been there since day one and you believe in this work.

Collin Pisarra
Digital Photos and Illustrations
Thank you for working with me on this book. You always make time for me
even though you are so busy. Your graphics add beauty to this book.

Winston Johnson
Illustrations
You are an amazing artist. Thank you for all your help in creating the beautiful diagrams.

Maria Carbardo and Cindy Ondrick
Book Designers
You are the best; you have supported me with all three books. You are both miracle workers. Your
work is gorgeous and you are a true artists and true friends. Thank you for all your support through-
out all these years. It is wonderful to have you in my life.

Dr. Moritz
Foreword
You support my work and me in the most beautiful of ways. Thank you for
allowing me to have the birth of my dreams and for delivering my daughter safely
in my hands. You are a great friend. Thank you for writing the foreword. You rock!!

To my Renew PT Team and Contributing Authors:
Rachel Schneiderman, Justine Picciano, and Catherine Garro.
Thank you for your contributions to the book. Thank you for being part of my team and working
hard for the divine feminine. You guys do amazing work and you do it with grace.

Marissa Klapwald:
Main Editor
Best editor in the world. This is our third book together. You know how to tease
the words and make them work so the message is loud and clear. Thank you.

This book is dedicated to my beautiful and amazing daughter,
Ella-Jade, and to my loving and awesome husband David.
I am grateful to you both. You guys are the best part of my life.
You hold space for me and support me in the most loving of ways.
Thank you for letting me write at all hours of the day and night—
including getaways and vacations! Your sacrifices are deeply appreciated
and do not go unnoticed. I will cherish you forever.
To Crusita Soto, my mom, who showed me that birth is beautiful,
natural and nothing to be afraid of.

Ending Pain in Pregnancy author Isa Herrera would like to give special thanks for the amazing work from her contributing authors:

Rachel Schneiderman, DPT, ATC
Chapter 3: Pregnancy Exercise Guidelines and
Listening to Your Body's Messages

Chapter 5: Be Your Own Healer: Align Your Pelvis, Stay Out of Pain
and Keep Your Baby in the Best Position

Justine Picciano, DPT
Chapter 4: Stop Destructive Forces Now: Avoid Injury and Pain with Our Trade Secrets

Chapter 6: Relieving Back Pain, Sciatica
and Sacroiliac Joint Pain: How to Create a Stable Body
and Avoid Pain with the Magical 8

Isa Herrera, MSPT, CSCS, Rachel Schneiderman, DPT, ATC, and Justine Picciano, DPT
Chapter 11: Twenty-Five Things You May Not Want to
Know about Birth—and the Truth That Will Set You Free

Isa Herrera, MSPT, CSCS, and Catherine Garro, Clinical Aromatherapist
Chapter 15: Aromatherapy for Today's Pregnant Woman

Contents

Contents, Continued

FOREWORD BY DR. JACQUES MORITZ

Director, Division of Gynecology, Mount Sinai Roosevelt Hospital

Every once in a while a book comes along that is an expert manual. A book that teaches us a different way of being and helps us to conquer our health conditions and create well-being. It does not surprise me that Isa has decided to write a book of this caliber. *Ending Pain in Pregnancy* is a mind-body-spirit book filled with educational strategies that every pregnant women should know about. This book, like her last book *Ending Female Pain,* is a powerhouse that helps women overcome many of the common physical symptoms and pain experienced in pregnancy.

I have treated pregnant women for over twenty-five years and I see them come in various states of health and many times they come in with extreme pain and aches. Unable to walk and sit and do simple day-to-day things. Pregnancy can take women by surprise because many are not prepared for the physical challenges that the body has to undergo to grow a baby. There is little help that my field of medicine can offer these women in pain. I have learned over the years that these women need to be referred to physical therapy for help.

Many of my colleagues might not share this point of view but I have seen over and over where physiotherapy can get women out of pain and functioning again while pregnant. Isa has taken this type of therapy to the next level. Her treatments are powerful and produce extraordinary pain relief. Not only does her therapy work but I also often find that the women who come back from seeing her have learned how to take care and heal themselves. These women undergo a profound transformation and they feel empowered and ready to move through the pregnancy into the next phase, childbirth. I invite you to enjoy the fruits of her labor, as you learn how to heal and empower yourself using the tools and techniques in this great resource.

PART ONE:

PREGNANCY POWER: BUILDING A POWERFUL BODY AND AN AWESOME PREGNANCY EXPERIENCE WITH TIME-PROVEN STRATEGIES

*"To be pregnant is to be
vitally alive, thoroughly woman,
and undoubtedly inhabited."*

– Anne Buchanan & Debra Klingsporn

Chapter I

INTRODUCTION

Does the world really need another pregnancy book? The answer is *yes* because there is no other pregnancy resource like *Ending Pain in Pregnancy*. This book is designed to awaken the healer within and to put you on the right path to a pain-free pregnancy, an amazing birth experience, and a speedy postpartum recovery.

My first exposure to pregnancy pain came when I taught prenatal and postnatal exercise classes in New York City. I was interested in what my prenatal students had to say about the pain they were feeling. They would tell me: "I just can't walk anymore because I have pain in my pubic bone," "I can't lift or play with my younger child because my back is killing me," "Every time I cough or laugh I leak on myself," or "I feel pressure inside my vagina and don't know what to do about it." I wanted to help these women, but as a prenatal and postnatal fitness instructor I lacked the specific tools and knowledge. In physical therapy school little is taught about pregnancy and rehabilitation. I found that postgraduate study was required to develop skills in these areas, so I developed a plan to educate myself. I learned and learned not just from books but from great teachers like Elizabeth Noble and Holly Herman. After treating thousands of pregnant women at my healing center, Renew Physical Therapy, I came up with a set of tools, techniques and exercises that, when incorporated into a pregnant woman's day-to-day routine, brings profound pain relief, restores function, rebuilds strength, improves stability and most importantly transforms the body so that you are ready to push, give birth and ultimately recover.

I am here to tell women not to be afraid to talk about their issues with pregnancy-related pain and discomfort. Although these issues are common among the women that I treat, they are not discussed freely. I am also here to let you know that there are things you can do to help yourself. The medical community may tell you to live with these aches and pains, that they are an inescapable part of pregnancy. But this is absolutely not true. You can help yourself and you don't have to live with pain.

Ending Pain in Pregnancy (EPP) is much more than a book filled with fluffy exercises and narratives; it is written with you in mind. Some of the exercises and tools in this book are normally taught to physical therapists, osteopaths and rehabilitation doctors. Many other exercises are from my clinical experience in treating pregnant women for more than two decades. My aim is to share with you what we do at our healing center: we help pregnant women stay pain free and we help those experiencing pain to eliminate it. My book can be your personal healing guru.

EPP is written from the point of view of a physical therapist. As an expert in women's health and prenatal care, I am in a unique position to help and guide you throughout your pregnancy. This guidance incorporates specialized tools such as pelvic alignment, pelvic floor training, abdominal exercises and pain-relieving techniques.

Today pregnant women are inundated with information from all sectors of the healing and exercise industry. But all this information cannot magically enlighten pregnant women as to how to manage their pregnancy pain, how to take care of themselves during pregnancy, during labor and delivery, or during postpartum recovery. *EPP*, my one-of-a-kind book, will help you to navigate—and make sense of—much of the information that is currently on the market.

I encourage you to be proactive in your own healing and to seek practitioners who will partner with you in your pregnancy journey. Partnership healthcare is the only way to go. Work with caregivers who specialize in the field of pregnancy pain and always follow your instincts when choosing your healthcare team. You must trust and believe in them and they should listen to what you are saying and remain open to your vision. Select caregivers who are willing to try different methods and techniques to give you the birth and pregnancy experience you want. Make sure they take the time to hear what you are saying and feeling, and be sure they answer your questions no matter how trivial they may seem. For instance, if you want a VBAC (vaginal birth after Cesarean) then choose a caregiver that is open to this. If you don't want an episiotomy then choose a caregiver that rarely performs them or has a low episiotomy rate. You are the consumer; shop wisely.

Most importantly, you must keep your head up and avoid negative self-talk. Never give up on yourself. Search for your answers with intelligence and sensitivity. Always follow your own heart and intuition. If something doesn't feel right or hurts, that's an internal cue. Do not ignore what your body is telling you.

This concept of listening to your body is especially important when you perform any of the exercises and techniques in this book. If you feel pain, stop and reassess whether this technique or exercise is the right one for you. Ask yourself: "Am I being too aggressive with the tools? If I do this technique gently and slowly, will it hurt less and give me pain relief?" Oftentimes, the techniques you try will cause some pain as you take back control of your pregnant body, but just remember to listen to the messages your body is sending you. Keep track of the tools and exercises that you do and become your own expert on what helps to relieve your pregnancy pain. Understand that when you use the tools in this book you will have setbacks. At times, you may experience more pain. This is normal. Wait a few days and see how you feel. If symptoms flare up due to the exercises, you may feel worse for twenty-four to seventy-two hours, but eventually, you will feel better. It's similar to the muscle soreness you experience when you work out at the gym. If an exercise is not working for you, move on and try a different exercise or tool. If you need help with the exercises, seek out a trained women's health physical therapist and show them this book. The main point is to listen to your body; if it doesn't feel right then something is not right. Pain is always a signal to stop and assess what you are doing or stop what you are doing altogether until your body is ready.

Now that I have covered the overall background to my mission and have primed you to get started, remember that ultimately you hold the key to your own healing. Go through this book carefully and with an open mind. There are two roads before you: the road to getting your body back by eliminating your pregnancy pain with *EPP* or the road to staying as you are by doing nothing. Read *Ending Pain in Pregnancy* and make yourself the heroine of your own story.

CHAPTER TWO

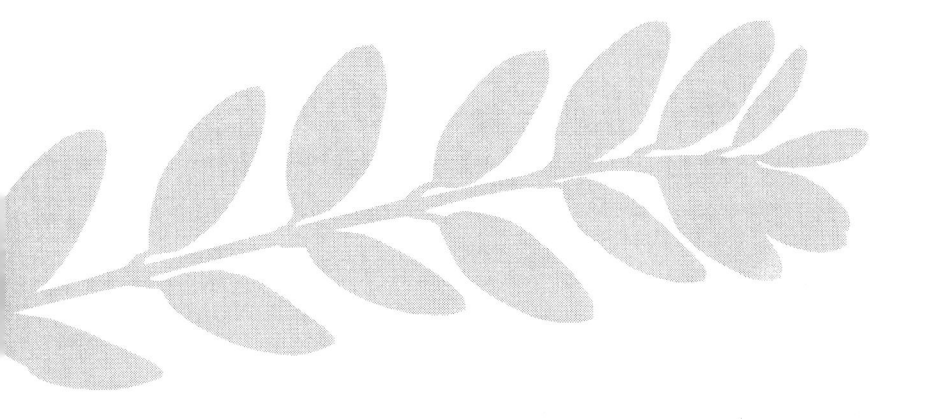

*"Three grand essentials to happiness
in this life are something to do,
something to love,
and something to hope for."*

– Joseph Addison

Chapter 2

HOW TO USE THIS BOOK

Ending Pain in Pregnancy represents a fusion of exercises, pain-relief techniques, and mind/body methods that I've put together to help my patients defeat their pregnancy pain. Working with pregnant women suffering from pelvic and low back pain, I discovered a core group of exercises and techniques that, when incorporated into their self-care program, enabled them to reduce their pain, walk longer, and function better. Ultimately they gained back their lives. These simple-to-learn and easy-to-implement techniques, which are rolled up into "The Renew Program for Women™," rescued many of my prenatal patients.

The tools are a set of holistic, natural and non-medical methods for the treatment of pregnancy pelvic and low back pain. This unique approach incorporates several protocols that I have developed, helping many of my pregnant patients enjoy their pregnancy journey, whether it's their first pregnancy or they've experienced pregnancy previously.

The large selection of techniques in this book are based on the latest medical research and on my real-life, practical experience in treating pregnant women. The techniques include massage, trigger point release, perineal stretching, abdominal exercises, pelvic floor relaxation exercises, pelvic alignment techniques, and others. Above all I consider myself a coach in the lives of my patients, carefully tailoring a holistic mind/body program that works for them.

You will find that after reading this book you will become an active participant in your own self-care and treatment. You will learn how to manage and control your pain on your own, and you will feel more hopeful in your pregnancy journey. *Ending Pain in Pregnancy*, with its innovative methods and scientifically-based exercises, will put you on the right track to a pain-free and wonderful pregnancy and a safe labor and delivery. You will be able to perform your daily chores with ease, develop a more positive outlook, and realize there are ways that you can help yourself when you experience pain flare-ups. Overall, your quality of life will improve and you will be able to move into motherhood with the confidence that your body is strong and healed.

What I do is physiotherapy, and what I tell my patients is that they must participate physically, emotionally, and spiritually in their treatments in order to achieve their goal of pain-free pregnancy. By teaching my patients specific exercise techniques, healing methods, and behavioral changes, they learn to care for themselves with the knowledge that they need to be self-sufficient and in control of their pain. At first, many of my patients feel insecure about doing the exercises and techniques on their own. With time they come to find that practice makes perfect.

Exercise alone will not set you on the road to pain-free pregnancy. You must also address your mindset and perform mental hygiene on a daily basis. I have observed that the women I treat who are suffering from pregnancy pain conditions tend to be anxious, fearful and depressed. They feel hopeless because their journey has been a difficult and trying one and they are worried about the future and how they will handle the stress of a new baby and a new life. Pregnant women today have busy lives that may include juggling full-time work and taking care of younger children. Many didn't seek help when suffering with their first pregnancy and now they are battling to get their bodies back before the second baby arrives. I believe strongly that you are what you think. Adopting a more positive outlook will help put you on the road to full recovery. Women with younger children may also need to seek out help if caring for themselves and their younger children becomes too challenging or overwhelming. I find that some mothers are guilt-ridden and forget that getting help is not a sign of weakness but a sign of strength. You can't be all things to all people. First you must take care of yourself and then—*and only then*—will you be able to take care of others.

Remember that many of the pregnant women I treat had pain *before* they got pregnant and many have suffered for years with pain. Many have gone from doctor to doctor in search of answers. Many have been told the pain is all in their head, or even worse, that there is nothing you can do about pregnancy pain but accept it. Without any relief to their pain, these women are left feeling anxious, depressed and hopeless. All these emotional experiences can accumulate and add to catastrophic thinking that results in negative behaviors. You are not alone. Use this book as a springboard to the realization that there are many other pregnant women out there who are feeling the same things you are. Throughout this book I have included stories from my patients so you can see the results that can be achieved if you work hard enough and put yourself first on your own list. Here is a story from one of my patients.

In Their Own Words – Finding Relief for Pubic Bone Pain

"With my first baby I had pubic pain that was so bad I didn't know what to do about it. I went to see my OB and he said: 'This is pregnancy; there's nothing we can do for you.' So I lived with it and suffered beyond belief. During my labor I went to the hospital and labored on my back with my legs spread out. I didn't know then that this is the worst position to give birth for women who have pubic bone symphysis pain. I barely walked out of the hospital. I had to use a cane. I did nothing about this pain because I thought it would go away on its own. I had pain for a very long time after the birth of my first child.

"For my second child I started to experience the same pubic bone pain early in the pregnancy. I panicked and cried. I felt alone. I didn't know how I would manage with two kids. Then I found Isa. She saved me. Isa gave me exercises that helped control my pubic bone pain. She also gave me a belt that wrapped around my pelvis. I never went anywhere without this belt because it reduced my pain by a lot. She showed me how to carry my first child and how to use my body correctly. Honestly I don't know what I would have done without this kind of help. Isa educated me on proper labor positions and how to pick one that was safe for me. I switched my doctor and went to someone who listened to me and let me labor in any position that I desired. After the baby was born I went right back to physical therapy to work not only on my pubic bone pain but also my pelvic floor muscles. I had no idea I even needed to train my muscles down there. Who knew? Isa told me that this kind of therapy for the pelvic floor muscles is common in many countries but not the United States. So today I can tell you that if you do these exercises you recover faster after that baby comes; better yet you will be able to enjoy a pain-free pregnancy."

Typical Renew Program for Women™ Routine

Ending Pain in Pregnancy is best used as a foundation to your self-care and healing journey. Read the whole book before creating your first mind/body routine. By reading all four parts of the book first, you will be better able to integrate the tools and techniques into a life-changing strategy to help you take control of your pregnancy pain. Remember to be gentle with yourself. If you fall off the exercise wagon, don't beat yourself up. Instead, make a decision to transform your condition and to change your outlook toward your condition from sufferer to empowered woman.

What can you expect to feel when you begin your program? You may experience emotional release and short-term muscle soreness. You may feel some or all of these symptoms before your momentum builds up and you begin to defeat your pain. Your typical routine should be based on a Monday-to-Sunday approach. Your program needs to include activities every day of the week to combat and defeat whichever condition or combination of conditions that have led you to read this book. You will have to dedicate thirty minutes to one hour a day to yourself to overcome your painful pregnancy condition. Break your routine into smaller parts during the course of the day, or set aside a bock of time in the evening and complete your whole routine at the same time. Incorporate your routine into your daily life: practice your Kegels while waiting on line or brushing your teeth; stretch at work; do your abdominal exercise while checking your emails; meditate over coffee; and end your day with a thigh massage and warm bath. You should not become overwhelmed by the tools and exercises in this book; instead, the goal is for you to make them a part of your daily life without being stressed out doing and making time for them. In the beginning a bigger commitment is needed, but as you get stronger, more stable and build up your endurance, your exercise and self-treatment time will reduce.

Use the charts below to track your progress with your self-care therapy.

Table 2.1: How to Create Your Pain-Relief Routine

SCHEDULE	ACTION ITEM	WHERE TO FIND INFO
Daily	Walking	Chapter 3
Daily	Pelvic floor training Perineal massage (Starts at thirty-four weeks of pregnancy)	Chapter 9
Daily	Follow exercise guidelines	Chapter 3
Daily	Control stress and negative thinking	Chapter 14
Daily-several times a day	Symphysis Pubic Dysfunction	Chapter 7
Daily or every other day	Determine your type of pain (back pain, sciatica pain, sacroiliac pain) and follow exercise guidelines and healing tools listed in chapters	Chapter 4, Chapter 5, Chapter 6, Chapter 8
Daily	STOP destructive forces: What are you doing that is causing you pain?	Chapter 4
As needed	Check your pelvic alignment; do you need a belt?	Chapter 5, Chapter 8

Table 2.1 (cont.): How to Create Your Pain-Relief Routine

SCHEDULE	ACTION ITEM	WHERE TO FIND INFO
Monday, Wednesday and Friday	Abdominals program	Chapter 12
Monday, Wednesday and Friday	IF NO PREGNANCY PAIN: Exercises that work in every trimester: Maintenance program	Chapter 13
Thirty-Plus Weeks of Pregnancy	Preparing for labor and picking out the right labor position for your body type; comfort measures and birth plan sample	Chapter 10

Table 2.2: Mind/Body Routine Tracking

TYPE OF MIND/BODY EXERCISE	MON.	TUES.	WED.	THURS.	FRI.	SAT.	SUN.

Table 2.3: Mapping Your Pelvic Alignment

TYPE OF PELVIC MALALIGNMENT	MON.	TUES.	WED.	THURS.	FRI.	SAT.	SUN.

Table 2.4: Weekly Pain and Progress Diary

DATE	LOCATION OF PAIN	PAIN LEVEL 0-10 (0=NO PAIN, 10=WORST PAIN EVER)	TECHNIQUES USED FOR PAIN RELIEF	PAIN LEVEL AFTER SELF-CARE THERAPY

Now that you understand how to use this book, we will tackle pregnancy exercise guidelines. The next chapter is filled with important information that will serve as the building block of your "get out of pain" programs. Read it carefully. If you are in doubt about the guidelines please show this book to your midwife or OB/GYN. Ultimately they will give you not only the guidance that you need, but also the medical clearance that some of the tools and/or exercises in this book require. Let's get started.

CHAPTER THREE

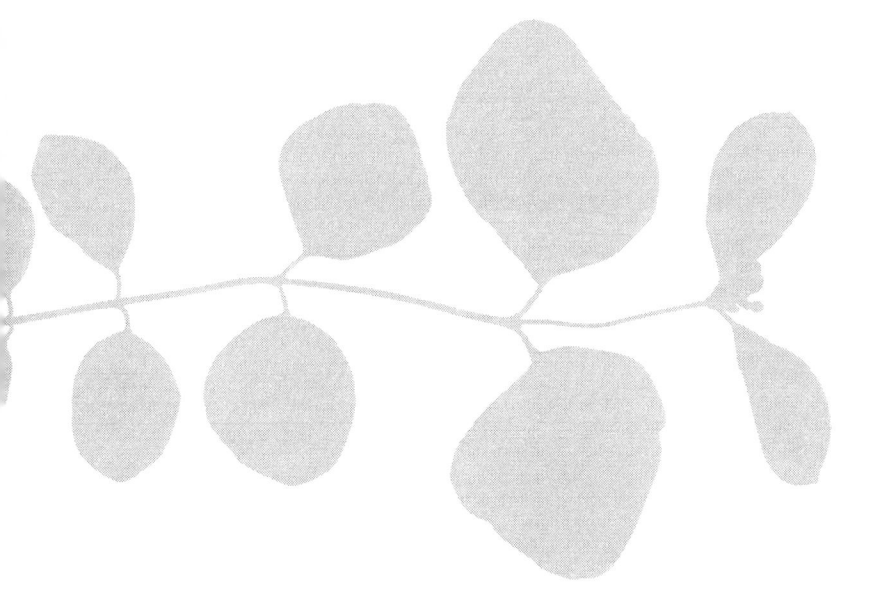

*"You have to learn the rules
of the game and then you have
to play better than anyone else."*

— Albert Einstein

Chapter 3

PREGNANCY EXERCISE GUIDELINES AND
LISTENING TO YOUR BODY'S MESSAGES

All expectant mothers desire what is best for their growing babies. There is little doubt that exercise provides a great number of benefits to both the pregnant woman and the growing baby. However, there are many misconceptions in the popular culture regarding what types of exercise are safe and beneficial during pregnancy.

Every week at our healing center we care for pregnant women who want to be stronger, who are not sure whether they are doing the appropriate exercise or who have injured themselves during prenatal exercise. In this chapter, we will present the benefits of exercise, the precautions for exercise and the importance of listening to your body when choosing an appropriate exercise routine. We encourage you to take control of your health and be your own healer during your pregnancy!

Exercising during pregnancy will prepare you for the most physically challenging time of your life. Most studies relating to pregnancy and exercise conclude that exercise is not only safe during pregnancy, but that it is actually better for both the mother and baby for the pregnant woman to engage in exercise throughout the pregnancy.

The Effects of Pregnancy on the Maternal Body

Your pregnant body undergoes many physiological, hormonal and physical changes while making more and more room for the baby. As your baby gets bigger, your hormonal, muscular and skeletal systems are altered in subtle and not-so-subtle ways. Overall, the ligaments and joints become loose due to a pregnancy-related hormone called relaxin. This joint looseness, or hypermobility, can lead to joint sprains and muscle strains. Other hormonal changes can also make pregnancy a time of intense emotional upheaval as body systems are put in a constant state of change.

The body's natural center of gravity also tends to shift forward, which challenges a woman's posture, balance and coordination. The weight of each breast increases by about one pound by the end of the pregnancy. This increase in weight can pull your shoulders forward, overstretching your mid-back muscles and possibly leading to upper back and neck pain. The additional frontal weight on the body sometimes causes women to overcompensate by leaning backward, adding stress to the lumbar spine and sacroiliac joint. Your overall metabolic system also speeds up, requiring an additional 300 calories a day in order to maintain metabolic homeostasis. As we move through the book you will have to learn the names of muscles so that you can better listen to your body. The next two diagrams label all the muscles that we target with the exercises in this book. Make sure to use these diagrams and our extensive glossary as a reference point.

Diagram 3.1: Anterior Female Muscles

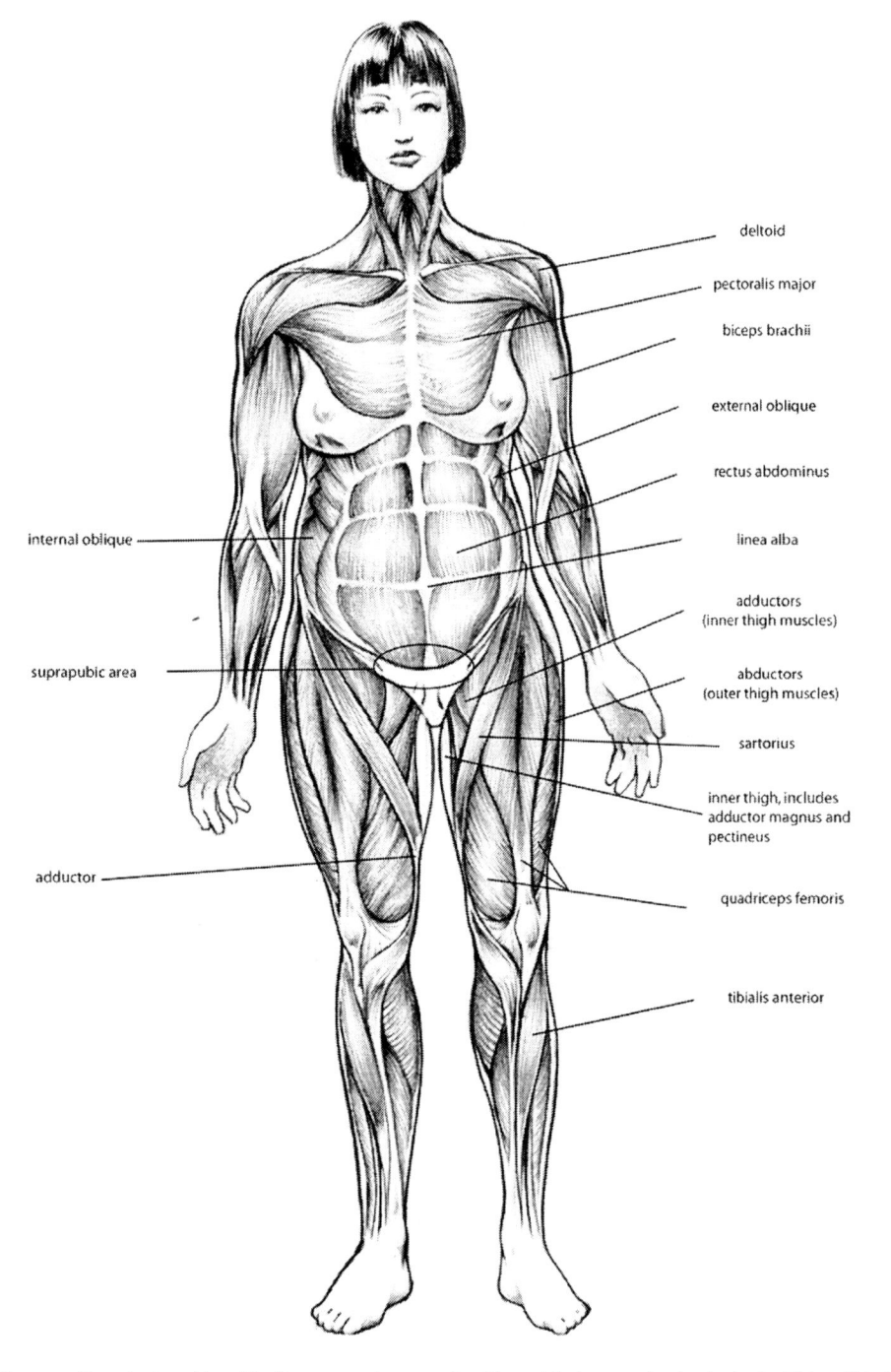

deltoid

pectoralis major

biceps brachii

external oblique

rectus abdominus

linea alba

adductors
(inner thigh muscles)

abductors
(outer thigh muscles)

sartorius

inner thigh, includes
adductor magnus and
pectineus

quadriceps femoris

tibialis anterior

internal oblique

suprapubic area

adductor

Diagram Description: Use this diagram to become familiar with the muscles in the body. This will help you with the exercises, tools and techniques in this book. Source: Winston Johnson

Diagram 3.2: Posterior Female Muscles

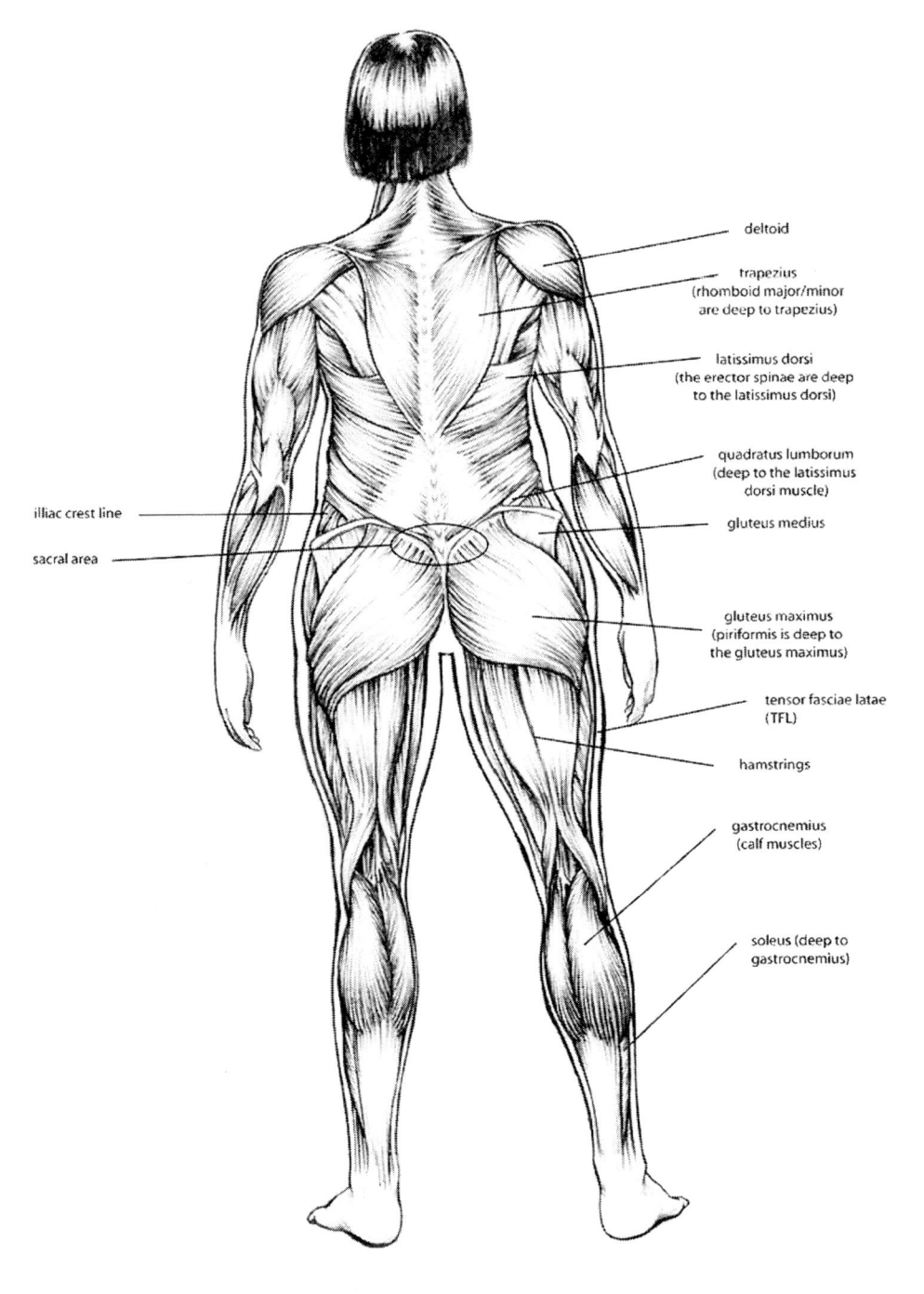

deltoid

trapezius
(rhomboid major/minor
are deep to trapezius)

latissimus dorsi
(the erector spinae are deep
to the latissimus dorsi)

quadratus lumborum
(deep to the latissimus
dorsi muscle)

gluteus medius

gluteus maximus
(piriformis is deep to
the gluteus maximus)

tensor fasciae latae
(TFL)

hamstrings

gastrocnemius
(calf muscles)

soleus (deep to
gastrocnemius)

illiac crest line

sacral area

Diagram Description: Use this diagram to become familiar with the muscles in the body. This will help you with the exercises, tools and techniques in this book. Source: Winston Johnson

In the lower body, hamstrings and hip flexors get tighter, which can lead to groin pain. A woman's abdominal muscles are especially challenged during pregnancy. Without proper exercise, a gap can develop in the front of abdominals, a condition called diastasis recti abdominis (see Chapter 12). If the muscles of the pelvic floor are weak, you can experience stress incontinence, or urine leakage with activity, during pregnancy. There is also a second type of incontinence called urge incontinence. The growing uterus puts pressure on the bladder, making you feel an intense urge to use the bathroom. Sometimes the urge is so great that it is difficult to make it to the bathroom in time. During one forty-five-minute physical therapy session, many pregnant women go to the bathroom two times.

Diagram 3.3: Diastasis Recti Abdominis

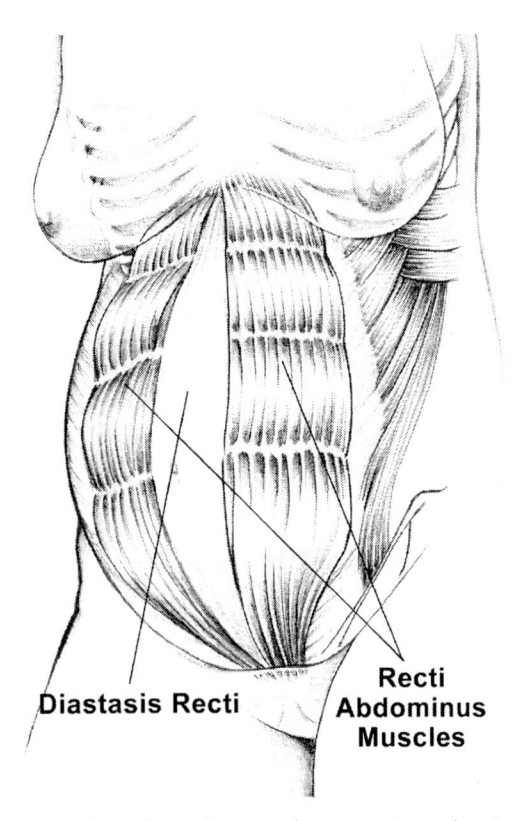

Diastasis Recti

Recti Abdominus Muscles

Diagram Description: Notice the wide gap between the two recti muscles. Source: Winston Johnson

Diagram 3.4: Layer of the Pelvic Floor Muscles

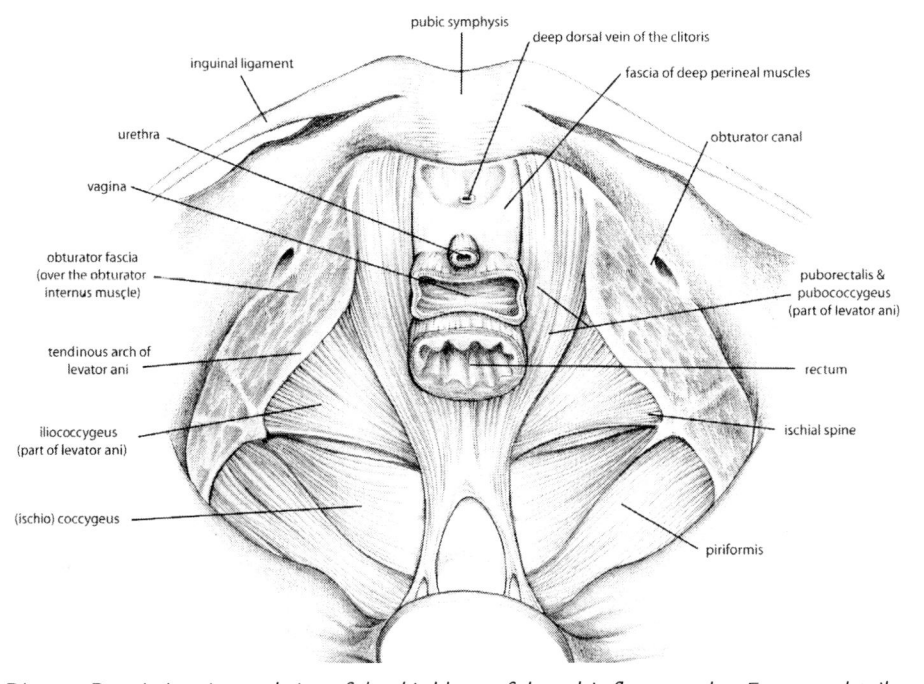

Diagram Description: Internal view of the third layer of the pelvic floor muscles. For more details on these very important muscles see Chapter 9. Source: Winston Johnson

In the abdomen, the digestive system slows down so that it can absorb more nutrients. This slowing down can lead to constipation, a common complaint among pregnant women. The stomach is pushed up by the growing uterus, especially during the second and third trimesters. As a result, there is less room for food in the stomach, and women often experience acid reflux or heartburn. The growing uterus also displaces the diaphragm upward into the space normally occupied by the lungs, causing the pregnant woman to breathe more often in order to take in the needed amount of oxygen. This physiological change often causes shortness of breath. In the circulatory system, the amount of blood increases 40 to 50 percent by the thirty-fourth week, causing exhaustion and nausea, especially in the first trimester. As the amount of blood increases, there is a greater chance of blood pooling and varicose veins.

The good news is that many pregnancy-related discomforts and problems can be alleviated and prevented by staying fit. Performing specific Dyna-Band exercises, flexibility and cardiovascular exercises will make your body stronger and better prepared for the physical and hormonal changes that occur during your pregnancy.

Table 3.1: Benefits of Exercise during the Prenatal Period

1. Exercise strengthens the muscles most affected by pregnancy and reduces the effects of pregnancy-related discomforts, such as hip pain, upper and lower backaches, and pelvic pain.
2. Exercise may help prevent or treat gestational diabetes.
3. Women who are fit have shorter and less complicated labors and tend to recover faster after giving birth.
4. Exercise improves body mechanics and posture. Women who exercise are better able to adapt to their growing belly and weight gain.
5. Women who exercise have larger placentas and pass more nutrients to their babies.
6. Exercise improves your mood by increasing endorphins.
7. A moderate-intensity exercise program reduces your chances of a Cesarean section and instrumental (forceps/vacuum) delivery.
8. A moderate-intensity exercise program reduces your chances of an abnormally large baby (macrosomia). This may then reduce your risk of Cesarean section.
9. Exercise helps promote bowel movement, decreasing the risk of constipation.
10. Exercise helps you sleep better; poor sleep quality is a common complaint during pregnancy.
11. Exercise can improve circulation, helping to prevent the instance of varicose veins.
12. Exercise improves muscle tone, strength and endurance, which are especially important during labor and delivery.

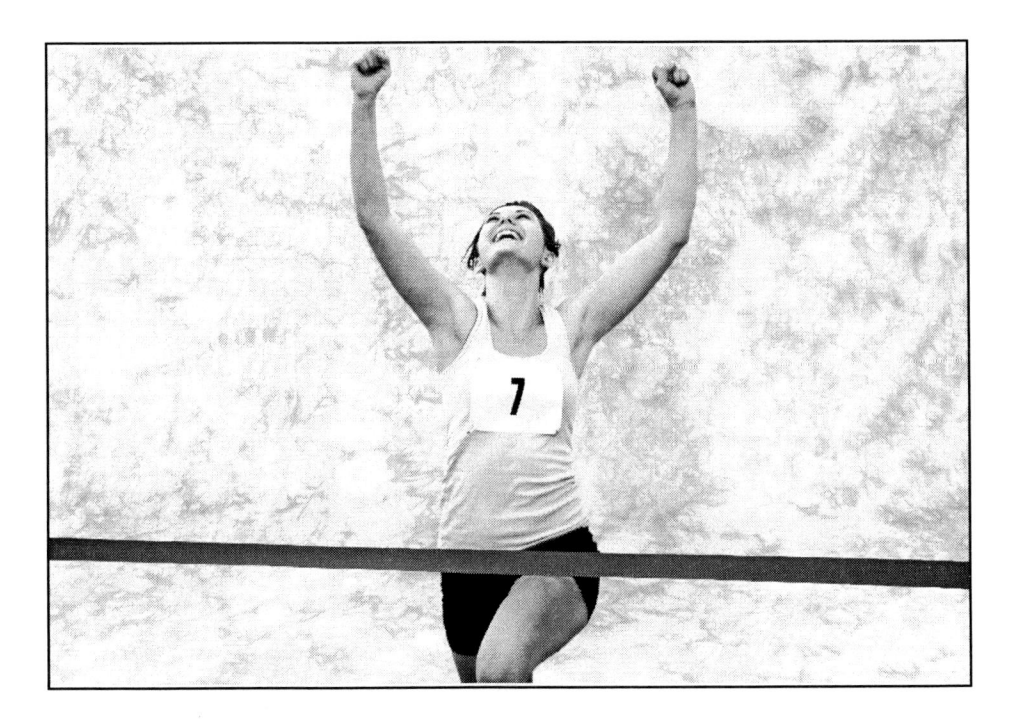

Exercise Guidelines during Pregnancy

Although exercise has many benefits, there are a number of guidelines that are very important to understand and adhere to in order to prevent injury and avoid pregnancy-related complications. Many women assume that their general exercise knowledge is sufficient for guiding their exercise during pregnancy. Unfortunately, that belief often leads to overtraining, injury or even unintended complications in the pregnancy. All exercise programs should be discussed with your physician or midwife.

Table 3.2: General Guidelines for a Safe and Healthy Exercise Program

1. Previously inactive women and those with medical or obstetric complications should be evaluated before recommendations for physical activity during pregnancy are made.
2. If it has been some time since you have exercised, start slowly. Begin with as little as five minutes of exercise a day and add five minutes each week until you can stay active for thirty minutes a day.
3. Prepregnancy exercise routines can be continued during pregnancy, but intensity levels should be kept at a mild to moderate level. Remember to listen to your body talk and rest when you are tired. To reap the benefits of exercise, regular exercise is better than sporadic exercise.
4. A physically active woman with a history of or risk for preterm labor or fetal growth restriction should be advised to reduce her activity in the second and third trimesters.
5. After the first trimester of pregnancy, avoid doing any exercises flat on your back. Exercising in this position can reduce blood flow to the uterus and can also lead to decreased cardiac output (the amount of blood pumped by the heart). Exercising in the supine (flat on back) position can also lead to supine hypotension and dizziness. The pregnant woman should switch positions frequently during work and exercise activities in order to avoid blood pooling in the legs, decreased cardiac output and supine hypotension.
6. Pregnant women should avoid standing motionless for long periods of time and avoid heavy lifting. Women whose jobs require heavy lifting and prolonged standing have been shown to deliver smaller babies and deliver earlier than their due dates.
7. There are some risks from becoming overheated during pregnancy, especially in the first trimester. Drink plenty of water to keep from overheating and dehydrating. Avoid brisk exercise in hot, humid weather or when you have a fever. Wear comfortable clothing that will help you to remain cool.
8. Exercising during pregnancy increases how many calories you need to eat. You should eat an additional 300 to 500 calories per day if you exercise regularly during your pregnancy.
9. During pregnancy, your center of gravity shifts, putting you at a greater risk of falls, especially in the last trimester when your belly is at its biggest. Avoid exercises that put you at risk for falling and exercises that could cause abdominal trauma. These include horseback riding, rollerblading, ice-skating, skiing, snowboarding and gymnastics.

Table 3.2 (cont.): General Guidelines for a Safe and Healthy Exercise Program

10. Avoid exercising in altitudes of 6,000 feet or more. Exercising at high altitudes can lead to altitude sickness. Symptoms include headache, nausea, vomiting and dizziness. Severe symptoms include inability to walk, decreased mental function and fluid build-up in the lungs. Altitude sickness can be detrimental to your baby, as the baby gets less oxygen. This can lead to fetal distress.

11. In general, you can continue your weight-bearing exercises, such as weight training, walking, dancing, aerobics and yoga. You should, however, avoid activities that call for quick changes in direction that may strain your joints, muscles and ligaments. Non-weight-bearing exercises, such as swimming, are less stressful for your body and can be continued throughout your pregnancy.

12. If you are weight training, avoid overhead or military presses. Lifting a heavy weight overhead may cause a woman to hold her breath and become dizzy. Since dizziness is common during pregnancy, it is best to avoid the risk of lifting a weight above your head. This exercise is also a common contributor to shoulder impingement and rotator cuff injuries.

13. Wear comfortable and sturdy shoes to avoid twisting your ankle or falling. Sturdy shoes may also help prevent pain from developing in the arch of the foot, which often stretches due to weight gain and increased ligament laxity.

14. Never exercise to the point of exhaustion or breathlessness during pregnancy. See the "Intensity Guidelines" later in this chapter for guidance on how to find the proper exercise intensity.

15. Never exercise through pain. If an exercise produces pain, stop immediately. Particular attention should be paid to abdominal, pubic bone and pelvic pain, which can be signs of serious problems. If the pain does not go away, contact your physician or midwife immediately.

16. For every hour of exertion, you should plan an hour of rest in the same day. Pregnancy is not the time to push yourself through long days and exercise regimens without allowing the body to rest and recharge.

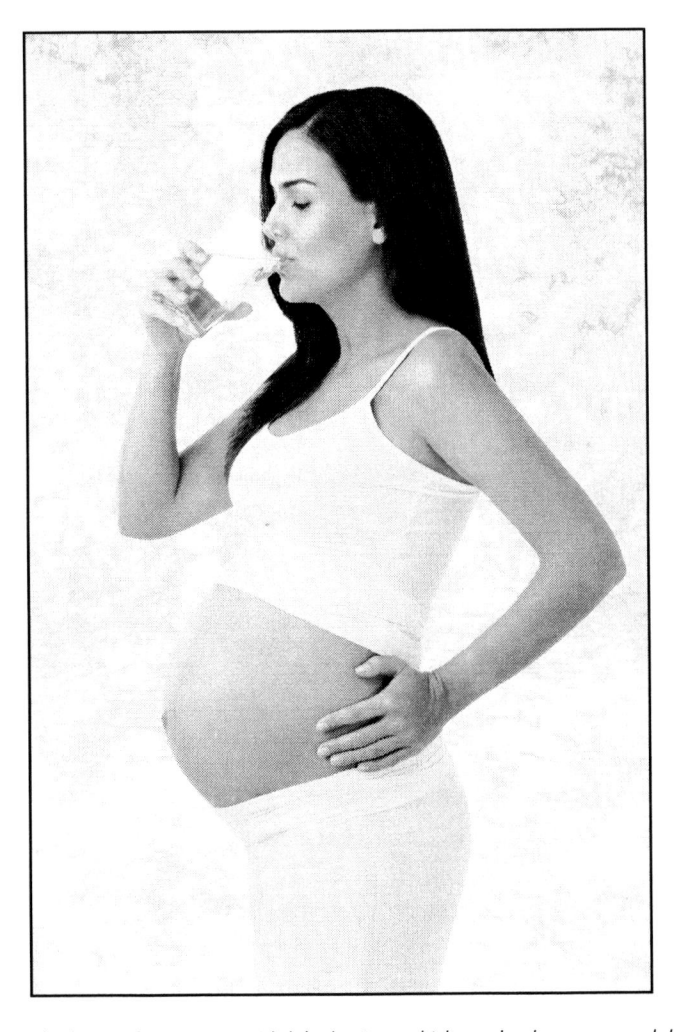

Description: Drink plenty of water to avoid dehydration, which can lead to pre-term labor.

Additional Safety Considerations for Exercising during Pregnancy

Although exercise has many benefits, there are times when a pregnant woman needs to proceed with caution or eliminate working out altogether. There are two categories of exercise contraindications:

Absolute contraindications: Under no circumstances are you allowed to exercise if you have any of the specified conditions or medical problems. (See Table 3.3.)

Relative contraindications: You can exercise, but you should modify your exercise program and be monitored closely by a healthcare professional. (See Table 3.4.)

Table 3.3: Absolute Contraindications to Aerobic Exercise during Pregnancy

1. If you suffer from chronic or pregnancy-induced high blood pressure/preeclampsia, heart disease, restrictive lung disease, or other serious conditions affecting glandular, cardiac, respiratory or pulmonary diseases, you should not be exercising.
2. If your cervix is weak or incompetent, or you have had a cervical cerclage, you should not be exercising. An incompetent cervix is one that dilates before your baby is ready to be born. This condition puts you at high risk for premature labor. A cervical cerclage is a surgical procedure in which a stitch is placed in the cervix to prevent premature labor in the presence of a weak or incompetent cervix.
3. If you are carrying multiples and are at risk of premature labor, you are classified high risk and should not be participating in aerobic exercise. Consult with your physician or midwife regarding your ability to participate in a modified exercise program.
4. Vaginal bleeding is a warning sign that should be taken very seriously. If you start to bleed at any time during your pregnancy, call your physician or midwife immediately. All exercise should be stopped until your caregiver gives you the clearance to start again. Persistent second- or third-trimester bleeding is an absolute contraindication to exercise.
5. Placenta previa, after twenty-six weeks of gestation, and placenta abruption are both absolute contraindications to exercise. Placenta previa is a condition in which the placenta covers the cervix. Placenta abruption is the separation of the placenta from its attachment to the uterus wall before the baby is delivered.
6. Premature labor during the current pregnancy is an absolute contraindication to exercise.
7. If your membranes are ruptured, exercising is contraindicated. Early rupture of the membranes will put you at high risk for premature labor.
8. If you have a history of miscarriages, especially three or more, you should not exercise until your second trimester, and then only with the approval of your physician or midwife.

Table 3.4: Relative Contraindications to Aerobic Exercise During Pregnancy

1. If you have hypertension, hyperthyroidism, anemia, seizure disorder, chronic bronchitis and/or type 1 diabetes, you must consult your physician or midwife before exercising. You may not be allowed to exercise until the condition is under control.

2. Irregular heart beat or heart palpitations are serious concerns and must be evaluated before you engage in an exercise program. Your care provider may provide modifications to your program.

3. If you are overweight, underweight (BMI <12) or have never exercised before, you absolutely need to get the approval of your physician or midwife before starting any exercise program.

4. Intrauterine growth restriction in current pregnancy. Poor fetal growth should be taken very seriously. If your baby is not growing properly, you need to be cleared by your care provider before engaging in exercise. Sometimes poor fetal growth is a result of over-exercising and not eating properly.

5. If you are physically injured, you should eliminate all exercise until your condition is evaluated by a medical professional. Exercising while injured will put you at even greater risk for more problems. Physical injuries such as broken bones, extreme sacroiliac joint pain, sciatica, pubic bone separation, hernias and muscle strains or pulls must not be taken lightly. It is best to see a physical therapist trained in pregnancy to help reduce your pain.

6. If your baby is in the breech position in the last trimester of pregnancy, your caregiver may modify your exercise program. Breech position occurs when the baby's feet are down, instead of the head.

In addition to the absolute and relative contraindications listed above, there are certain situations that require all exercise to stop immediately and for the woman to contact her physician or midwife. When a seemingly healthy pregnant woman experiences a sudden change in her physical condition—even if there is no previous history of medical complications—this is a red flag. See Table 3.5 below for the warning signs to cease exercising immediately.

Table 3.5: Warning Signs That Exercise Must Be Stopped Immediately and Care Provider Must Be Called

1. Vaginal bleeding of any kind.
2. Shortness of breath prior to start of exercise or extreme shortness of breath with or after exercise.
3. Dizziness, faintness, light-headedness or visual disturbances of any kind.
4. Headache, chest pain or muscle weakness.
5. Calf pain, redness or swelling.
6. Persistent uterine cramping after exercise may signal preterm labor. If uterine cramping continues for twenty to thirty minutes after you have stopped exercising, call your caregiver immediately.
7. Decreased, or absence of, fetal movement.
8. Sudden change in feelings of well-being or extreme fatigue.
9. Amniotic fluid leakage. A gush of fluid from the vagina should not be ignored. This can indicate a rupture of membranes.

How to Prevent Injury and Overtraining

As discussed earlier in the chapter, exercising during pregnancy offers numerous benefits to both mother and baby. Many women, however, fail to listen to their bodies and push themselves through exercise regimens that are too intense or that lead to pelvic and low back pain. Some women continue to participate in sports that have high risks of falling, such as skiing, not realizing that this goes against the recommendation of most obstetricians in the United States.

Table 3.6: American College of Obstetricians and Gynecologists (ACOG) Guidelines: Forms of Exercise That Should Be Avoided

1. Contact sports, such as hockey, basketball, and soccer. These sports can result in harm to you and your baby.
2. Sports with an increased risk of falling, such as skiing, horseback riding, gymnastics and vigorous racquet sports.
3. Scuba diving, which can put your baby at risk of decompression sickness.

A study published in 2010 evaluated the pregnancies of 1,469 women and found that although the overall incidence of injury during pregnancy was small, a majority of all injuries reported were due to falls. The authors of the study stated that while women should be encouraged to exercise during their pregnancies, they should be made aware of the risks, particularly the risk of falling. In the following section, you will be guided through the importance of "Body Talk," guidelines for exercise intensity, signs of overtraining and recommendations on appropriate weight gain in pregnancy.

Listen to Your Body Talk

A key concept taught at Renew is called "Body Talk." It is based on intuition. Intuition is sometimes called the sixth sense, and it is the ability to make sound decisions without always having concrete information. During a woman's pregnancy, intuitive powers, both emotionally and physically, are enhanced. Emotionally, you can sense when things are not right; this is probably due to high levels of pregnancy hormones. Physically, you are more in tune with the changes in your body as your baby grows inside you. Keeping yourself and your baby healthy and free of injury are your main priorities.

When the "Right" Exercise Feels Wrong: Take Precautions with Prenatal Yoga, Spinning, Swimming, Pilates, Running and Gym Workouts

You should always follow your instincts and listen to your body talk while exercising. That means if something doesn't feel right to you physically, stop doing it. To tune in to your body talk you must pay attention and listen to what your body is saying to you at all times. If you are experiencing any pain in your joints, abdominal or pelvic areas, modify your exercise or stop that exercise altogether. Many times women tell us that they "knew something didn't feel right" in their exercise class, but they continued anyway. This scenario is common with women who experience low back or pelvic pain during pregnancy.

A study published in 2005 reported the prevalence of low back and pelvic pain during pregnancy to be 72 percent, with most participants reporting both posterior (low back) and anterior (pubic joint/groin) pain. A history of joint hypermobility was found to be a risk factor for pain. Our experience at Renew Physical Therapy closely matches the results of the above study. Many of our patients who experience low back or pelvic pain report a history of being "very flexible," "double jointed" or having experienced sacroiliac joint dysfunction in the past. We would likely classify these women as having "hypermobile" joints.

A history of hypermobility becomes an issue during pregnancy, as the hormone relaxin further increases the mobility or "looseness" of the pelvis.

The role of relaxin and hypermobility requires extra attention when choosing an appropriate exercise program. Levels of relaxin peak during the first trimester and again during labor. Many women experience increased back and pelvic pain after participating in exercises that "open the pelvis," require the legs to be wide apart and/or require women to bear weight through one leg at a time. These exercises include prenatal yoga, Pilates, breaststroke with a wide frog-kick, running, spinning and one-legged resistance exercises.

Although the above exercises have many great benefits, they must be approached with caution during pregnancy, as sometimes the pelvis is simply not stable enough to maintain proper alignment in these challenging situations. These activities may require modification or close supervision of proper form to prevent low back and pelvic pain. Sometimes, the above activities need to be stopped completely in order to resolve low back pain or pelvic pain during pregnancy. Many women do not need to "open their pelvis" during pregnancy, but instead would benefit greatly from focused core and hip strengthening.

Many pregnant women come to Renew Physical Therapy believing that they are "supposed to" be doing yoga, climbing the stairs, or walking briskly as exercise. They feel guilty or abnormal if they are unable to perform a certain type of exercise. Unfortunately, not all pregnant women can safely perform the same type of exercises, especially if they are experiencing pain. For example, a woman who is experiencing pubic symphysis dysfunction will only increase her pain by walking up and down stairs and taking long strides with brisk walking. A woman who is experiencing sciatic pain from a herniated disc would be increasing the tension on the injured nerve and disc by doing many poses in her prenatal yoga class.

As you endeavor into your exercise program, please listen to *your* body talk and tune out all of the external chatter of what your pregnancy "should" look or feel like. You will see amazing results!

Determine Your Exercise Intensity: How Much Is Too Much?

Exercise intensity can be determined by using your heart rate, the talk test, or the rate of perceived exertion table. Heart rate alone as a measure of exercise intensity during pregnancy is not the best method to use because your resting heart rate increases by several beats (up to fifteen) during pregnancy. Still, knowing how to figure out your exercising heart rate is important because your caregiver might want you to keep your heart rate within a certain range. Personally, I recommend the talk test or rate of perceived exertion to women during pregnancy. These two methods are easy to use and accurate in determining exercise intensity.

The Talk Test

You should be able to walk and carry on a conversation during your exercise sessions. If you're exercising alone, you should be able to sing a song out loud. If you are out of breath, huffing or puffing, or unable to carry on a conversation, you are probably exercising too strenuously and need to slow down your pace.

Rate of Perceived Exertion (RPE)

Rate how much you are exerting yourself during your exercise sessions on a scale of 1 to 10 (see Table 3.7). On average, your intensity level should be within a range of comfort. For most pregnant women, that range should be between 3 (moderate) and 5 (strong). On the RPE scale, 10 represents the maximum activity level, and for most pregnant women this is an inappropriate exercise level. Remember to listen to your body talk and never exercise to fatigue.

Table 3.7: Rate of Perceived Exertion

0	Nothing at all
0.5	Very, very weak
1	Very weak
2	Weak
3	Moderate
4	Somewhat strong
5	Strong
6	
7	Very strong
8	
9	
10	Very, very strong – maximal exertion

Heart Rate

Your doctor will sometimes recommend that you stay within a certain heart rate range while exercising. To find your pulse, place your second and third fingers (not your thumb since it has its own pulse) at your wrist alongside the tendon that lies on the same side as your thumb. Count the number of pulses that you feel for ten seconds. Multiply this number by six to calculate your exercising heart rate.

If you're having trouble finding your heart rate using your wrist, you can use your carotid (neck) artery pulse instead. Gently place your second and third fingers on the side of your neck and feel for your pulse. Count your pulse for ten seconds and multiply by six to calculate your exercising heart rate. Avoid pressing hard against your carotid artery, as this will give you an inaccurate reading.

A heart rate monitor provides another way of calculating your exercising heart rate. The monitor consists of a chest transmitter, which you place around your chest in alignment with your heart, and a wristwatch that is programmable. The chest transmitter sends the electrical impulses from your heart to your watch. Your watch will then display your exercising heart rate.

Signs of Overtraining: How to Recognize When You Are Overdoing It

Overtraining not only increases your risk for injury and other problems, but it may also negatively affect your baby. Poor fetal growth rate, a decrease in the baby's movement after exercise, and a severe increase or decrease in the fetal heart rate are all signs that you are overdoing your exercise sessions. Overtraining and experiencing an injury will not only impact your exercise program, but will also impact your ability to perform your everyday home and/or work-related tasks. Listen to your body talk and err on the side of safety so that you can continue your exercise sessions throughout the nine months of your pregnancy. The following table describes the signs of overtraining.

Table 3.8: Signs of Overtraining

Reduce the volume, frequency and intensity of your exercise program if you experience any of the following:

1. *Pain while you exercise.* If an exercise produces pain or doesn't feel right, stop what you are doing immediately. If you experience pain in your abdominal or pelvic area, contact your physician or midwife immediately.
2. *Feeling exhausted or depleted.* Make sure that you are not doing too much and that you are eating properly. Proper diet and rest will give you the fuel you need to exercise.
3. *Colds and other upper respiratory infections.* If you have a fever, you should not be exercising.
4. *Losing interest in your workouts.* If the workouts become a chore instead of fun and your workout performance is not up to par, this can be a sign of overtraining. Stop exercising and rest.
5. *Excessive muscle soreness and muscle cramps.* Some low-level soreness can be expected, but the kind of soreness that makes your muscles ache and hurt is no good.
6. *Slow fetal growth rate.* The baby is not growing as it should. Your baby's growth rate is usually determined by your physician or midwife during a sonogram.
7. *Baby does not move after exercise.* Your baby should move two to three times within thirty minutes after you finish working out. If the baby stops moving, call your physician or midwife immediately.

Fuel Your Body

Gain the amount of weight your physician or midwife has recommended. Inadequate weight gain can result in a low-birth-weight baby. Dieting while pregnant is an extreme no-no. If your body and growing baby do not get enough nutrients, you can develop ketosis, a dangerous condition that occurs when the body does not have enough glucose to burn for energy. Your body instead uses your fat and protein stores as fuel. This chemical process happens when you are not eating enough nutrients or as a result of severe morning sickness. The end product of this chemical process is the development of ketones. Ketones pass into the placenta, and if your baby is exposed to them for a long period, they can cause serious harm. The following will help you determine appropriate weight gain during your pregnancy:

Your prepregnancy Body Mass Index (BMI) determines the amount of weight you should gain throughout your pregnancy. (BMI measures your weight in relation to your height). To calculate your BMI, use the formula weight (kilograms) in relation to your height (meters).

1. Weight (lbs) _____ divided by 2.2 = _____ kilograms (A).

2. Height (inches) _____ multiplied by 2.45 = _____ centimeters; divide by 100 = meters. Now multiply the result by itself = _____ (B).

3. Divide A by B to get your BMI.

Once you have calculated your BMI, the following chart will give you a good idea of how much weight you ought to gain.

Table 3.9: Prepregnancy BMI and Pregnancy Weight Gain

PREPREGNANCY BMI	CATEGORY	TOTAL AMOUNT TO GAIN IN POUNDS	FIRST TRIMESTER TOTAL POUNDS	SECOND AND THIRD TRIMESTER POUNDS PER WEEK
19 or under	Underweight	28-40	5	1.07
19-24	Healthy weight	25-35	3.5	1
25-30	Overweight	15-25	2	0.67
>30	Obese	At least 15	0-2	0.5

Eat Every Three Hours

Eat before and after your workouts to replenish your energy stores. Never skip breakfast. Always be prepared by keeping food (especially carbohydrates and proteins) nearby. Keep nuts, fruits, dry cereal, bread, vegetables, and/or pasta in the bag you normally carry. This type of timed eating will also help keep your blood sugar from dropping too low. During early pregnancy, a drop in your blood sugar level can negatively affect the growth development of your baby. Eating every three hours and having a bedtime snack can also help reduce nausea and morning sickness during your first trimester. Increase your caloric intake by an additional 300 to 500 calories in order to cover the demands of your exercise sessions. A list of 300-calorie snacks follows.

Table 3.10: 300-Calorie Delights

1. One slice whole-wheat bread with one tablespoon peanut butter. Drink one cup skim milk.
2. One low-fat vanilla yogurt with one chopped banana.
3. One medium baked potato topped with two tablespoons low-fat sour cream. Add chopped chives or scallions for flavor.
4. Fresh fruit cup: half a cantaloupe with one-half cup blueberries, one kiwi, half a banana and one-half cup grapes.
5. Yogurt shake: one-half cup frozen low fat vanilla yogurt with one cup fresh strawberries and one cup skim milk.
6. Pasta salad: one cup bowtie or shell pasta with one cup vegetables, tossed with one teaspoon olive oil and balsamic vinegar dressing.
7. One can (six ounces) solid white tuna in water with five saltines and one tablespoon light mayo.
8. Two graham crackers with one cup frozen yogurt in between the crackers.
9. Two cups assorted chopped raw vegetables (carrot, broccoli, red peppers, cucumbers) with one cup spinach sour cream dip.
10. One half cup guacamole with ten tortilla chips.
11. One mango with one ounce almonds (twenty-two pieces).
12. Two slices whole-wheat bread with four slices turkey breast and one tablespoon light mayo.
13. Two hard-boiled eggs with ten saltines.
14. One banana with two tablespoons peanut butter spread on it.

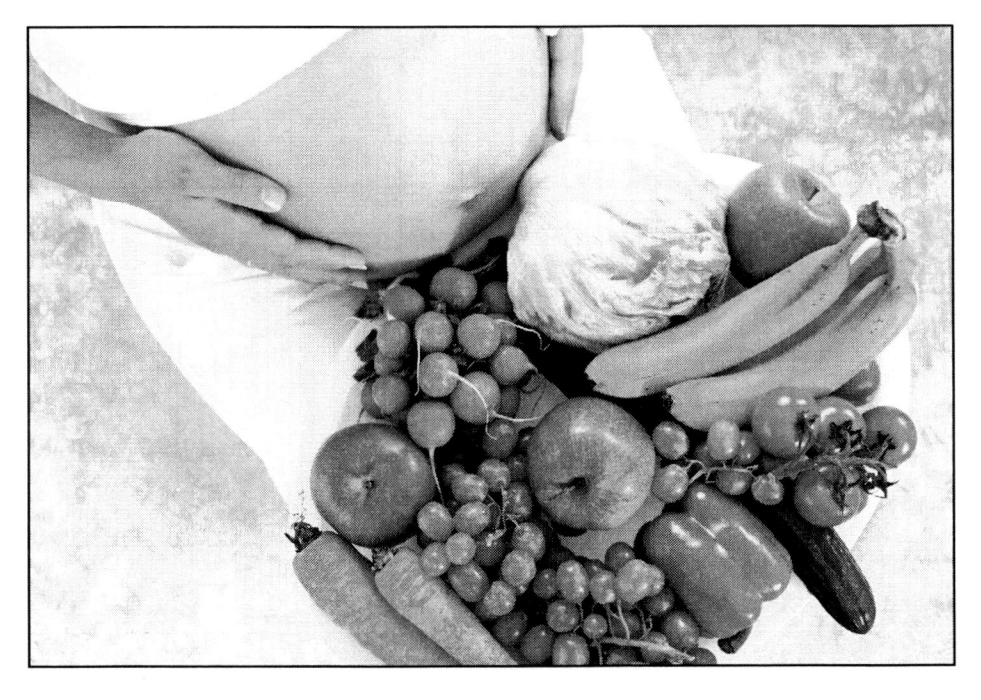

Description: Choose foods that are good for you. Avoid processed and genetically-modified foods. Eat organic foods whenever possible.

Pregnancy is an extraordinary time to tune in and listen to your body. Take care to nourish yourself and your growing baby with smart exercise, adequate rest and proper nutrition. Use your intuition and the knowledge gained from this book to be your own healer throughout your pregnancy. You do not have to participate in the workouts or activities that everyone else thinks you "should" be doing while pregnant. Focus on staying strong and safe and your body will thank you.

So far we have covered the basics. Next, we will look at some everyday things many pregnant women are doing that may need to be modified. Read on and we will share our top trade secrets with you and show you how to stop destructive forces that can be contributing to your pregnancy pain.

PART TWO:

BE YOUR OWN HEALER AND THERAPIST: TRADE SECRETS THAT KEEP YOU PAIN-FREE AND HAPPY

"A life spent making mistakes is not only more honorable, but more useful than a life spent doing nothing."

— George Bernard Shaw

Chapter 4

STOP DESTRUCTIVE FORCES NOW:
AVOID INJURY AND PAIN WITH OUR TRADE SECRETS

Many pregnant women come to Renew Physical Therapy because they are in pain and don't know how to get themselves out of pain. They want to be healthy and fit but are inundated with confusing and conflicting information from the healthcare community and marketing companies. After experimenting with many different kinds of modalities such as Pilates, yoga, chiropractic care, spinning classes and running, they come to us seeking clarity and help. All exercise is not necessarily beneficial and just because an exercise or class is labeled prenatal does not mean that it is appropriate or safe. We have treated many pregnant women who have injured themselves in prenatal classes. We find that if women are not instructed properly with regard to exercise they are at risk for injuries to the pubic bone, low back and upper back. What we have noticed at our center is that basic safety information is not given to pregnant women and most of the time they are not shown how and what to do to be safe. Oftentimes basic exercise principles are not covered in many prenatal exercise classes.

Based on our experience treating women with injuries of the pubic bone, hips, low back, and upper back, we recommend that all newly pregnant women should be seen by a women's health physical therapist to discuss safe and effective exercise principles, guidelines, and injury prevention strategies. At our healing center in New York City, we find that women who are evaluated and given our trade secret list in the first and second trimesters of their pregnancy are able to maintain active lifestyles longer, grow stronger with improved body awareness, gain confidence in their physical and mental abilities, and implement safe exercise strategies throughout their pregnancies.

In Chapter 3 we covered exercise basics; in this chapter we will equip you with the knowledge that you need to be safe in any class environment. Destructive forces that can wreak havoc on your body will be discussed at length so that you can prevent injuries, have a pain-free pregnancy, and enjoy the incredible nine-month journey ahead. This chapter will outline exactly what these destructive forces are, why they cause harm to your body, and how you can use simple physical therapy tools and modifications to avoid them. We will also advise you on the things you should be doing to keep your body strong, healthy, and out of harm's way.

Many of our patients find that making simple modifications can significantly decrease their pain, improve their daily function, and allow them to do all the activities they love to do from week one to week forty and beyond. By using our trade secrets you can prevent many injuries and ailments including, but not limited to, sciatic pain, upper back pain, neck pain, hip and pelvic pain, incontinence, prolapse, and pelvic floor dysfunction. Keep in mind that these strategies should also be used in the immediate postpartum recovery period and even beyond, as they will keep you safe, healthy, and strong while taking care of your new baby. Therefore, we encourage you to use the trade secret list (see Table 4.1) as a guideline to stop and modify the destructive forces that you face on a day-to-day basis. Implementing our recommendations will create a new path of wellness and strength and restore your power so that you go into motherhood pain free and prepared to take care of your baby.

The Trade Secret List

At Renew Physical Therapy, one of the first educational materials we give our patients is a comprehensive list, which encompasses the basic rules and precautions all pregnant women need to know to stay healthy, strong, and prevent injury. As you read through this list, examine your daily habits to get a better picture of what destructive forces may be impacting your body. We will give you suggestions along the way on how to modify the destructive forces so that you can stay pain free and avoid the pitfalls that other women will undergo if they don't heed this advice. We truly believe that following these simple rules will help you lay a strong foundation for your body to thrive during your pregnancy.

Table 4.1: Strategies for a Pain-Free Pregnancy: The Trade Secret List

WHAT TO AVOID	TRADE SECRETS TO USE
Jackknife out of bed	Log roll out of bed
"Valsalva" maneuver breath holding	Breathe naturally focusing on exhale
Push with urination or defecation	Use the proper potty posture
Just in Case (JIC) Urination	Avoid all JIC voids and keep a bladder diary
Bend forward from the waist when lifting heavy objects	Use proper lifting mechanics
Heavy lifting	Only lift your baby or five to ten pounds maximum
Poor sitting posture	Use correct sitting posture
Poor standing posture	Use correct standing posture
Avoid impact exercises	Walk and listen to your body
Don't let it all hang out	Use the "Pelvic Brace" (a simultaneous transverse abdominal contraction and low-level Kegel contraction)

Avoid Jackknifing Out of Bed

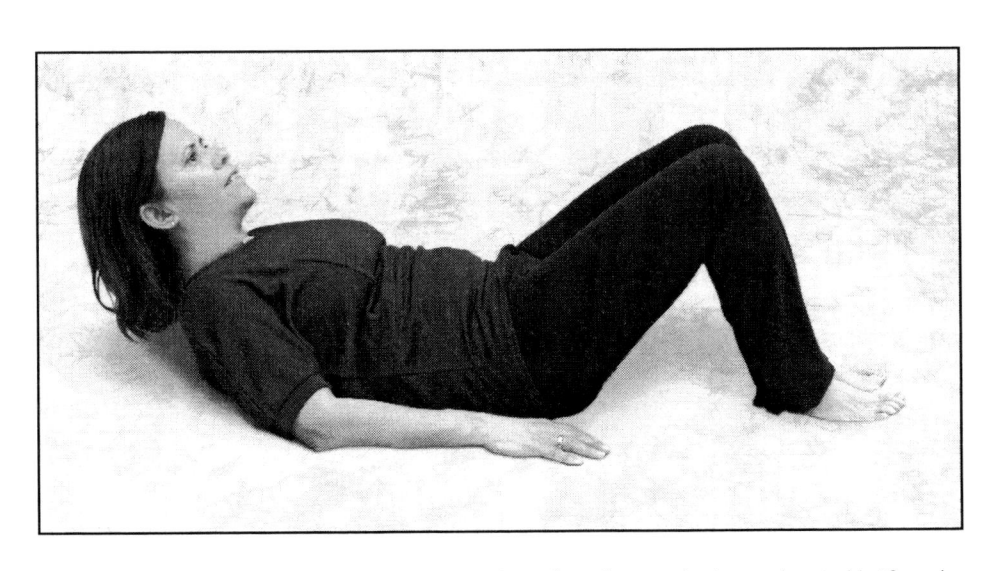

Description: Notice the tension in the abdominal, neck and upper back muscles. Jackknifing also strains the abdominals and causes them to open up like a zipper at the linea alba.

Jackknifing is the act of sitting up straight out of bed as if you were doing a crunch. This action places a large amount of stress through the abdominal muscles and can lead to a condition called diastasis recti. The rectus abdominis, or our "six-pack abs," are joined at the middle by a connective tissue sheath called the linea alba. In pregnancy, the linea alba and abdominal muscles are forced to stretch to accommodate the growth of the baby, which leads to weakness and instability. It is normal to have a slight separation of the abdominals during pregnancy. However, jackknifing out of bed, or performing any movement requiring shortening of the trunk, such as crunches, can lead to further separation of the abdominal muscles and cause significant weakness. See Chapter 12 for an in-depth analysis of how to test and correct for diastasis recti abdominis (DRA). If you have ever seen a bulge that looks like a little tent in the middle of your belly, especially during transitional movements, this typically indicates you have DRA.

Trade Secret to Use: Log Rolling

A simple alternative to jackknifing is log rolling out of bed. A log roll occurs when you roll your body completely to the side first, and then use your arms to help you sit up along the edge of the bed. This movement places less stress through the abdominal muscles and will help prevent the diastasis from getting any larger. **Additional tip:** If you are suffering from pubic bone or groin pain, squeeze a pillow between your knees while you roll to the side. This helps to stabilize the pelvis and hip bones and can significantly reduce pain during these difficult transitional movements. See more tips for symphysis pubic dysfunction in Chapter 7.

Avoid Holding Your Breath

Holding your breath, or using a "Valsalva" maneuver, can place increased stress on the abdomen, pelvic organs, and pelvic floor muscles. The Valsalva maneuver can be defined as a forced expiration of air through a closed glottis. If you have ever seen anyone lifting a heavy box who struggles to breathe, turns red, or uses grunts and groans to lift, you have most likely witnessed someone doing the Valsalva maneuver. In pregnancy, it is very important to minimize stresses through the pelvis at all costs because of the ever-increasing pressure and force that occurs in the pelvis through the growth of the baby. Holding your breath, especially when lifting objects or having a bowel movement, can cause your pelvic organs to descend placing increased pressure through the pelvic floor muscles. This causes these important structures to stretch and weaken. There are also cardiovascular risks associated with the Valsalva maneuver, including increased blood pressure, decreased blood flow to the heart, dizziness, fainting, and even stroke.

Trade Secret to Use: Focus on the Exhale

The alternative to holding your breath during strenuous activities would be to exhale. Exhaling allows your abdominal pressure to normalize, decreasing force through the pelvis and preventing cardiovascular stress from occurring. A strategy we often use with our patients, especially when teaching abdominal and core exercises, is to have the individual count out loud while exercising. This ensures the patient is not holding her breath and prevents her from doing a Valsalva maneuver. You may find this strategy helpful during exercise, lifting, or even having bowel movements. Our patients have also reported that using soothing or hissing sounds like "*Oooo*," "*Shhh*," and "*Ahhhh*" during bowel movements can make going to the bathroom easier and prevents them from holding their breath or straining.

Avoid Pushing to Urinate or Defecate

Do you ever feel as if you need to push or strain when you have a bowel movement or urinate? This destructive force can be detrimental to your pelvic floor muscles. When you push or strain to go to the bathroom, the abdominal organs actually descend downward resulting in a large amount of stress through the muscles of the pelvic floor. We tell many of our patients that the only thing you want to "push" out is your baby. The cumulative effect of pushing and straining when going to the bathroom can make you susceptible to pelvic organ prolapse, weakened pelvic floor muscles, incontinence, and pelvic pain. It is extremely important to limit the amount of stress through the pelvic floor and limit pushing as much as possible.

Trade Secret to Use: Potty Posture

There are a few options that can help you limit the amount of pushing and straining you do when using the bathroom. The first is using proper "potty posture." American toilets put our descending colon, or sigmoid colon, at a kink. This makes it much more challenging to have a smooth, strain-free bowel movement. The potty posture, pictured below, provides a way to help align the spine and internal organs and relax your pelvic floor muscles so that you are able to eliminate without strain or stress on the pelvic floor muscles. Proper potty posture includes the following steps:

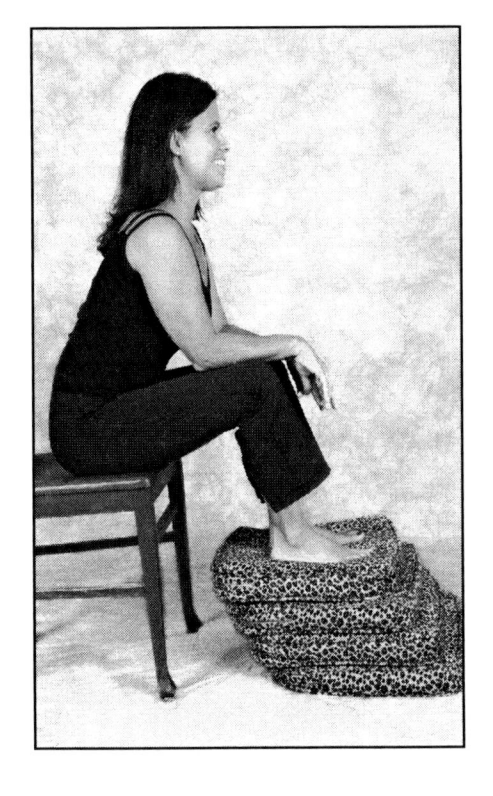

1. Sit with your knees above hips, legs wide apart and feet plantar flexed, which means on your toes. For women less than five feet tall, use a footstool or book if necessary. Taller women may not need to elevate feet to maintain the position.

2. Lean forward and place your elbows on your thighs. Keep the arch in your back and avoid slumping or rounding the lower back.

3. Gently bulge out your abdominals while simultaneously widening your waist as if to "brace" yourself from a blow to the abdomen.

4. Once you can bulge and brace simultaneously this can be used as a toilet technique, as it will help relax the pelvic floor muscles and facilitate defecation.

5. Avoid straining. Do not hold your breath. As mentioned earlier, play with sounds such as "*Ohhh,*" "*Ahhh,*" and "*Shhh,*" which will help further relax your pelvic floor muscles. Correcting your potty posture takes time, but with practice you will master it.

Constipation is another destructive force that can wreak havoc on the body. The digestive system slows down so that it can absorb more nutrients during pregnancy, which makes pregnant women more susceptible to constipation. It is extremely important to manage constipation and avoid it at all costs so that you can prevent straining to eliminate stool. Some tips for managing constipation include making sure you are getting an adequate amount of fiber, drinking plenty of water, and always using the potty posture as described previously. Discuss with your doctor, midwife, or healthcare provider additional safe and effective ways to manage your constipation so that you can keep your pelvic floor muscles happy and prevent additional pressure and strain through these very important structures.

Avoid Just in Case (JIC) Urination

"Just in Case" urination, or "JIC," can negatively influence the way your bladder functions causing you to have to use the bathroom frequently. JIC can also lead to excessive nocturia or waking up at night to use the bathroom. What is JIC? Have you ever found yourself saying, "I am going to go to the grocery store, so just in case, I'm going to go to the bathroom first"? This would be a first-degree JIC offense. When your bladder fills to capacity, a signal gets sent to your brain which then prompts your body to urinate by getting an urge. If you go to the bathroom before you get the urge to urinate, your brain gets faulty signals thinking that the bladder was full when in reality it was not. Over time, this leads to "shrinkage" of the bladder, or a premature signal being sent to the brain, telling you that you have to go to the bathroom when your bladder can really accept more fluid. This disorder can be referred to as urinary frequency. Normal bladder function is typically six to eight voids per day, with each episode of urination lasting for approximately eight to ten seconds. If you notice you have to use the bathroom more than once every three to four hours, you may have urinary frequency. Urinary frequency can become a burden, affecting your daily life, work, and social activities with frequent and oftentimes unnecessary visits to the bathroom.

Trade Secret to Use: Use Time Voiding, Bladder Diary and Waiting for Proper Urge

Normalizing bladder function early in your pregnancy can help you regain control of your bathroom habits and make your postpartum recovery much smoother. During the late stages of your pregnancy, urinary frequency is challenging, if not impossible, to manage due to the pressure of the baby pressing down on the bladder. Because of this, you may find you need to void frequently in your postpartum recovery as well. However, if you simply vow to avoid just-in-case urination, this will help build a strong foundation for normalizing bladder habits and allow the brain-bladder connection to function properly.

You should only urinate when you get the urge to go, not before. You may find it helpful to fill out a bladder diary, pictured in Table 4.2, to determine your voiding interval and help to retrain your bladder back to normal function. Many of our postpartum patients find this tool very beneficial because it allows them to see their progress, and can also help identify bladder irritants, such as foods or liquids, which may be triggers for getting a premature urge to urinate. We recommend keeping a bladder diary every two to four weeks to track your progress. This will allow you to resume your normal daily functions without having to worry where the nearest bathroom may be.

Table 4.2: Bladder Diary

PDF version of this table available at http://www.RenewPT.com, in the free info center.

TIME OF DAY	FOOD/LIQUID (OTHER THAN WATER) INTAKE: STATE TYPE OF FOOD AND DRINK	WATER INTAKE (OUNCES)	AMOUNT URINATED (COUNTED IN MISSISSIPPIS)	URGE PRESENT (LOW, MEDIUM OR HIGH URGE) LEAKING? (Y/N?) IF YES, WHAT WERE YOU DOING?
6AM				
7AM				
8AM				
9AM				
10AM				
11AM				
12PM				
1PM				
2PM				
3PM				
4PM				
5PM				
6PM				
7PM				
8PM				
9PM				
10PM				
11PM				
12AM				
Overnight				

Avoid Bending Forward from the Waist

Body mechanics, or the way an individual moves her body when carrying and lifting objects, can have a huge impact on the joints and muscles in your neck, back, hips, and legs. Improper mechanics over time can lead to conditions such as cervical or lumbar disc herniation, sacroiliac joint pain and instability, hip bursitis, muscle spasms, and generalized low back and hip pain. Bending forward from the waist with a rounded low back places increased stress on the intervertebral discs in the lumbar spine.

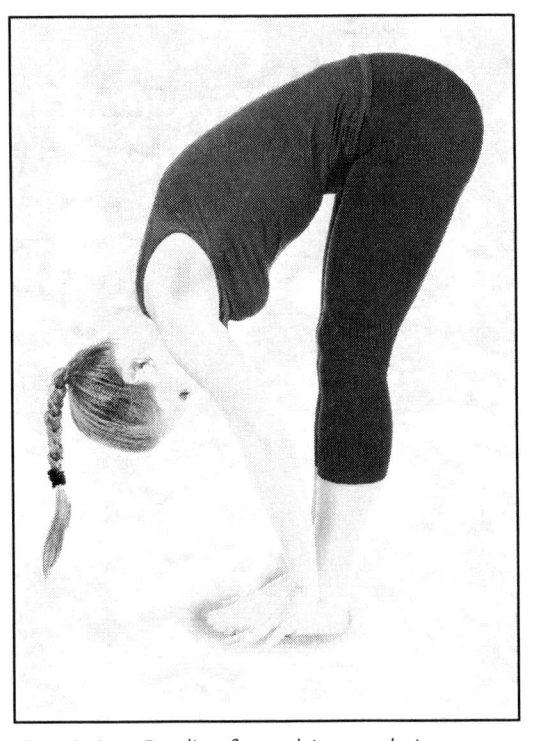

Description: Bending forward incorrectly increases the mechanical forces on the spine and increases the likelihood of injury.

The intervertebral disc lies between each lumbar vertebra, or bone, in the back and functions as a cushion to support the back and absorb impact forces. It is sometimes compared to a jelly donut. There is an outer ring, called the annulus fibrosus, which is made up of tough connective tissue and helps to contain the nucleus pulposus. The annulus fibrosus is the outer shell of the donut which surrounds the jelly. The nucleus pulposus, or the jelly in the donut, is a water-based substance which acts as the cushion in the system and helps to absorb and distribute forces. When you bend forward and round your back, it is like smushing one side of a donut against the plate. If you do this once in a while and without too much force, the donut may bounce back to its original form and be just fine. However, what happens if you do this over and over, or smash the donut against the plate? The jelly squirts out the other end and your donut is ruined. This is similar to what can happen to our lumbar discs if we repetitively bend forward from the waist, or attempt to lift a very heavy object with improper body mechanics. A disc affected in this way is described as herniated; herniated discs can cause severe pain in the back, and can even impinge the nerves in our spine sending pain, and sometimes numbness or tingling, into the legs. Some refer to this phenomenon as sciatica. You should never bend forward from the waist to lift or pick up objects due to the stress that is placed on your intervertebral discs and the risk for disc herniation and resultant nerve irritation.

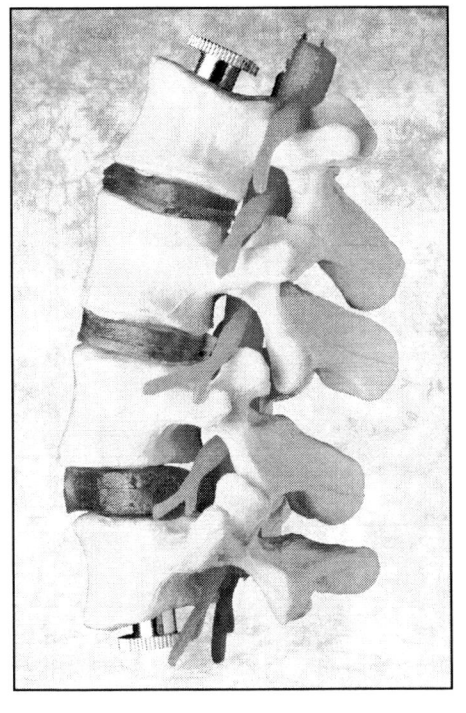 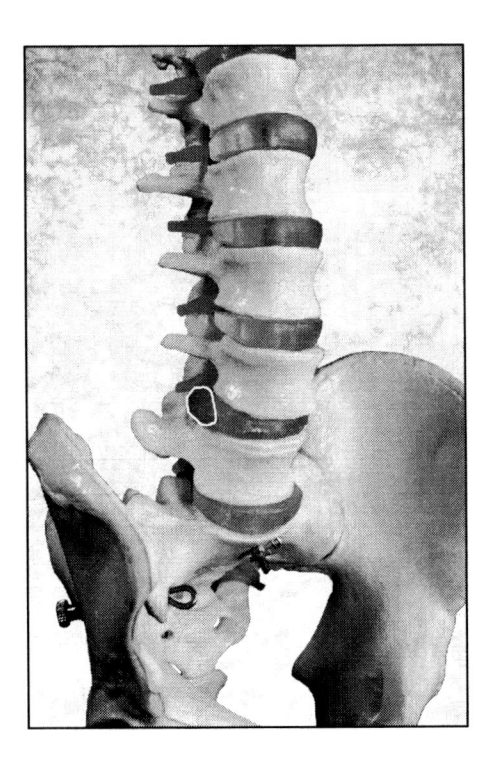

Description: On the left is an intact lumbar spine, showing the vertebrae, intervertebral discs, and spinal nerves. On the right, notice the pea-sized structure circled here. This is what a typical herniated disc looks like. Notice how the disc herniation compresses or impinges upon the nerve.

Trade Secret to Use: Proper Body Mechanics

Proper lifting mechanics can feel awkward at first and may be challenging to your body. However, it is extremely important to practice proper mechanics before, during, and after your pregnancy to keep your body healthy and protect your back and hips. Instead of bending forward from the waist to pick up objects, you should follow these simple guidelines to help minimize the stress on your back and hips. The sooner you begin to practice proper lifting mechanics, the better your body will be prepared to lift, carry, and swaddle your new baby lovingly without putting yourself at risk for back or hip injury.

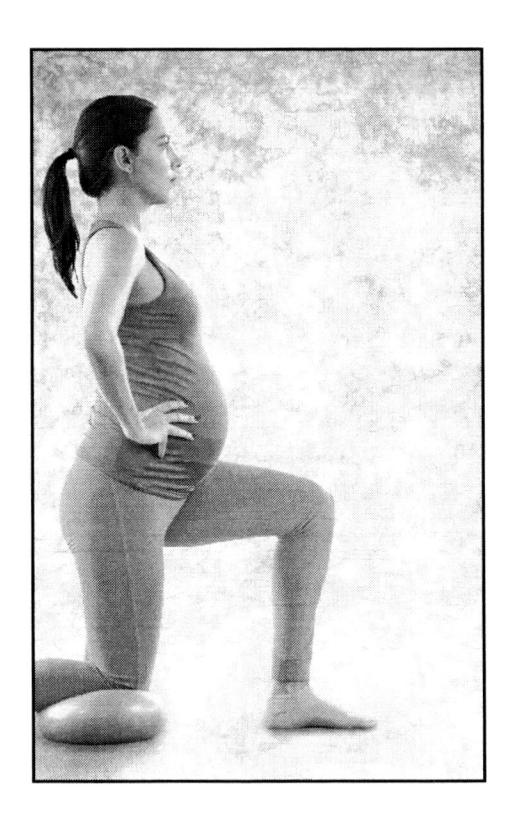

Description: Improper body mechanics can place undue stress on the back and hips and increase risk for intervertebral disc herniation. Do not bend forward from the waist. Instead bend from the knees and use proper biomechanics.

Table 4.3: How to Lift Properly and How to Use Proper Body Mechanics

Bring the Load/ Object Close	Bring your body as close to the load/object you are about to lift as possible. This will prevent you from reaching too far forward to grab the object, placing increased stress on the low back. You want the object almost directly underneath your body before you lift it.
Wide Base of Support	You want a wide base of support when you lift objects to improve your balance and allow you to reach the object without straining the back or legs. Widen your stance and try to keep your toes pointed forward or slightly turned out, as if you are about to straddle the object. For women with pubic bone or groin pain, your stance should be no wider than hip-width apart to minimize stress on the pubic symphysis.
Squat Down and Bend Your Knees	To reach the object, you will need to squat down by bending your knees. The most important aspect of squatting down is maintaining a flat back with a slight lumbar curve or arch. This is what helps the jelly in the donut stay centered, placing less stress through the intervertebral discs.
Keep the Load Close	When you grasp the object, bring the load close into your body and stand up with your back remaining straight up and down. If you have a younger child make sure your child is close to your body so you are not over-reaching and putting undue stress on your spine.
Take Steps: Do Not Rotate	Do not rotate, or twist, your trunk to place the object on a different surface. Instead, take small steps with your legs to reposition your body. Set this object down using these same principles. Proper body mechanics take practice, but with time, you will master this skill and prevent serious injury to your body. In the early postpartum period women are the most vulnerable to injury especially when changing diapers. Make sure you have everything you need close to the changing table and keep your body as upright as possible when changing diapers.

Avoid Heavy Lifting

Many women will ask us if it is okay to lift weights during pregnancy. We never advise patients to do heavy lifting during pregnancy due to the shift in the center of mass, decrease in balance, and increased risk for falls and further irritation of unstable joints. Additionally lifting heavy weights such as several bags of groceries puts a lot of downward pressure on the pelvic floor muscles and organs. Many women develop organ prolapse during pregnancy or in the postpartum period because they are carrying heavy weights or their older children.

Trade Secret to Use: Don't Lift Anything Heavier Than the Baby or Anything Over Ten Pounds

Our rule is simple: if you have a child already, try not to lift any objects heavier than your child. If you do not have a child, limit your lifting as much as possible to avoid straining your back, hips, and pubic bone. Listen to your body. If you are unable to maintain proper body mechanics, feel pain with lifting, or notice you have to hold your breath when you lift, you are most likely lifting an object that is too heavy and you should lighten the load. Avoid carrying heavy groceries or any thing over ten pounds.

Avoid Poor Sitting Posture

How many times have you been told to sit up straight or stop slouching? In today's society, more and more people have assumed desk jobs requiring them to sit for prolonged periods. Slouching, or bad posture, can be a destructive force on your body especially during pregnancy. Research suggests that there is a relation between posture and complaints of back pain during pregnancy. Sitting postures in general result in the largest amount of pressure through the lumbar intervertebral discs, as compared to lying down and standing. Slouching or slumping in your chair further increases the amount of pressure in the discs in the low back, which can exacerbate low back pain and sciatica, and cause the upper back and neck muscles to become overstretched. Therefore, it is particularly important to improve your sitting posture to minimize stress through the vulnerable joints in your body and avoid exacerbation of postural-related aches and pains in pregnancy.

Trade Secret to Use: Proper Sitting Posture

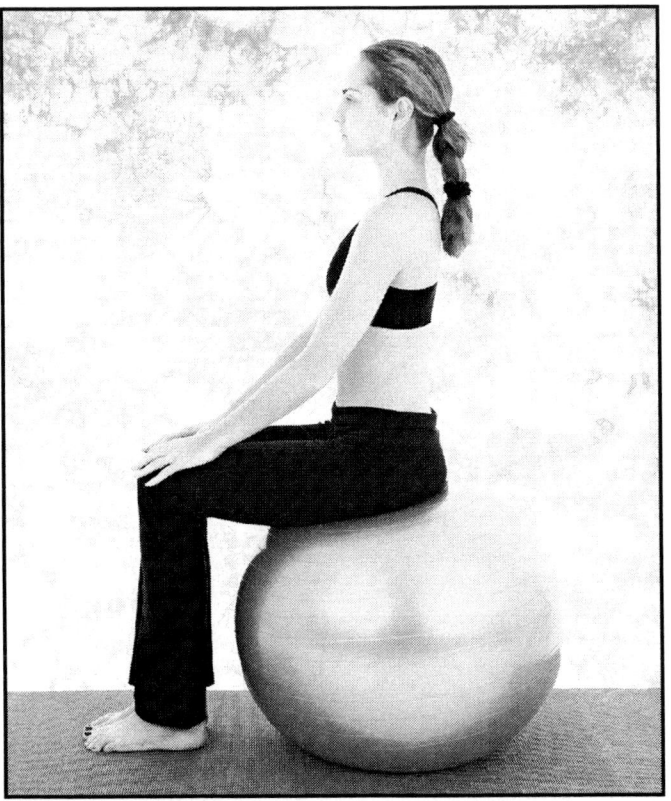

Description: This woman is in excellent sitting posture. Notice how the ears are aligned with the shoulders and the shoulders are aligned with the hips. The knees are aligned with hips creating a right angle and feet are flat on the floor. Her spine is also in neutral alignment. This is optimal sitting posture.

Sitting in proper posture is very challenging for many women in pregnancy, but there are a few simple ways you can modify your home or work environment to decrease stresses through the spine, hips, knees, and feet while sitting. The following chart gives you great tips on how to improve sitting posture. Please look it over and implement recommended changes into your everyday life and into your workstation.

Table 4.4: Recommended Trade Secrets for Proper Sitting Posture and for the Work Environment

Maintain a Neutral Spine	The spine naturally should have a slight arch, or lordosis, when sitting. However, not enough arch, or an excessive arch, can place undue stress on the ligaments, discs, and joints in the spine. Neutral spine can be achieved by rocking your pelvis back and forth as if sticking your bottom out and then tucking your tailbone under. Do this several times, and then find the midpoint between the two extremes to achieve a neutral spine. Neutral spine is our recommended position for the lower back.
Use a Lumbar Roll	Roll a towel into a cylinder and place it in the small of your back to help you maintain neutral spine and take some of the load off the back while sitting. It may take some trial and error to find the right size and texture towel to fit your spine properly. A lumbar roll can also be purchased online or in an office supply store.
Proper Hip, Knee, and Foot Positioning	The hips, knees, and feet should all be at a 90 degree, or right, angle with the feet resting flat on the floor. If your feet do not reach the floor because your chair is too high, consider resting your feet on a step stool in order to maintain contact with the floor and place less stress through the hips and knees.
No Leg Crossing Allowed: Keep Your Feet Flat on the Floor or on a Stool	Crossing your legs can cause you to lose neutral spine and create asymmetry through the pelvis. This can cause sacroiliac joint malalignment, as well as muscle spasms and pain. Plant your feet flat on the floor with equal weight through both sit bones to minimize shearing forces and allow you to maintain neutral spine.

Table 4.4 (cont.): Recommended Trade Secrets for Proper Sitting Posture and for the Work Environment

Keyboard or Computer Position	The position of your keyboard should allow you to have relaxed shoulders, elbows at 90 degrees tucked close to your waist, and most importantly, a neutral wrist position. Pregnant women are particularly susceptible to carpal tunnel syndrome, a condition which causes compression of the median nerve that travels through the wrist resulting in numbness, tingling, and weakness in the hand. A kink in the wrist can increase pressure in the carpal tunnel leading to nerve compression and irritation. Therefore, you should keep your wrists flat when typing or using the mouse.
Preventing Neck and Upper Back Pain	Forward head posture and rounded shoulders are two major causes of upper back, shoulder, and neck pain. Keep your neck centered over your shoulders and chin tucked in to avoid overstretching the muscles in the back of your neck and placing increased stress through the cervical intervertebral discs. For proper shoulder position, envision your shoulder blades going down and back, as if you are going to put them into the back pockets of your jeans or pants.
Do Not Sit for Long Periods of Time	Do not sit for longer than thirty minutes at a time. It is difficult to maintain proper sitting posture for this amount of time and places a lot of stress on the neck, back, and hips. Stand up, do a chest stretch, or take a walk to the water fountain as an opportunity to take pressure off the back and reset your muscles.

Avoid Poor Standing Posture: Tucked Back and Sway Back

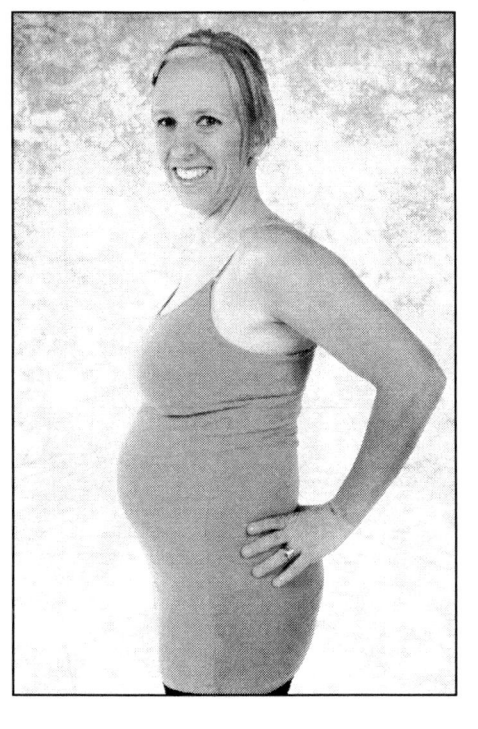 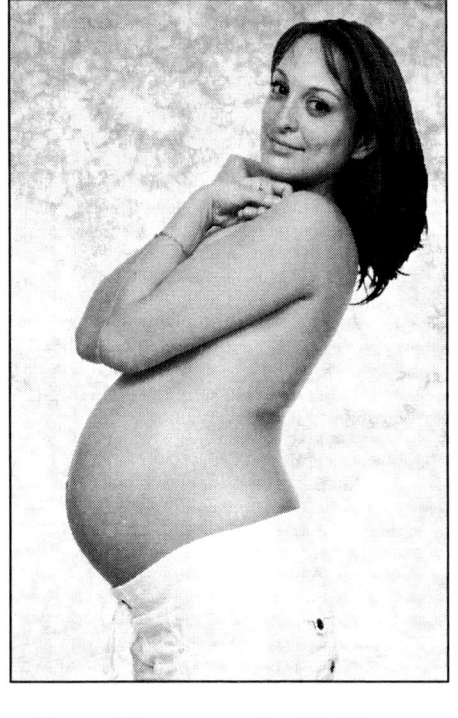

Description: The woman on the left is in a tucked-in position and the woman on the right is in a sway-back posture.

While the baby grows, your body's center of gravity shifts anteriorly, or forward. This shift forward forces your body to compensate in order to maintain your balance and prevent you from falling. There are two major postures that most women will assume during their pregnancy to compensate for the physiologic changes that occur: "swayback" or "tucked tush." The swayback posture, or increased lumbar lordosis, occurs when a woman assumes an excessive arch in the low back to maintain her balance. The tucked tush posture, on the other hand, occurs when a woman essentially squeezes the butt muscles to bring the center of gravity over the base of support in order to prevent falls. Both of these postures add stress to the lumbar spine, sacroiliac joint, and hip muscles and ligaments, which are particularly vulnerable due to hormonal changes. The hormone relaxin results in the ligaments of the pelvis loosening, causing sacroiliac joint instability, malalignment of the pelvis, and additional muscular compensations. These muscular compensations can cause painful spasms, trigger points, and inflexibility leading to a vicious cycle of pain and pelvic malalignment. In addition, the weight of each breast increases by about one pound by the end of pregnancy, and can pull your shoulders forward, overstretching your mid-back muscles, and possibly leading to mid-back as well as neck pain.

Trade Secret to Use: Proper Standing Posture

Our big trade secret for standing posture is don't lock your knees. Why? Locking the knees throws you into a swayback posture and increases stress on your joints. Bring awareness to how you are standing and correct yourself every time you lock your knees. Keep your knees slightly bent. Another trade secret is to keep your chest lifted and your shoulders pulled back. Imagine that you are wearing a beautiful necklace and you want to show it off to everyone. Keep your head aligned with your neck; avoid forward head posture and keep your chin tucked in. The lower back should be in neutral spine position. Posture is cultivated by what we do every day. It may seem

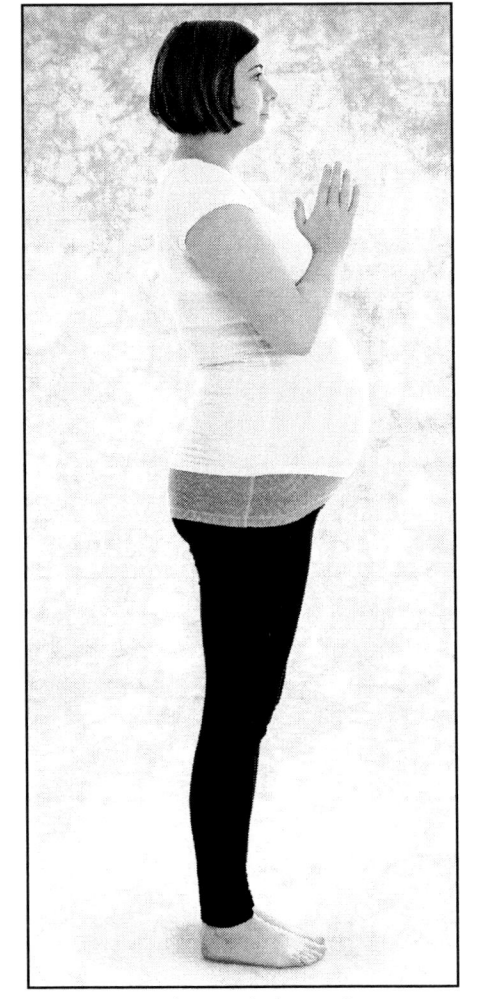

Description: This is ideal standing posture. Notice the bend in the knees and the neck and hip alignment.

easier to stand in poor posture, but at the end of the day your body will not be happy and pain will set in. Do yourself a favor and stand up straight.

Avoid Impact Exercises

Impact exercise, such as running and jumping exercises, can sometimes be harmful to the body during pregnancy. As previously discussed, the changes in your body will make you more susceptible to experiencing loss of balance, falls, instability, and generalized weakness. These changes can make impact exercises unsafe for some women and place mother and baby at risk for injury. If something just doesn't feel right, or if you are experiencing pain with impact exercises, you should not continue to do these activities during your pregnancy.

Trade Secret to Use: Walking and Listening to Your Body's Signals

Women who have sciatica, pubic symphysis dysfunction, sacroiliac joint instability, diastasis recti abdominis, or pelvic pain should proceed cautiously with impact exercises and refer to Chapter 3 for specific exercise recommendations. Women who learn that their usual body-sculpt, boot camp, Pilates, yoga, spinning, or aerobics classes may be causing and/or exacerbating their pain are sometimes disheartened. However, there are many alternative exercises that will help keep you active, healthy, and pain free, and most importantly are safe for you and your growing baby. One fantastic low-impact alternative to running or jumping activities is walking. A moderate-intensity walking and exercise program can help improve muscle tone, strength, and endurance, promote healthy bowel movements, increase circulation, decrease risk for Cesarean section and vacuum/forceps deliveries, and can improve mood, energy, and sleep. Other low-impact alternatives include swimming, recumbent biking, and light weight training.

Chapter 3 discusses what we refer to as "Body Talk," or the ability to listen to your body's signals and make safe decisions when exercising. Again, if something just doesn't feel right, listen to your body talk and discontinue the activity you are doing. Not all exercise benefits everyone, and we encourage you to become your own healer and discover what works best for your body and your baby. This principle cannot be stressed enough and is extremely important when developing your own exercise regimen. At our healing center, we help women who desire to continue their current exercise routines make modifications, offer alternative exercise strategies, and develop personalized yoga, Pilates, and cardiovascular routines that are challenging but follow the necessary precautions and safety considerations discussed in this chapter. The journey toward a safe and healthy exercise program during pregnancy can be challenging; however, if you listen to your body and the exercise guidelines outlined in Chapter 3, you will be on your way to awakening the powerful goddess within you.

Avoid Letting It All Hang Out

In pregnancy, the abdominal muscles become stretched and weakened. As the baby grows your abdominals offer less support for your spine, back and hips. Many pregnant women have no idea how to utilize their deep core muscle (transverse abdominal TrA) as "medicine" for the spine, hips and back. Many women over-activate their abdominals by over-tightening their bellies. This is WRONG. When you try too hard to get your abdominals to kick in you use the external oblique muscles rather than the deep core muscles. Instead of letting it all hang out (or over-activating your core), use our trade secret and see your body shift into a more powerful position and experience less pain with your everyday living.

Trade Secret to Use: Pelvic Brace (Combination of a TrA Hold plus Kegel Contraction)

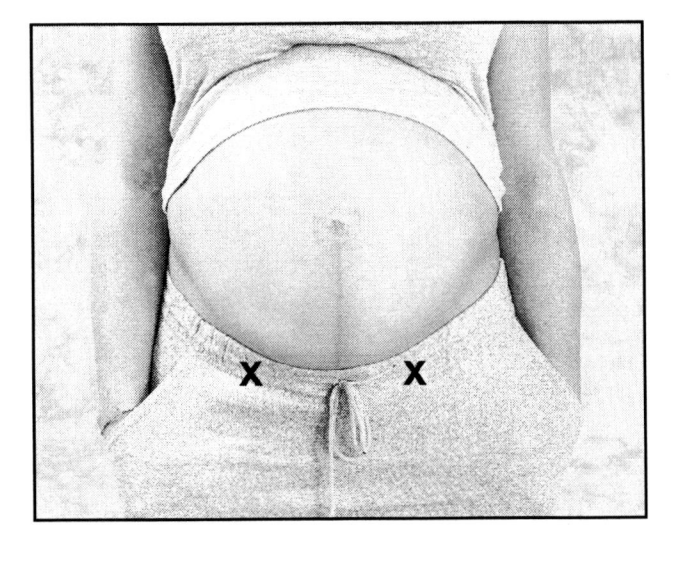

Description: The X's mark where the transverse abdominal muscles can be felt when properly activated.

The pelvic brace is your secret weapon. A pelvic brace is a combination of a TrA contraction and a low-level Kegel contraction. This mighty combo exercise can help decrease back pain, stabilize the sacroiliac joint, minimize DRA, and prevent pelvic floor muscle dysfunction including pelvic organ prolapse and incontinence. All pregnant women should learn to activate their transversus abdominis muscle, or use this pelvic brace, in order to minimize strain through the abdomen and pelvic floor. Activating the TrA is a skill that requires practice, precision, and coordination. The TrA muscle is anatomically wired to activate with the pelvic floor muscles, making these two structures a dynamic duo in core strengthening and stabilization exercises. For example, when log rolling out of bed, do a pelvic brace first before you roll. Or, before you lift an object or transition from sitting to standing, do a pelvic brace. This pelvic brace will help prepare the body for movements which place increased strain on the low back and pelvis, and keep your body supported and safe. You can do amazing things with your body during pregnancy with time, practice, and diligence. By tuning into the pelvic brace early on, you can help prevent injury during difficult transitional movements throughout the day and lay the foundation upon which to build a safe and rewarding core training program. For additional recommendations and amazing strategies to safely train your core during pregnancy, see Chapter 12.

Follow these steps to learn how to do a pelvic brace:

1. As you exhale, do a Kegel, or squeeze your pelvic floor muscles as if you are trying to stop the flow of urine. This ensures you will not push down on the pelvic floor muscles, and instead will initiate a lifting motion from the pelvic floor up to the TrA.

2. Draw your belly closer and more firmly toward the spine. As you pull in your abdominals try to imagine that you are trying to squeeze into an old pair of jeans that don't fit. Your belly should actually lift upward toward your nose if you perform the exercise correctly.

3. Avoid over-contracting the superficial abdominals, like the external obliques or rectus abdominis. Try to think of the TrA contraction as 20 percent of your maximal effort; it is very subtle and precise.

   - Do not hold your breath. Exhale as you perform the contraction.

   - Once you establish the above movement, hold for five seconds and repeat ten times. Do one to three sets per day to master this skill.

Stopping your destructive forces will be easy with our trade secrets. All you have to do is increase your awareness of body positioning, posture and body mechanics. Once you start to implement our trade secrets your pain, aches and discomfort will start to melt away and you will be able to remain active and pain free. In the next phase of healing you will learn to correct your bony alignment with more trade secrets that include correcting misalignment of the pubic symphysis, lumbar spine and innominate bones.

CHAPTER FIVE

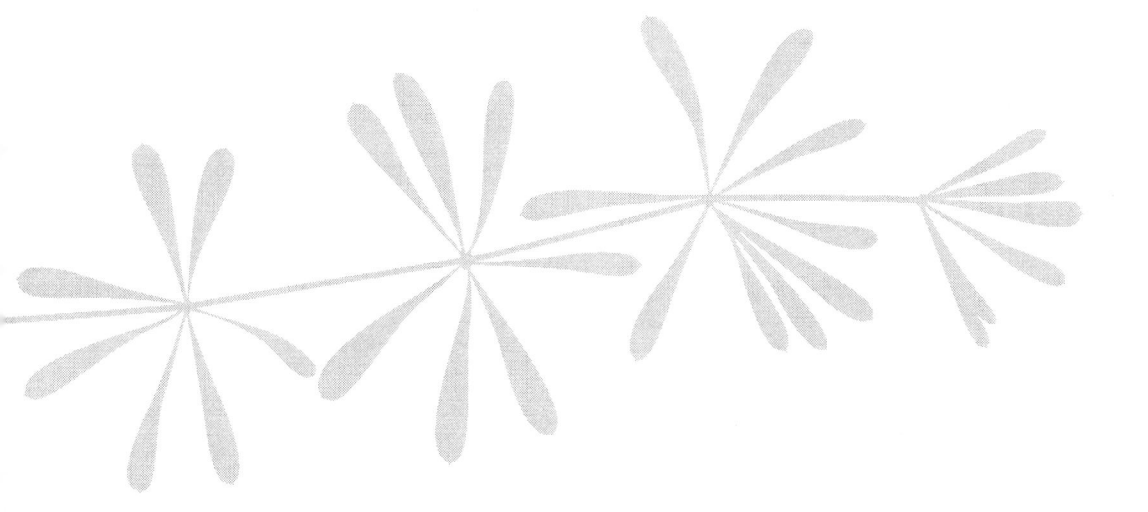

"Healing is a matter of time, but it is sometimes also a matter of opportunity."

– Hippocrates

Chapter 5

BE YOUR OWN HEALER: ALIGN YOUR PELVIS, STAY OUT OF PAIN AND
KEEP YOUR BABY IN THE BEST POSITION

Many of our patients come to Renew Physical Therapy in search of answers they are not getting from their MDs or midwives. They tell us: "I feel like something is out of place and my bones just don't feel right" or "Every time I take a step it's painful and I feel vulnerable and wobbly." Healthcare providers often dismiss these complaints as an unavoidable part of being pregnant. Physicians rarely offer pregnant women corrective strategies or referrals to physical therapy to alleviate these kinds of pain. In this chapter we put the power back into the hands of pregnant women. We show that issues relating to bones and their alignment can easily be addressed by the pregnant woman when she is shown the proper way to do so. The trade secrets we share here—secrets that are usually reserved for physical therapists, osteopaths and other rehabilitation experts—will arm you with pelvic corrections guaranteed to get you out of pain fast.

As discussed in the previous chapter, you absolutely can take steps to control your pain. Better yet, you may be able to prevent pain altogether or greatly reduce pain by using the tools in *EPP*. In this chapter, we will teach you safe and effective ways for correcting your own alignment. When your bones are in optimal alignment you will experience less pain and function better. Your muscles will get stronger faster because they are in an ideal position to contract and relax. *And your baby will also be in the ideal position for labor and delivery.* You will learn how to evaluate your alignment by using simple bony landmarks. (You will first need to learn all the bony landmarks covered in this chapter to be successful with your own adjustments.) We'll begin with a review of the anatomy and function of the pelvic girdle bones.

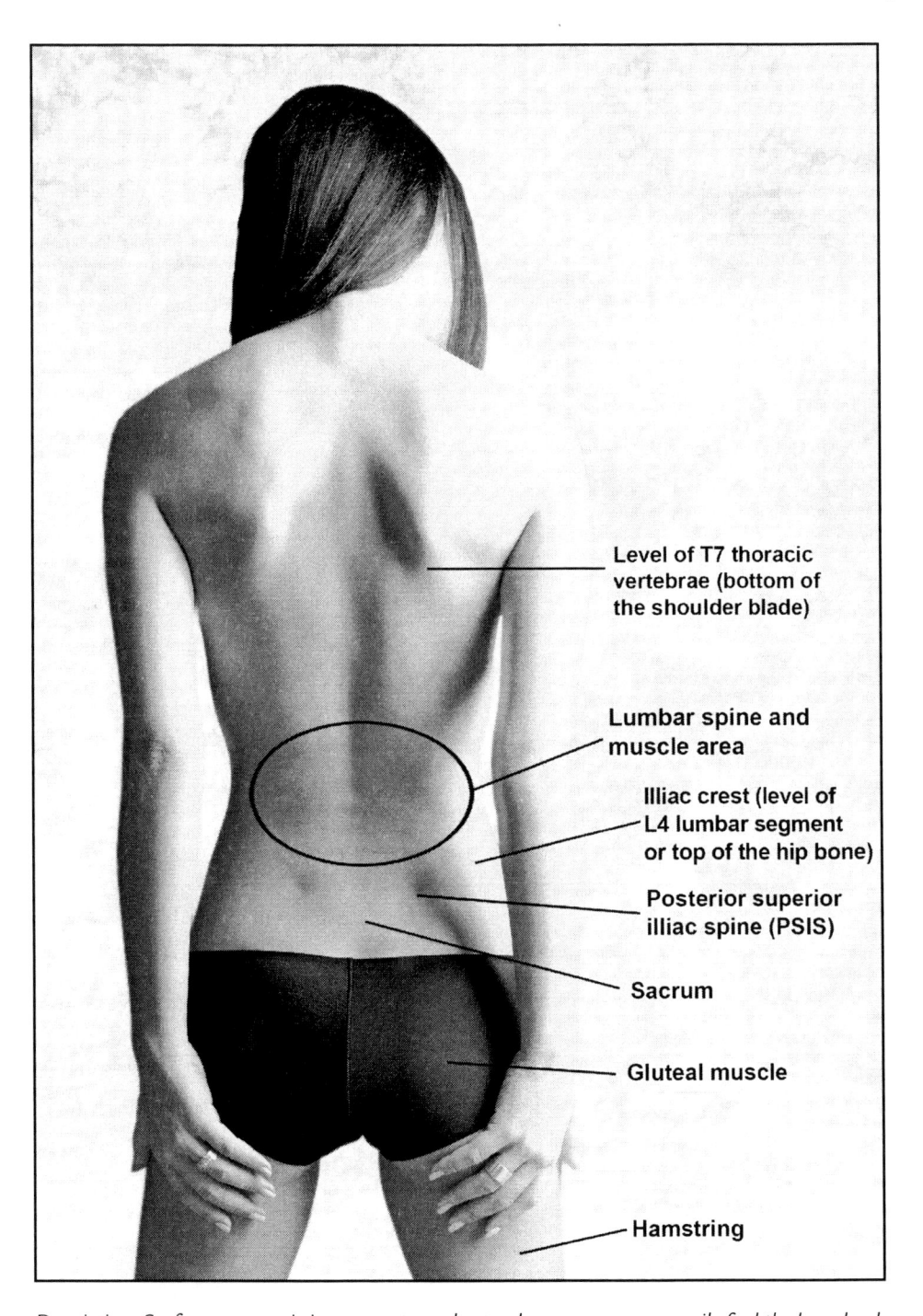

Level of T7 thoracic vertebrae (bottom of the shoulder blade)

Lumbar spine and muscle area

Illiac crest (level of L4 lumbar segment or top of the hip bone)

Posterior superior illiac spine (PSIS)

Sacrum

Gluteal muscle

Hamstring

Description: Surface anatomy is important to understand so you can more easily find the bony landmarks. Please take note of the different areas and keep them in mind as you read this very important chapter on how to correct your own alignment.

Pelvic Girdle Anatomy and Function

The human pelvis is often referred to as the pelvic girdle. The pelvic girdle is a three-part bony ring composed of one sacrum and two innominates. The sacrum is a triangular-shaped bone that forms the back of the pelvis. It is actually a continuation of the spine; however, instead of having individual vertebrae that move and flex, the sacrum is made up of five fused vertebrae. This fusion of the vertebrae results in a solid piece of bone. The sacrum acts as the keystone of the pelvic ring and is wedged tightly in between the two innominates.

Diagrm 5.1: Bones of the Pelvis: Anterior View of Sacrum and Innominate

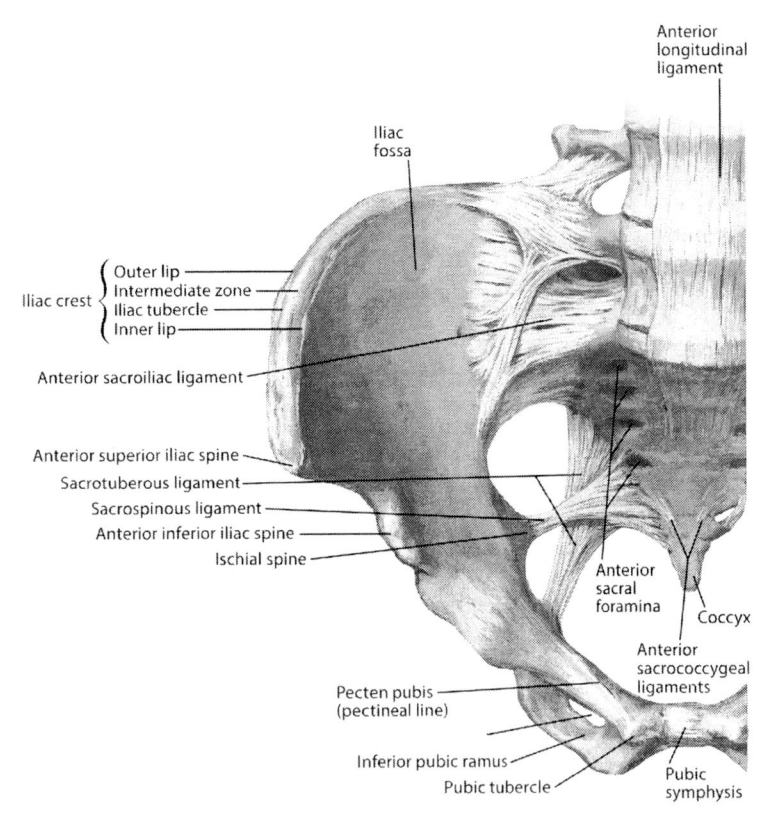

Diagram Description: This is an anterior view of the pelvic girdle. Notice the triangular-shaped sacrum. The larger bone is called the innominate and consists of three bones fused together. There is a right and left innominate bone. These bones can frequently get out of alignment because of the hormonal shifts and other challenges of pregnancy. Source: Netter Images.

Diagram 5.2: Bones of the Pelvis: Posterior View of Sacrum and Innominate

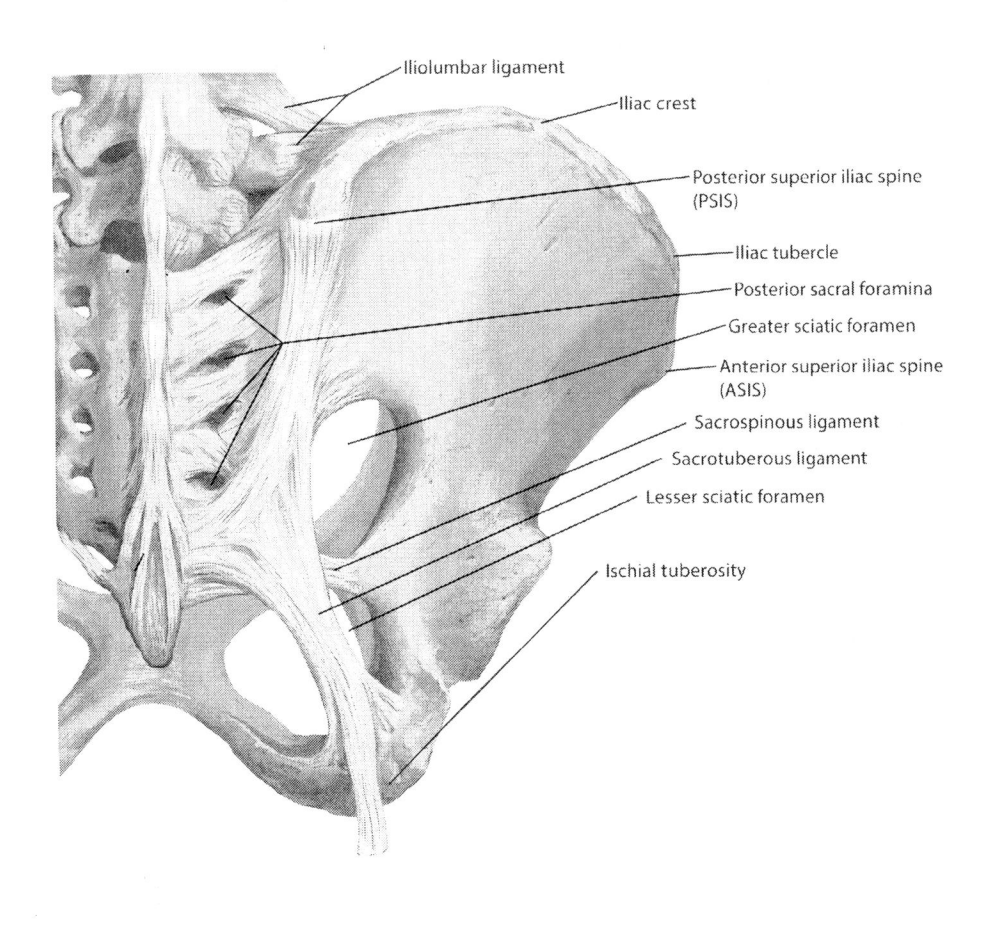

Iliolumbar ligament

Iliac crest

Posterior superior iliac spine (PSIS)

Iliac tubercle

Posterior sacral foramina

Greater sciatic foramen

Anterior superior iliac spine (ASIS)

Sacrospinous ligament

Sacrotuberous ligament

Lesser sciatic foramen

Ischial tuberosity

Diagram Description: This is a posterior view of the pelvic girdle. Notice the ligaments that surround and connect the sacrum and innominate. The connection between these two bones creates the sacroiliac joint. There is a left and right sacroiliac joint. It is common for pregnant women to experience pain in this joint and for this joint to get out of alignment. Source: Netter Images.

The innominates form the sides of the pelvis and are made up of three different bones that are fused (permanently joined) together: the ilium, the ischium and the pubis. The right and left innominates meet the sacrum to form the right and left sacroiliac joints (SI). The tight-fitting SI joints are designed primarily for stability and help transfer weight between the spine, legs and the ground. The strength of the entire pelvic ring is highly dependent on the stability of the SI joints.

In addition to stability, the SI joint plays a secondary role in allowing slight motion within the pelvic ring. As we walk, each side of the pelvis rotates out of sync with the opposite side of the pelvis. This opposite rotation of the innominate bones produces a torque, or torsion, within the pelvic ring. Without some flexibility of the SI joint, the pelvic ring would be too rigid to allow for walking. The faster we walk, the greater the torsions within our pelvis and the harder SI joints work to keep us moving without pain. Dysfunction at the SI joints causes pain with moving in bed, transferring from sitting to standing, walking and stair climbing.

In the front of the pelvic ring, the right and left innominates join at the pubic symphysis. Commonly referred to as the pubic "bone," the pubic symphysis is actually a joint made up of two bones, one cushioning disc and numerous ligaments. During walking, the pubic symphysis serves as the front axis for the alternating movement of the legs. Similar to the sacroiliac joints, the pubic symphysis helps to decrease pressure within the pelvic ring during walking. Dysfunction at the pubic symphysis alters the mechanics of walking and can cause pain in the groin, inner thighs or abdominal muscles.

The pelvic ring, or pelvic girdle, serves as a transfer station for movement. When we change positions, shift our weight, take a step, or stand on one foot, the weight of our bodies is transferred through the SI joints and pubic symphysis. As we read earlier, the SI joints and pubic symphysis must simultaneously provide stability and allow for motion. For simple activities, such as sitting and standing, most of our stability is provided by the bony architecture of the sacrum fitting tightly in between the two innominates. For more difficult activities, such as walking, stair climbing or running, the tight fit of the SI joints is not enough to stabilize the pelvic girdle. For these demanding activities, the pelvic girdle relies heavily on its muscles and surrounding ligaments.

The Pelvic Girdle during Pregnancy

In pregnancy, the ligaments that provide stability for the pelvic girdle become lax, or loose, due to an increase in the hormone relaxin. Although the pelvic girdle is designed to provide both stability and motion, the loosening of the ligaments may cause excessive motion, or hypermobility, in the SI joints and at the pubic symphysis. During pregnancy, excessive or unequal force placed through the SI and pubic joints can disrupt their alignment and cause pain in the joints and ligaments of the pelvis. Without the stability of the ligaments, the muscles of the pelvic girdle are then asked to take on more of the stabilizing work. Oftentimes, these muscles are simply too weak for their new work load, which leads to muscle pain and spasms.

How Pelvic Alignment Affects the Position of the Fetus

When planning for childbirth, there are many factors that we attempt to control: the location of the birth, the people who will be attending the birth and the person who will be delivering or catching the baby. However, there is another factor that will highly influence the birth: the position of the baby in the uterus. A baby who is in a breech position may need to be delivered via Cesarean section. Many women are told during labor that their pelvic opening (pelvic outlet) is simply not large enough for the baby to be delivered vaginally. These women also may be given a Cesarean section.

The optimal position for a developing fetus is the head-down, or vertex, position. One of the reasons that a baby may not assume this head-down position is due to external forces on the uterus that may not allow the baby enough room to turn. This is referred to as intrauterine constraint. Many women are surprised to learn that the alignment of the sacrum can impact intrauterine constraint and breech positioning. In fact, there are two uterosacral ligaments that directly connect the uterus to the sacrum. When the sacrum rotates out of its optimal alignment, it may pull the uterus out of its proper position via tension on these ligaments. When the uterus is tensioned out of its proper positioning, a breech baby may not assume the head-down position prior to birth.

Pelvic alignment not only affects the position of the uterus, but also the positioning of the pelvic opening, or outlet. When the innominates and sacrum are in a neutral position, the pelvic outlet forms a symmetrical and round opening. If the sacrum or innominates are rotated out of their neutral position, the pelvic outlet may become smaller and less symmetrical.

Many of our clients at Renew are surprised and grateful to learn that maintaining optimal pelvic alignment may help reduce the chances of a baby remaining in the breech position and may provide the widest and most symmetrical pelvic outlet for vaginal birth. You may use the pelvic alignment techniques in this chapter to maintain optimal pelvic alignment throughout your pregnancy.

How Pelvic Alignment Affects the Pelvic Floor Muscles

Optimal pelvic alignment not only affects a woman's ability to move without pain and deliver a baby, but alignment also affects the function of the very important pelvic floor muscles. The pelvic floor muscles consist of three layers of muscle that support your pelvis, control urination and defecation and allow for optimal sexual function. Many women become acutely aware of these muscles during pregnancy. Some women experience urinary incontinence due to pelvic floor weakness, while other women experience pelvic pain due to spasm of these very same pelvic muscles. Optimal pelvic floor muscle control during pregnancy can help prevent incontinence and pelvic pain, stabilize the low back and pelvis and aid the smooth delivery of the baby with minimal trauma to the perineum.

Maintaining good pelvic alignment is key to pelvic floor muscle function. The pelvic floor muscles are housed within the bony pelvis and form the secure foundation for pelvic floor muscle contraction and relaxation. For further insight on how to assess and prepare your pelvic floor muscles for birth, see Chapter 9.

Anatomical Landmarks and Surface Anatomy: The Pubic Symphysis, Anterior Superior Iliac Spine (ASIS), and Posterior Superior Iliac Spine (PSIS)

There are three important bony "landmarks" that we will use to assess your pelvic alignment: the pubic symphysis, the anterior superior iliac spine (ASIS) and the posterior superior iliac spine (PSIS).

Diagram 5.3: Finding the Pubic Symphysis

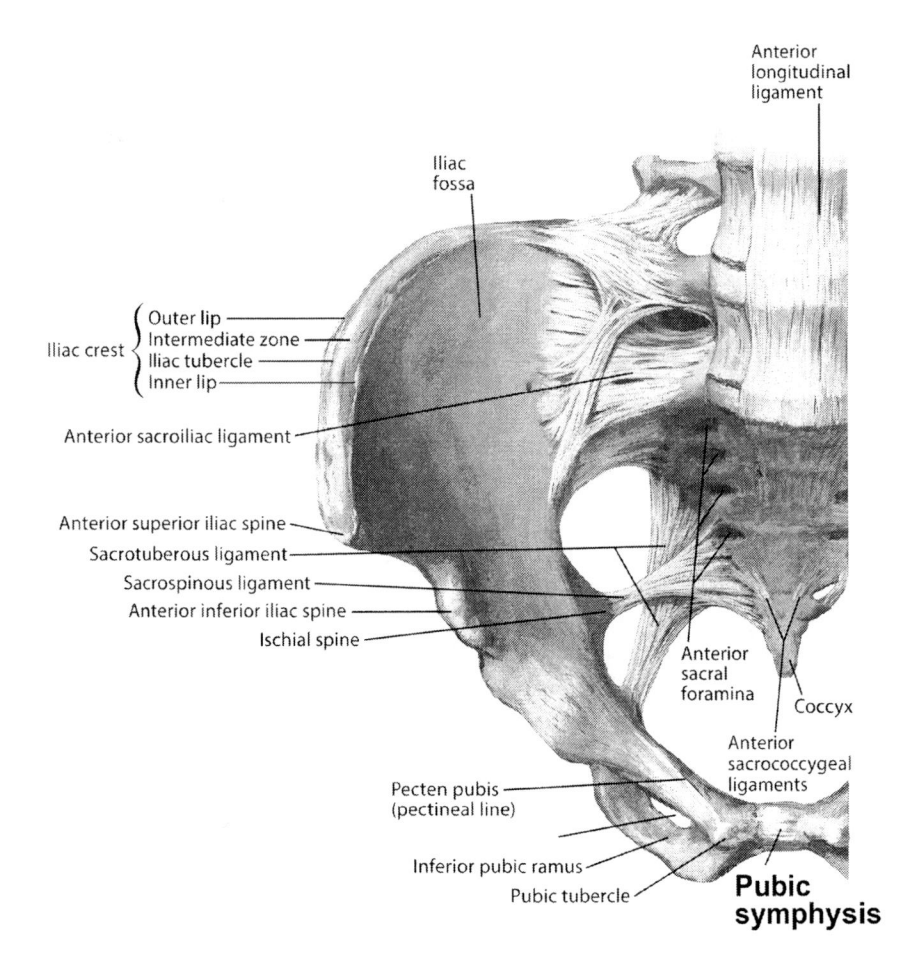

Diagram Description: Notice the pubic symphysis and the ligaments that surround and keep this joint in place. When there is a separation or misalignment of this joint pregnant women experience a great deal of pain. Source: Netter Images.

WHAT TO DO:

The pubic symphysis is best located while standing or lying down. Place the heel of one of your hands at your belly button, with your fingers facing down toward your feet. If you are early in your pregnancy, your fingers will drop down and contact the bones of your pubic symphysis. If you are further along in your pregnancy, gently slide your hands over or around your belly and toward your feet until you contact the bones of the pubic symphysis. Remember that the pubic symphysis is actually made up of two separate bones that are joined in the middle.

Finding the Anterior Superior Iliac Spine (ASIS)

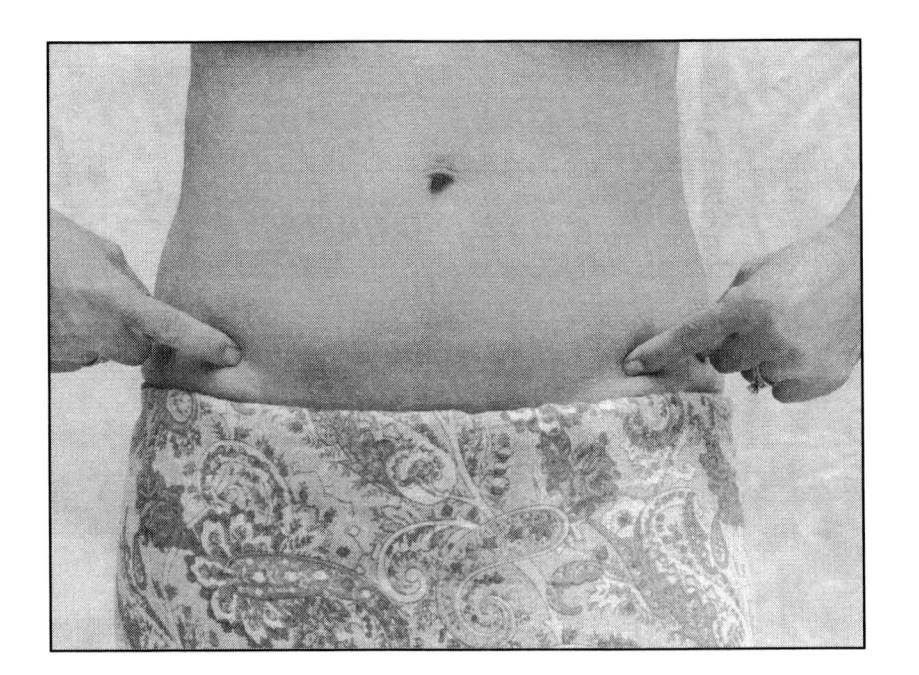

Description: The finger placement shows you the location of the ASIS. You can easily see it in this photograph as this bony prominence sticks out anteriorly. Practice finding ASIS on your body.

WHAT TO DO:

Start by placing your hands on the highest part of your pelvis. Most people naturally assume this position when placing their "hands on their hips." The highest point on your pelvic bones is called your iliac crest. Now trace your iliac crest forward until you come across two distinct, bony projections toward the front of your pelvis. These two rounded projections are your ASIS.

Diagram 5.4: Finding the Posterior Superior Iliac Spine (PSIS)

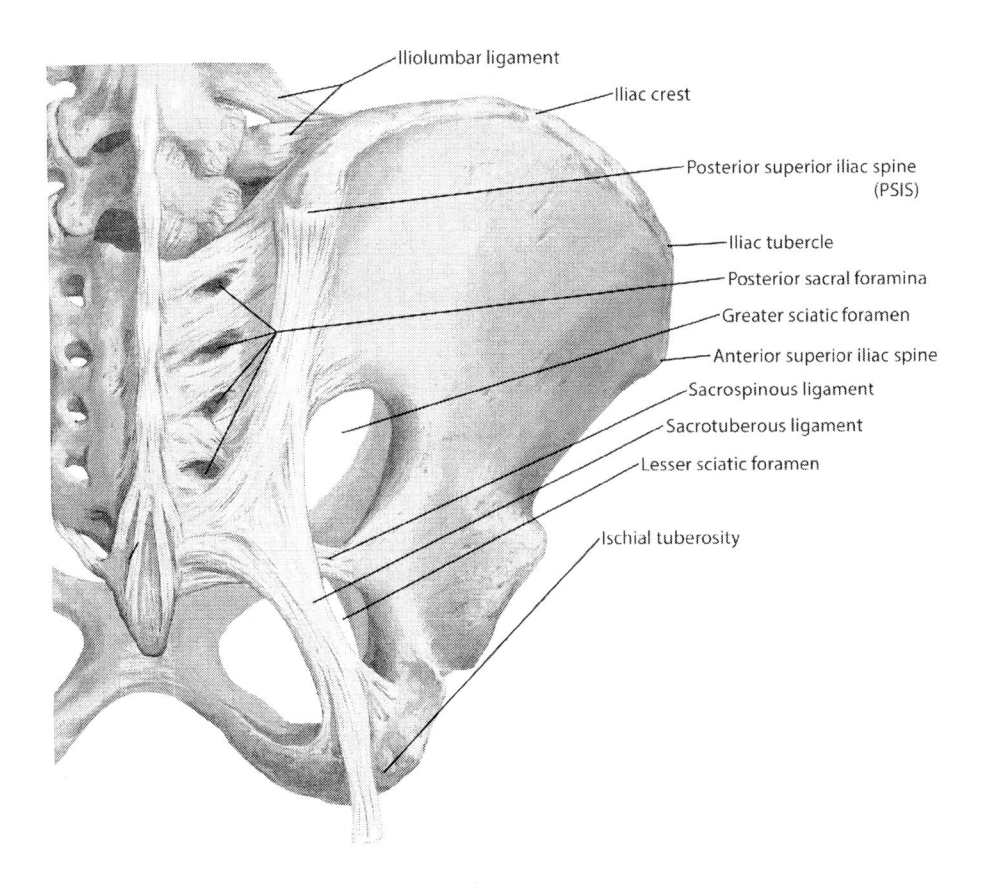

Diagram Description: Notice the large bony protrusion on the top. That is the PSIS and it can be easily found on most pregnant women. Source: Netter Images.

The Dimples of Venus and Its Relationship to PSIS

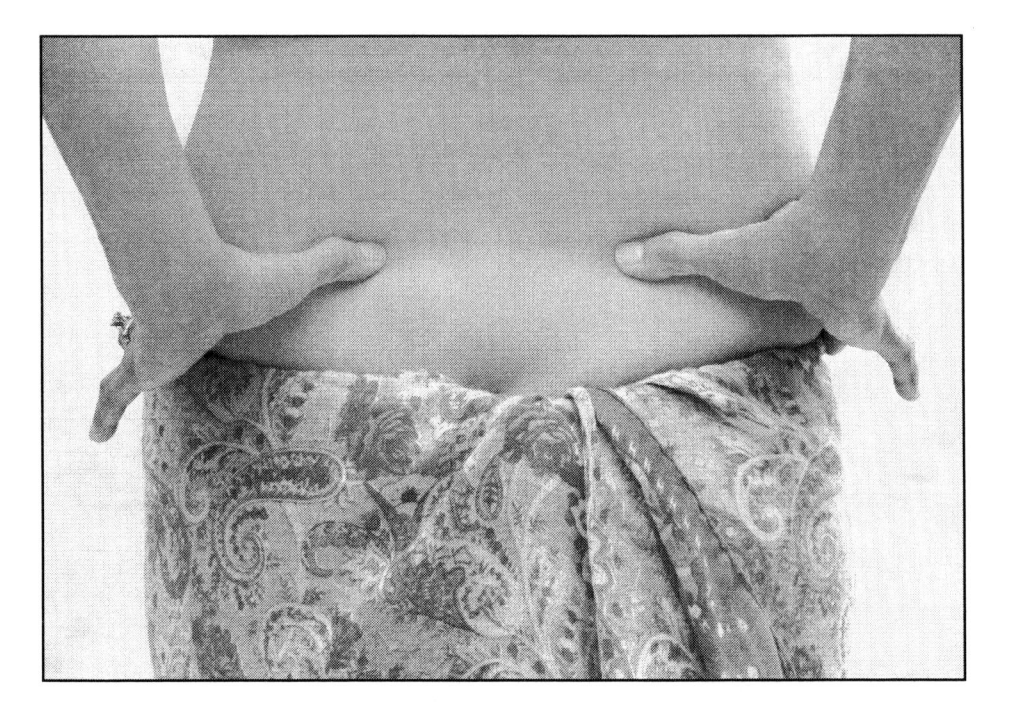

Diagram Description: Notice the indentations on the skin. These dimples are called the "Dimples of Venus" and right next to them you can find the PSIS. The finger location shows you the location of the PSIS.

WHAT TO DO:

Place your hands at the top of your iliac crest. Now trace your iliac crest toward your low back until you come across two rounded bony projections in the low back. These two rounded projections are your PSIS. Some people have small indentations, or dimples, next to their PSIS, making them easier to find. For most people, these are not as easy to find as ASIS.

How to Assess Your Alignment: The Pubic Symphysis

WHAT TO DO:

1. If you are early in your pregnancy, you may be able to directly assess whether the two sides of your pubic symphysis are in alignment. Start by identifying the two bones of your pubic symphysis as described above.

2. Find the very top, or most superior portion, of these bones and slide your thumbs on top of the right and left bone. Now assess whether your thumbs are level, or whether one thumb is higher than the other.

3. If you notice that one side of the pubic symphysis is higher than the other, you may benefit from the shotgun correction described later in this chapter.

4. If you are later in pregnancy, you may find it difficult to assess the relative heights of the pubic bones. If your belly is preventing you from assessing the pubic bones, move on to the next assessment for innominate rotations.

5. If you find an innominate rotation in the next assessment, then you can assume that the pubic symphysis is also out of alignment and you can proceed with the shotgun correction.

How to Assess Your Alignment: Anterior and Posterior Innominate Rotations

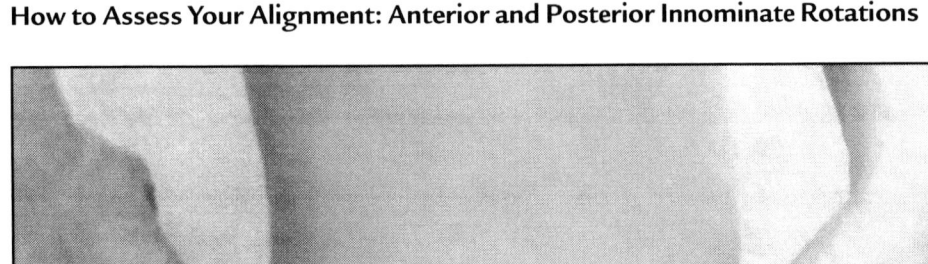

Description: Notice the ASIS and PSIS and the line connecting both. The inclination of this line determines whether you are suffering from a posterior innominate or anterior innominate misalignment. This is normal, optimal alignment.

WHAT TO DO:

1. Stand sideways in a mirror and identify your ASIS and PSIS on your right side. Picture an imaginary line going from your right PSIS to your right ASIS and take note of the angle that this line forms. Although this angle may vary from person to person, the line should slope downward from the PSIS to the ASIS. A recent research article found the average angle from PSIS to ASIS to be thirteen degrees sloped downward from the horizontal.

2. Repeat this procedure on your left side. Take careful notice of whether the line from PSIS to ASIS seems to be sloped more vertical or more horizontal than your right side.

3. If you find that one line is noticeably more horizontal, the innominate on this side may be rotated posteriorly, or backward, compared to the other side. We will refer to this later in the chapter as a posterior innominate.

4. If you find that one line is noticeably more vertical or sloped downward, the innominate on this side may be rotated anteriorly, or forward, compared to the other side. We will refer to this later in the chapter as an anterior innominate.

How to Correct Your Own Alignment Using Muscle Energy Technique (MET)

Muscle energy technique (MET) is a gentle, yet powerful, osteopathic treatment technique. Osteopathic techniques use the hands rather than machinery to diagnose, treat and prevent injury. MET is a specific technique that involves gentle muscle contraction performed against equal resistance in a specific direction. This type of contraction, in which a muscle contracts but does not shorten, is called an isometric contraction.

Muscle energy technique is simple to perform, yet yields powerful results. MET is used to gently mobilize, or move, joints in order to maintain optimal alignment and function. Due to the fact that MET utilizes voluntary muscle contraction, MET also strengthens muscle as it corrects the joint alignment. In addition to mobilizing and strengthening, MET can reduce localized swelling and venous congestion, as muscle contraction helps to "pump" fluid through the lymphatic and venous systems. All of these benefits are derived from a technique that can safely be performed by anyone anywhere.

One of the greatest benefits of using MET during pregnancy is the innate safety of the technique. When performing MET on yourself, you are the one who controls both the muscle contraction and the resistance to the contraction. In this respect, it is the pregnant woman who is responsible for the "dosage" of the corrective technique. Since the technique uses a woman's own muscle contraction, the techniques are widely considered to be extremely safe. In the next section, we will explore how to use MET to correct and maintain optimal pelvic girdle alignment throughout your pregnancy.

How to Correct Your Own Pelvis

We will now share five trade secrets with you; while we commonly perform these corrections on our patients, there are a number of low back and pelvic alignment corrections that a pregnant woman can safely perform on her own body. In order to be your own best healer, you must perform careful investigative work. Your body may need one, two or three of the self-corrections described below. As you move through the following section, perform each alignment assessment and write down your findings. Follow the corrections that are appropriate for your specific findings. Please note that your pelvic alignment may change over the course of days or weeks. Before performing an alignment correction, repeat the appropriate alignment assessment in order to determine the appropriate correction for your body at the specific time.

As you move through the alignment assessments below, you may discover that your body requires more than one alignment correction. In the osteopathic approach to treatment, the specific order that you perform corrections is important to achieving optimal alignment and maximal pain. Once you have identified the specific corrections that you need, refer to the table below for the proper order of the corrections. The lumbar shift and shotgun corrections can be performed as stand-alone corrections. The anterior and posterior innominate corrections should always be preceded by the shotgun correction.

Table 5.1: Trade Secrets: Order of Pelvic Girdle Corrections

1. Lumbar Shift Correction
2. Shotgun Correction
3. *Anterior Innominate Correction
4. *Posterior Innominate Correction
5. *Simultaneous Anterior/Posterior Correction

Anterior and Posterior Innominate Corrections should always be preceded by the Shotgun Correction.

Trade Secret #1: Lumbar Shift Correction

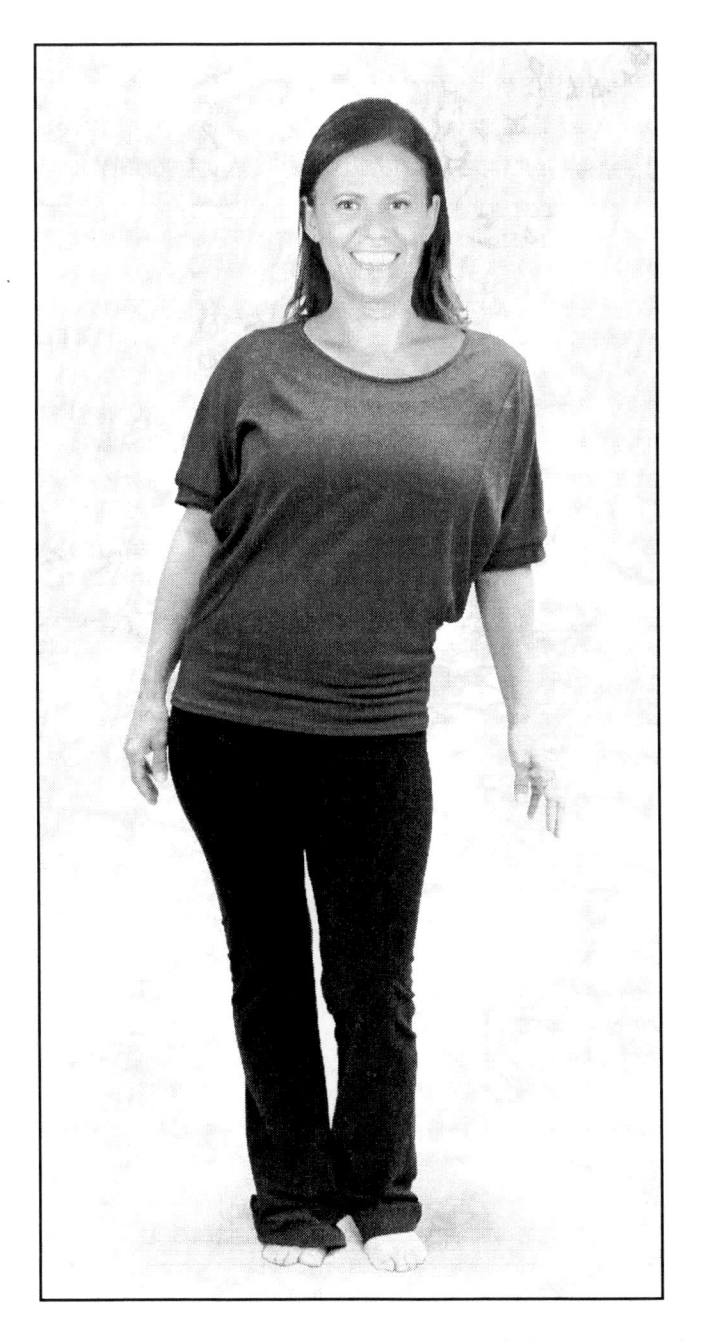

Description: Notice how the upper body shifts away from the lower body. Sometimes a lumbar shift is not this obvious so you really have to scan the body and take notice to determine the shift.

Prior to investigating and correcting dysfunctions of the pelvic girdle, we must first take a quick look at the lumbar spine, or low back region. There are some instances of low back pain when the upper body shifts away from the lower body in order to take pressure off a painful segment in the low back. It is very important to correct a lumbar shift to avoid further compensation and pain in the low back and legs.

HOW TO IDENTIFY

Stand facing a mirror in snug clothing that allows you to see the position of your hips and shoulders. If both of your shoulders are located directly over your hips, then you do not have an obvious lumbar shift and should move on to the next alignment assessment. If you do notice that your shoulders are off to one side when compared to your hips, then you likely have a lumbar shift.

Common Symptoms of Lumbar Shift

A lumbar shift is often seen as a result of back pain that radiates into the buttocks or leg. In many instances, the woman may experience a feeling of tingling or numbness in the leg, rather than pain. Many women report that their leg simply goes weak or collapses under them when they stand up from bed. Some women have no back pain at all, but only symptoms in their leg or foot. All of these symptoms may be due to dysfunction in the low back region. As we mentioned earlier, correcting a lumbar shift is essential to avoid further pain and compensation.

WHAT TO DO:

1. The motion used to perform the lumbar shift correction is similar to the motion made while playing with a hula hoop or performing a hula dance. First make sure to identify your hip position relative to your shoulders, as we are going to slide or "hula" your hips back under your trunk and shoulders.

2. Inhale to prepare for the correction. Exhale and gently engage your transversus abdominis (TrA) as you slide, or hula, your hips back under your shoulders (for instruction on how to properly engage your TrA, see Chapter 12). You may also simultaneously slide your shoulders back over your hips. Hold this position and your TrA contraction for five seconds. Then release the contraction and return to your starting position. Repeat the correction ten times.

WHAT TO WATCH OUT FOR:

1. Although you will be shifting into correct alignment, this new positioning may feel very awkward at first, especially if your body has been shifted for a long period of time. Performing this correction over time will help you to regain proper alignment.

2. Performing this correction may cause a brief increase in symptoms. Your symptoms should lessen as you move through the ten repetitions. If your pain increases with repeated repetitions, stop the exercise, as you may not benefit from this correction. You may have a more complex alignment issue and need to be evaluated by a skilled physical therapist.

BENEFITS:

1. Helps to resolve low back pain and sciatica.

2. Helps to strengthen transversus abdominis and maintain spinal alignment.

HOW TO MAINTAIN CORRECTION:

1. Avoid destructive forces to prevent low back pain (see Chapter 4).

2. Figure Four Stretch to elongate piriformis and prevent sciatica (see Chapter 11).

3. Abdominal strengthening to stabilize spine (see Chapter 12).

Trade Secret #2: Shotgun Correction for Alignment of Pubic Symphysis

The "shotgun" correction is a pelvic MET that aligns the joint of the pubic symphysis. This is the first correction that is performed if no obvious lumbar shift is noted in the section above. The shotgun correction is appropriate for pregnant women who are experiencing symptoms of pubic bone pain or sacroiliac joint pain. Pain at the pubic bone or pubic symphysis is often referred to as symphysis pubis dysfunction (SPD). If you are experiencing symphysis pubis dysfunction, this may be the only correction that you need. If you are experiencing symptoms of sacroiliac joint dysfunction, this will be the first in a series of corrections. For more information on symphysis pubis dysfunction and sacroiliac joint dysfunction, see Chapters 6 and 7.

HOW TO IDENTIFY

1. Assess your alignment at the pubic bone and innominates as described in the last section.

2. Continue on to the shotgun correction if you find that one side of the pubic symphysis is higher than the other side or if you find an anterior or posterior innominate rotation, as described in the previous section.

Common Symptoms of Symphysis Pubis Dysfunction (SPD)

1. Pain in the pubic joint, groin and/or inner thigh with turning over in bed, moving from sitting to standing, walking and going up and down stairs.

2. Inability to stand on one foot while dressing, bathing and/or exercising.

3. Lower abdominal pain, usually greater on one side than the other. The rectus abdominis muscles that form your "six-pack" attach into the pubic symphysis. If the pubic symphysis is in poor alignment, there may be increased tension on these muscles and lower abdominal pain may result.

All abdominal pain during pregnancy must be evaluated by your physician or midwife to rule out more serious causes of abdominal pain.

Shotgun Correction: Phase A (Resistive Abduction) and Phase B (Resistive Adduction)

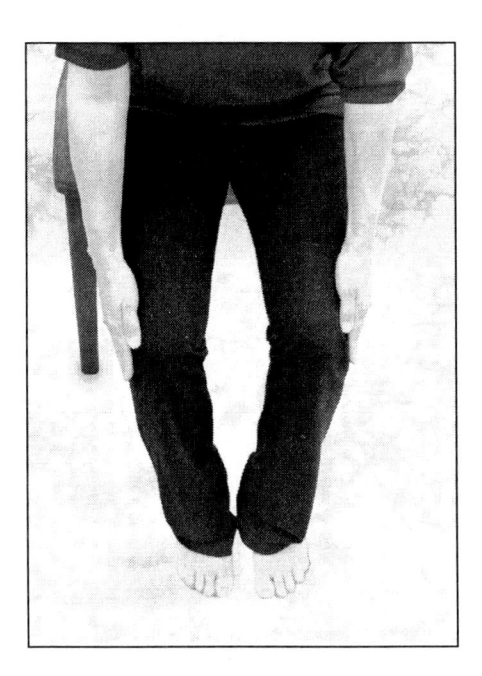

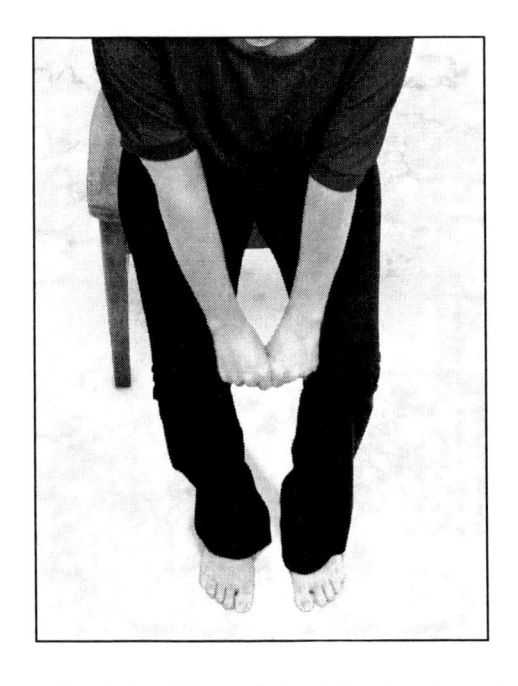

Description: This is called resistive abduction and it's the first phase of the shotgun correction.

Description: This is called resistive adduction and it's the second phase of the shotgun correction.

WHAT TO DO:

1. This correction can be performed while lying down or sitting up in a chair. If you are past your first trimester, you may be uncomfortable lying flat on your back. You may modify the lying position by placing a few pillows behind your back so that you are in a semi-reclined position. A woman can perform the correction on her own or with the help of a partner or friend.

2. If you are seated, scoot toward the edge of the chair and sit up tall. If you are lying down, bend your knees and place your feet flat on the floor or bed. Your knees should be slightly open and in line with your hips and feet.

3. Place your hands on the outside of your knees. While maintaining good posture, if sitting, open the knees and apply resistance to your hands. Press the thighs into your hands as if the legs are trying to rotate away from each other. As the thighs push out into the hands, the hands should apply equal pressure to the thighs, so that the legs do not actually move from their start position. This is called resistive abduction.

4. As you push the thighs into the hands, maintain this contraction for ten seconds. Do not hold your breath during the ten-second contraction. Try to maintain normal breathing, as breath-holding can increase blood pressure and pelvic pressure.

5. Repeat this exercise two more times, for a total of three ten-second contractions.

6. Next, place a firm object between your knees that you can squeeze. You may use a yoga block, firm ball or your own fist. While lying down or sitting in good posture, squeeze your knees against the object for ten seconds. Remember to breathe comfortably throughout the ten seconds. This is called resistive adduction.

7. Repeat the knee squeeze two more times, for a total of three ten-second contractions.

8. If you are using a sacroiliac support belt to treat SPD, you should apply the belt immediately after completing the shotgun correction. Refer to Chapter 8 for further instructions on how to choose and apply an appropriate sacroiliac support belt.

WHAT TO WATCH OUT FOR:

1. In the case of SPD, you may experience pain with the first repetition of the knee squeeze. Ask yourself to rate the pain on a scale of 0 to 10. Then continue to rate your pain during the next two knee squeezes. The pain should decrease during each repetition. If you are continuing to experience pain with the third repetition, then continue to repeat the ten-second knee squeeze until your pubic pain resolves. In our experience, some women need to perform the knee squeeze up to ten times in order to fully correct the joint alignment and resolve their pain.

2. It is possible that you may hear a "pop" as the pubic joint corrects into better alignment. This sound is neither dangerous nor necessary for the joint to achieve alignment.

3. If your pain increases, rather than decreases with repeated repetitions, stop the exercise. You may have a more complex alignment issue and need to be evaluated by a skilled physical therapist.

BENEFITS:

1. Helps to resolve SPD and sacroiliac joint pain.

2. Strengthening of the inner thigh and outer hip muscles, which are critical to stabilizing your spine and pelvis.

HOW TO MAINTAIN CORRECTION:

1. Avoid destructive forces (Chapter 4) and follow the precautions for SPD, as detailed in Chapter 7.

2. Use a sacroiliac support belt to maintain the correction, decrease pain and prevent recurrence of pubic symphysis malalignment (see Chapter 8).

3. Incorporate abdominal strengthening to stabilize the pelvis (see Chapter 12).

Trade Secret #3: Correction for an Anterior Innominate

HOW TO IDENTIFY

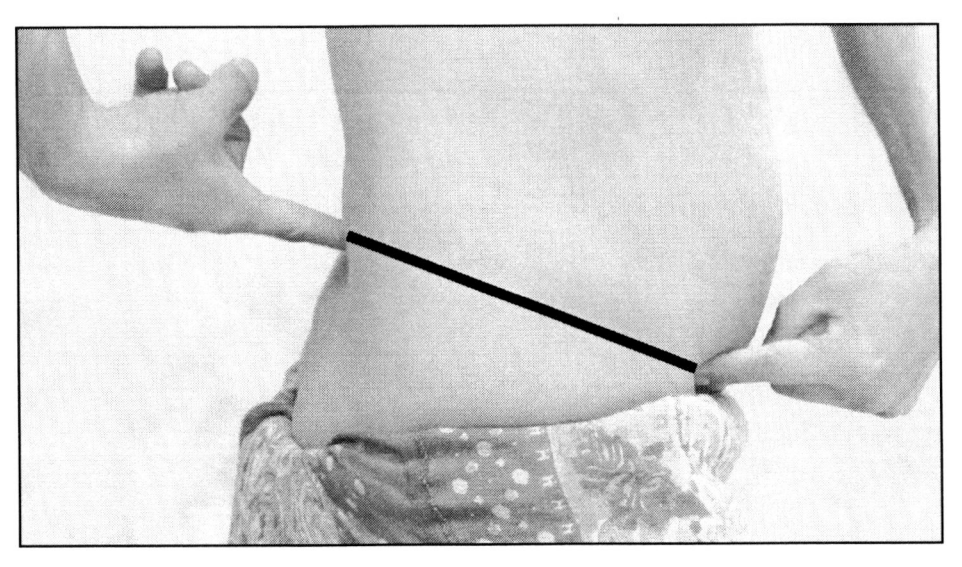

Description. Notice how the ASIS is lower than the PSIS. This is a typical presentation of an Anterior Innominate. Sometimes it's not as obvious as in the photo so you must look very closely.

Using the standing alignment assessment above, identify if one side of the pelvis forms a steeper line when drawn from the PSIS in the back to the ASIS in the front. If you find that one ASIS is significantly lower than the other, and you are experiencing one of the common symptoms listed below, you would likely benefit from an anterior innominate correction.

Common Symptoms of an Anterior Innominate Rotation

1. Pain in the front of the thigh, hip or lower abdomen on the side of the dysfunction.

2. An anterior innominate can also contribute to **round ligament pain**, which is a sharp, stabbing pain that occurs due to a sudden tightening of a ligament that travels from the uterus to the **labia majora**.

WHAT TO DO:

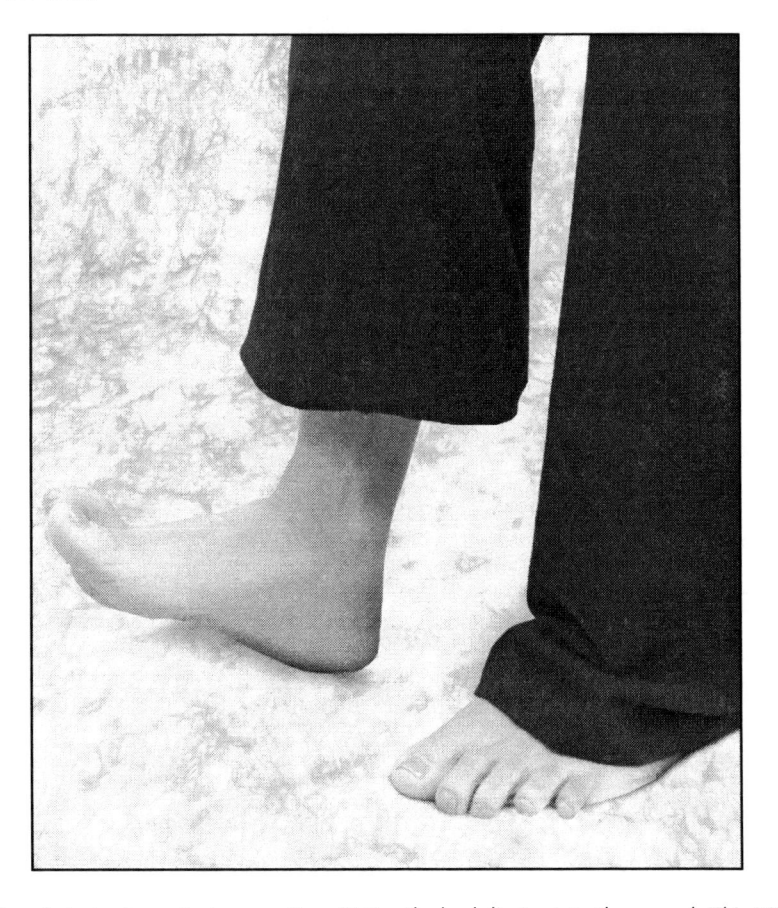

Description: Anterior Innominate correction. Notice the heel digging into the ground. This MET pulls the ilium back from an anterior rotation.

1. Make sure that you have completed the shotgun correction first and have identified the side of your pelvis that appears to be in an excessive anterior tilt.

2. You may be seated or lying down for this correction. If you are seated, sit toward the front of the chair in good posture. If you are lying down, bend both of your knees so that your feet are on the exercise surface.

3. Press the involved heel down into the floor and hold this isometric contraction for ten seconds. Continue to breathe throughout the contraction.

4. Repeat the ten-second contraction for a total of three repetitions.

5. If you are using a sacroiliac support belt, apply the belt now that you are in optimal alignment. Refer to Chapter 8 for belting instructions.

WHAT TO WATCH OUT FOR:

1. Do not hold your breath during the contractions, as this may increase your blood pressure.

2. It is best to perform this correction so that the heel presses into a firm surface, such as the floor if performing the correction while seated or a yoga mat if lying down. Some women find that they must perform this correction in bed before rolling to their side to get up. If you are performing this correction on a soft bed, you may be able to modify the correction by clasping your hands behind the involved thigh. You can then press the thigh down into your hands for ten seconds and three repetitions.

3. If after performing this correction, your pain or symptoms worsen, you may not benefit from this correction. You may have a more complex alignment issue and would benefit from seeing a skilled physical therapist.

BENEFITS:

1. Decreased pain with turning in bed, going from sitting to standing and walking.

2. Strengthening of your hip extensor muscles, including your gluteals, which can help stabilize your spine and pelvis.

HOW TO MAINTAIN CORRECTION:

1. Avoid destructive forces as described in Chapter 4.

2. Perform a standing hip flexor stretch on the involved side (with involved leg as the "back" leg in the stretch) two to three times per day (see Chapter 13).

3. Use a sacroiliac support belt to maintain the correction, decrease pain and prevent recurrence of the anterior innominate rotation (see Chapter 8).

4. Incorporate abdominal strengthening to stabilize the pelvis (see Chapter 12).

Trade Secret #4: Correction for a Posterior Innominate

HOW TO IDENTIFY

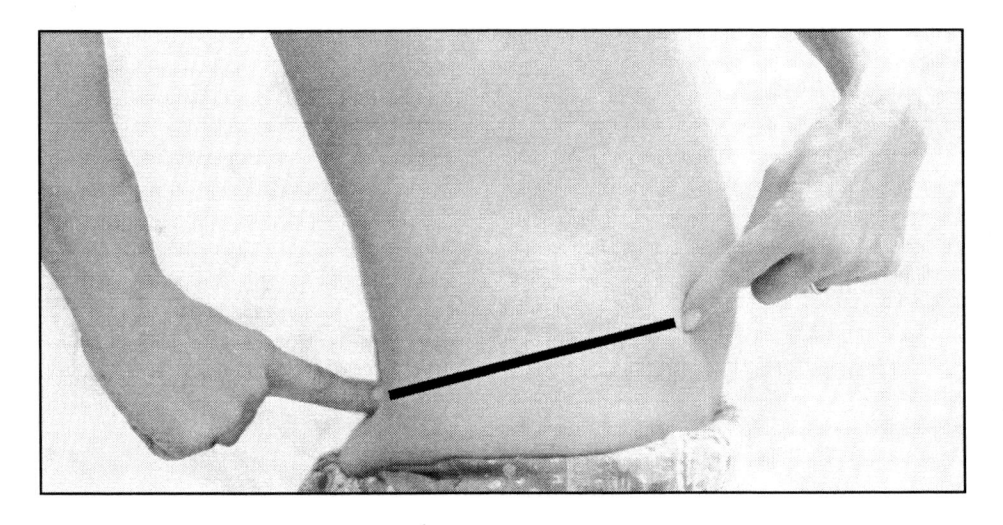

Description: Notice how the PSIS is lower than the ASIS. This is your typical presentation and posterior innominates can contribute to sacroiliac, gluteal and hip pain.

Using the standing alignment assessment above, identify if one side of the pelvis forms a flatter line when drawn from the PSIS in the back to the ASIS in the front. If you find that one PSIS is significantly lower than the other, and you are experiencing one of the common symptoms listed below, then you would likely benefit from a posterior innominate correction.

Common Symptoms of a Posterior Innominate

1. Pain in the lower back, buttock and/or occasionally pain down the back of the leg on the side of the dysfunction. Many people assume that pain traveling down the back of the leg must be a symptom of a herniated disc; however, a posterior innominate can cause tightness of the piriformis muscle, which can then place pressure on the sciatic nerve.

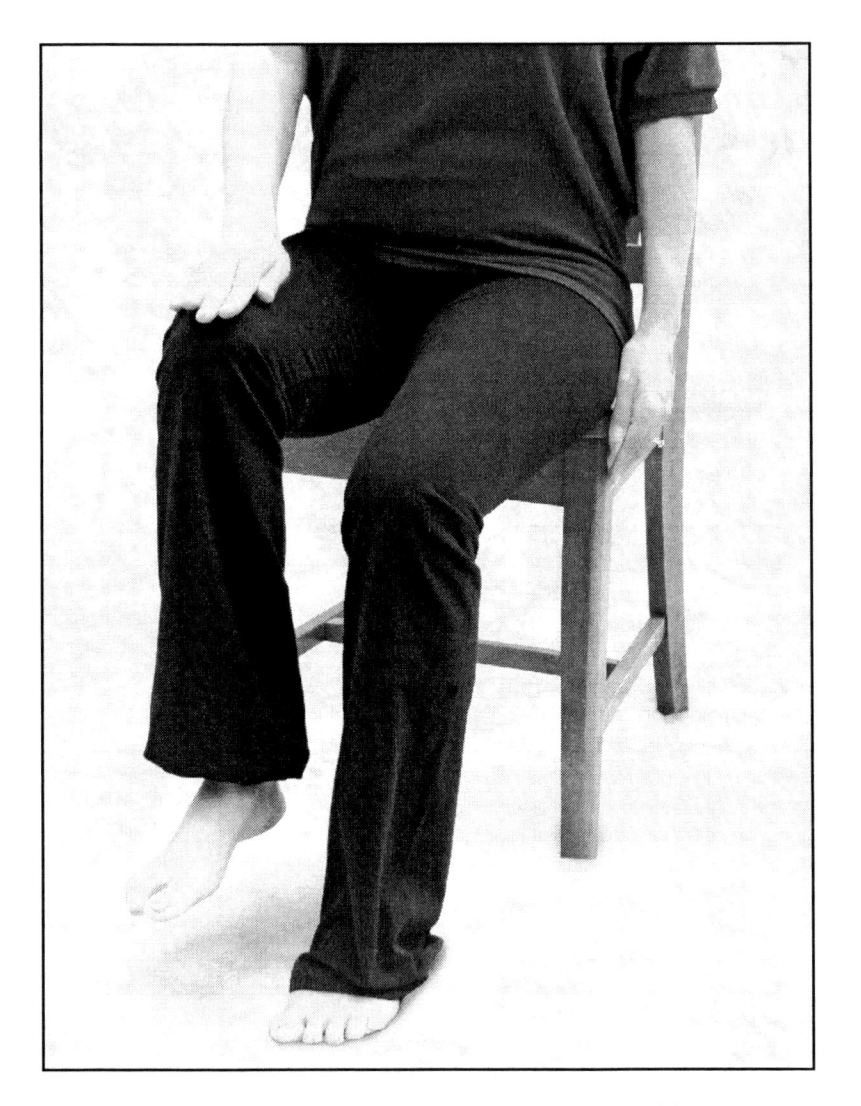

Description: Notice the hand on the thigh. This MET pulls the ilium forward from a posterior rotation.

WHAT TO DO:

1. Make sure that you have completed the shotgun correction first and have identified the side of your pelvis that appears to be in an excessive posterior tilt.

2. You may be seated or lying down for this correction. If you are seated, sit toward the front of the chair in good posture. If you are lying down, bend both of your knees so that your feet are on the exercise surface.

3. Lift the involved knee up to meet your hand. If you are lying down, your knee should form a right angle while in the air. Some women find it difficult to maintain their leg in the air and prefer to start the correction with both legs resting on a ball, as shown in the picture. Press the involved knee up into your hand. Your elbow should remain locked and your arm should meet your knee with an equal amount of pressure so that the knee does not actually move. Continue to hold this isometric contraction for ten seconds and continue to breathe throughout the contraction.

4. Repeat the ten-second contraction for a total of three repetitions.

5. If you are using a sacroiliac support belt, apply the belt now that you are in optimal alignment. Refer to Chapter 8 for belting instructions.

WHAT TO WATCH OUT FOR:

1. Do not hold your breath during the contractions, as this may increase your blood pressure.

2. Some women report cramping in the muscles at the front of the hip during this correction. If you experience spasms or cramping of the muscle, decrease the force with which you are pressing the knee into your hand.

3. If after performing this correction, your pain or symptoms worsen with walking, you may not benefit from this correction. You may have a more complex alignment issue and would benefit from seeing a skilled physical therapist.

BENEFITS:

1. Decreased pain with turning in bed, going from sitting to standing and walking.

2. Strengthening of your hip flexor muscles, including the psoas, which can help stabilize your spine and pelvis.

HOW TO MAINTAIN CORRECTION:

1. Avoid destructive forces as described in Chapter 4.

2. Perform a seated Figure Four Stretch on the involved side two to three times per day (see Chapter 6).

3. Use a sacroiliac support belt to maintain the correction, decrease pain and prevent recurrence of the posterior innominate rotation (see Chapter 8).

4. Incorporate abdominal strengthening to stabilize the pelvis (see Chapter 12).

Trade Secret #5: Simultaneous Correction of Anterior and Posterior Innominate – Lying Down Simultaneous Correction

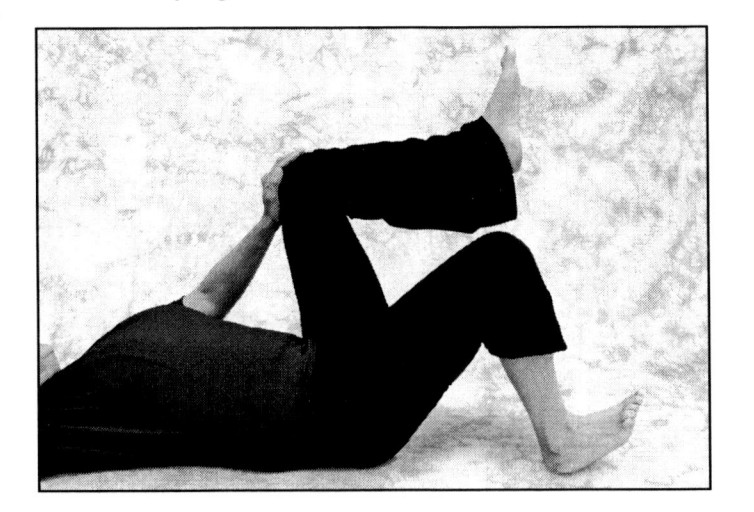

Description: Simultaneous corrections for posterior and anterior innominate can be performed in either a lying down position or seated position.

Seated Correction Simultaneous Correction

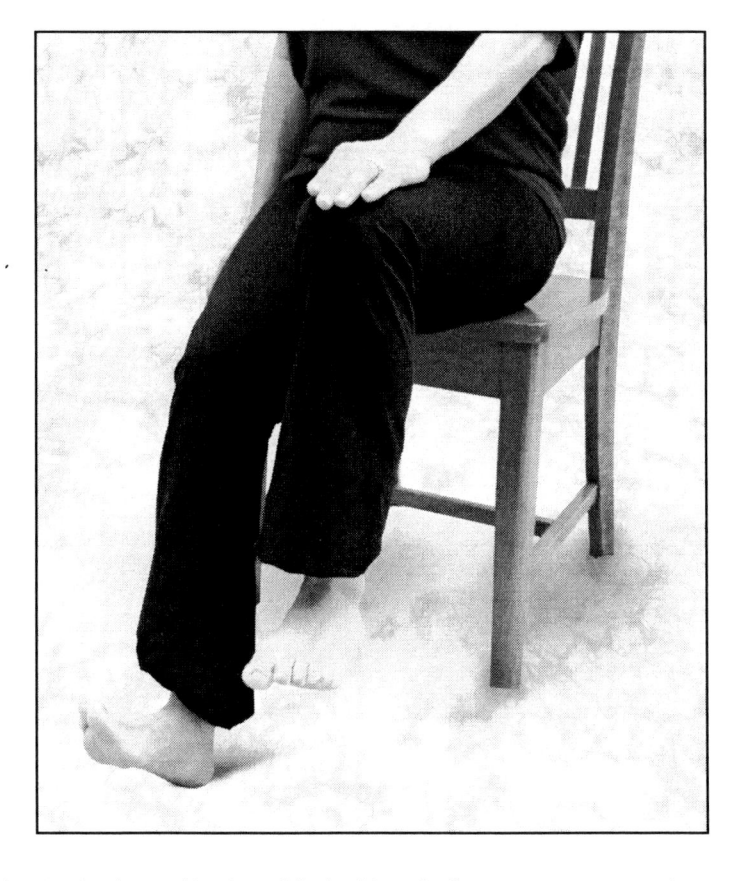

Description: Notice the combination of the heel into the floor to correct an anterior rotation and the thigh press to correct a posterior rotation. They are corrected simultaneously with this seated technique.

As we have just reviewed, anterior innominate correction is appropriate if you find an anterior rotation of the pelvis, while posterior innominate correction is appropriate if you find a posterior rotation of the pelvis. But what happens if you find that you have an anterior rotation on one side, a posterior rotation on the other side, and you do not know which side requires the correction?

Oftentimes, our symptoms will tell us which side is the "dysfunctional" side that requires a MET correction. For instance, if you find a posterior rotation on your left side and you have left low back and buttock pain, then you should perform posterior innominate correction for a left posterior rotation. Along the same line of thinking, if you find an anterior rotation on your right side and you have right hip and groin pain, then you should perform anterior innominate correction for an anterior rotation.

However, if you find an anterior rotation on one side, a posterior rotation on the other side, and you currently do not have pain, or your symptoms are unclear, then you can try a simultaneous correction as described below.

WHAT TO DO:

1. Make sure that you have completed the shotgun correction first and have identified the side of anterior rotation and the side of posterior rotation.

2. You may be seated or lying down for this correction. If you are seated, sit toward the front of the chair in good posture. If you are lying down, bend both of your knees so that your feet are on the exercise surface.

3. On the side of the anterior rotation, press your heel down into the floor. At the same time that you are pressing your heel down on one side, lift the opposite knee (on the side of the anterior rotation) and press the knee up into your hand. Hold both contractions for ten seconds and continue to breathe throughout the contraction.

4. Repeat the simultaneous correction, with one heel pressing down and one heel pressing up two more times, for a total of three repetitions.

5. If you are using a sacroiliac support belt, apply the belt following the three repetitions in order to maintain your corrected alignment. Refer to Chapter 8 for belting instructions.

WHAT TO WATCH OUT FOR:

1. Do not hold your breath during the contractions, as this may increase your blood pressure.

2. If after performing this correction, your pain or symptoms worsen, you may not benefit from this correction. You may have a more complex alignment issue and would benefit from seeing a skilled physical therapist.

BENEFITS:

1. Decreased pain with turning in bed, going from sitting to standing and walking.

2. Strengthening of your hip flexor and extensor muscles, which can help stabilize your spine and pelvis.

HOW TO MAINTAIN CORRECTION:

1. Avoid destructive forces as described in Chapter 4.

2. Perform a standing hip flexor stretch on the side of the anterior rotation two to three times per day. Refer to Chapter 13 and perform a seated Figure Four Stretch on the side of the posterior rotation two to three times per day (see Chapter 6).

3. Use a sacroiliac support belt to maintain the correction, decrease pain and prevent recurrence of the pelvic malalignment (see Chapter 8).

4. Incorporate abdominal strengthening to stabilize the pelvis (see Chapter 12).

Beyond the Pubic Symphysis and Innominates: Sacral Torsions

In addition to the pelvic alignment conditions and corrections covered above, there are numerous other spinal and pelvic alignment issues that are beyond the scope of this book. Due to its connection to the uterus, the alignment of the sacrum may pose a particular problem during pregnancy. If you are experiencing low back pain that increases with turning over in bed, moving from sitting to standing and walking, and your pain is not relieved with the pelvic corrections prescribed above, you may have a sacral torsion.

A sacral torsion is a rotation of the sacrum that disrupts the normal mechanics of the SI joint. Sacral torsions are often best evaluated and treated in-person by an experienced physical therapist. Since the sacrum has ligamentous attachments to the uterus, make sure to choose a practitioner who has extensive experience treating women during pregnancy.

Posture Is Everything: Good Posture Will Maintain Optimal Alignment

Now that you know how to correct your own alignment, let's dive into the exercises that will not only help you maintain it but will also provide comfort, strength and pain relief. Chapter 6 will highlight what we call the "Magical 8," eight exercises that—when performed correctly and regularly—bring magical pain relief with long-lasting effects for conditions such as sacroiliac joint pain, low back pain and sciatica.

CHAPTER SIX

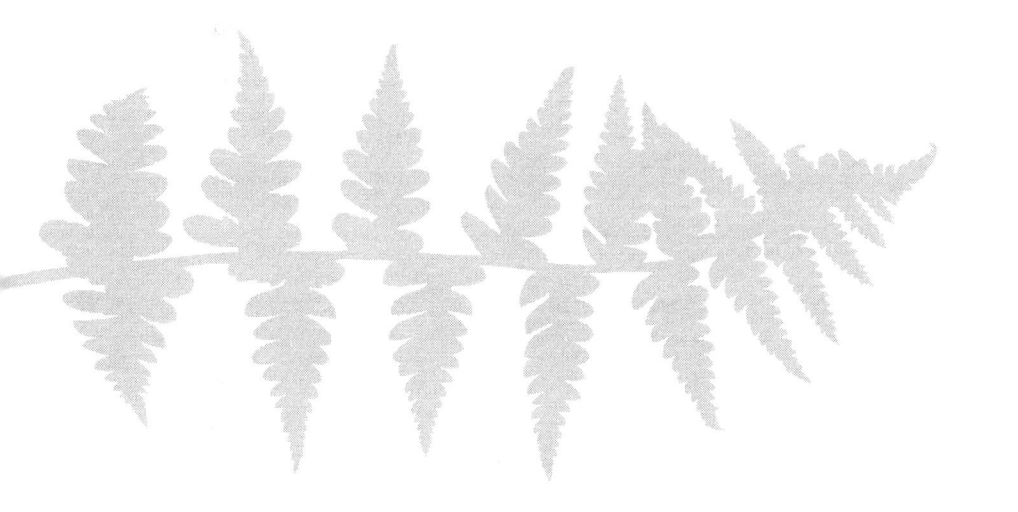

"Healing yourself is connected with healing others."

—*Yoko Ono*

Chapter 6

RELIEVING BACK PAIN, SCIATICA AND SACROILIAC JOINT PAIN: HOW TO
CREATE A STABLE BODY AND AVOID PAIN WITH THE MAGICAL 8

Experiencing pain in your low back, buttocks, or legs during pregnancy can be debilitating, frustrating, and downright confusing. Very often pregnant women are not given treatment options for pain by their healthcare providers and are left to fend for themselves when it comes to seeking pain relief. One study showed 85 percent of surveyed women were not offered treatment of their musculoskeletal pain during pregnancy. Just because pregnancy-related back and pelvic pain is common does not mean it is normal, or that it is untreatable. Our mission is for you to become an advocate for yourself and seek out appropriate treatment; you no longer have to suffer with these debilitating conditions.

Finding out what will work best for you, however, can be challenging. Have you ever felt overwhelmed with the amount of prenatal-based exercise classes and pain-relieving modalities out there? In New York City alone, there are thousands of prenatal exercise classes and modalities targeting pregnant women with core weakness, back pain, and pelvic pain. Prenatal yoga, Pilates, baby boot camp, Zumba, chiropractic care, aqua jogging, acupuncture, aerobics, and cycling are only some of the modalities out there claiming to either tone the abs, get you out of pain, or get mom and baby in shape and ready for labor. This information alone is enough to make your head spin. With the amount of options available today, it can be confusing and difficult to find which modality will be best for you and will help get you out of pain. Questions I get asked everyday include: "Do you think prenatal yoga would help me?" or "Can I still do my Pilates class?" or "Is it okay to go to my spinning class?" At our healing center in New York City, it is not uncommon for pregnant women to come to us in even more pain after trying a prenatal exercise class that was just not right for their bodies. In this chapter, we will dispel the mystery and give you simple exercises and tools to combat your pain at home and get you from week one to week forty feeling revitalized and ready for motherhood.

Where Is My Pain Coming From?

There is much controversy amongst the leading experts concerning definitions and causes of pregnancy-related pain syndromes. Knowing what your pain is and from where it originates will help you bring awareness to your body and empower you to find the best solution to your pain. Sacroiliac joint pain, low back pain, posterior pelvic pain, pelvic girdle pain, lumbopelvic pain, and sciatic pain describe only some of the pains or dysfunctions that originate on the posterior aspect of the female body in pregnancy. First, we will help diffuse the confusion by defining three of the most common terms used, describing their symptoms, and discussing their prevalence in pregnancy. We will then take you through a series of simple exercises that will help you safely combat the pain you are experiencing. Keep in mind that due to the multi-factorial nature of posterior pelvic and back pain in pregnancy it is not uncommon for several factors to contribute to your pain. As you try these exercises listen to your body and always seek the help of a women's health physical therapist if you are having difficulty finding the correct exercise regimen for you. The terms that will be discussed in this chapter include pregnancy-related lumbar pain (PLP), pelvic girdle pain (PGP), and sciatica.

These three different types of pain can be treated effectively with the same kind of exercises. For instance pregnancy-related lumbar pain (PLP) and pelvic girdle pain (sacroiliac joint pain) can be alleviated with the same group of exercises except that PLP has two additional exercises (the lean back exercise and the side stretch). (See Tables 6.1 and 6.2 for specific pain-relieving exercises.) Treatment for sciatica differs from PLP and PGP in that it requires that you do tennis massage on the gluteal muscles and that you perform a Figure Four stretch to get the piriformis muscle to release its hold on the sciatic nerve. In the upcoming sections I will detail each type of pain and include a description for each of these master pain busting exercises. We like the exercises listed in this chapter so much that at our center we call them the Magical 8. Why? Because the Magical 8 get rid of pain by restoring muscular imbalances and increasing hip, pelvic and spinal stability. When you do the Magical 8 you will see magical results.

Table 6.1: Pain-Relieving Exercises for Pregnancy-Related Lumbar Pain (PLP)

EXERCISE	POSITION	REPS AND SETS	PURPOSE
Transverse Abdominis (TrA)/Belly Holds	Seated, Standing, Supine, Semi-Recumbent	Beginner: five-second hold: ten reps/one to two sets Advanced: five-second hold: fifteen to twenty reps/two to three sets	Increases pelvic hip and spinal stability and strengthens the core. Protects the organs against adverse pressure.
Bridge with Chop	Supine	Beginner: five-second hold: ten reps/one to two sets Advanced: five-second hold: fifteen to twenty reps/two to three sets	Improves back, hamstring and gluteal strength and helps to maintain sacroiliac joint stability.
Seated Side Stretch	Seated	Beginner: ten to thirty second hold: ten reps/one to two sets Advanced: thirty to sixty second hold: fifteen to twenty reps/two to three sets	Allows the nerve to breathe. Side stretch away from the pain to open up the nerve and to help decrease pain. Stretches the intercostal muscle and facilitates breathing.
Seated Abduction	Seated	Beginner: five-second hold ten reps/one to two sets Advanced: five-second hold fifteen to twenty reps/two to three sets	Increases pelvic hip and spinal stability and strengthens the core. Protects the organs against adverse pressure.
Straight Arm Lat Pull Down	Seated or Standing	Beginner: three to five seconds: ten reps/one to two sets Advanced: three to five seconds: fifteen to twenty reps/two to three sets	Stabilizes sacroiliac joint via the thoracolumbar fascia.
Lean Backs	Seated or Standing	Beginner: five to ten seconds: ten reps/one to two sets Advanced: five to ten seconds: fifteen to twenty reps/two to three sets	Helps to centralize pain by moving pain from the leg up to the back.

Table 6.2: Pain-Relieving Exercises for Pelvic Girdle Pain (Sacroiliac Joint Pain)

EXERCISE	POSITION	REPS AND SETS	PURPOSE
Transverse Belly Holds	Seated, Standing, Supine, Semi-Recumbent	Beginner: five-second hold: ten reps/one to two sets Advanced: five-second hold: fifteen to twenty reps/two to three sets	Increases pelvic hip and spinal stability and strengthens the core. Protects the organs against adverse pressure.
Clams	Side lying	Beginner: ten reps/one to two sets Advanced: fifteen to twenty reps/two to three sets	Helps to increase pelvic, hip and lumbar stability. Improves hip strength and prevents the "waddle gait."
Bridge with Chop	Supine	Beginner: three to five second hold: ten reps/one to two sets Advanced: three to five second hold: fifteen to twenty reps/two to three sets	Improves back, hamstring and gluteal strength and helps to maintain sacroiliac joint stability.
Seated Adduction	Seated	Beginner: three to five second hold: ten reps/one to two sets Advanced: three to five second hold: fifteen to twenty reps/two to three sets	Helps strengthen the inner thigh and helps to maintain hip alignment.
Seated Abduction	Seated	Beginner: three to five second hold: ten reps/one to two sets Advanced: three to five second hold: fifteen to twenty reps/two to three sets	Increases pelvic hip and spinal stability and strengthens the core. Protects the organs against adverse pressure.
Straight Arm Lat Pull Down	Seated or Standing	Beginner: ten reps/one to two sets Advanced: fifteen to twenty reps/two to three sets	Stabilizes sacroiliac joint via the thoracolumbar fascia.

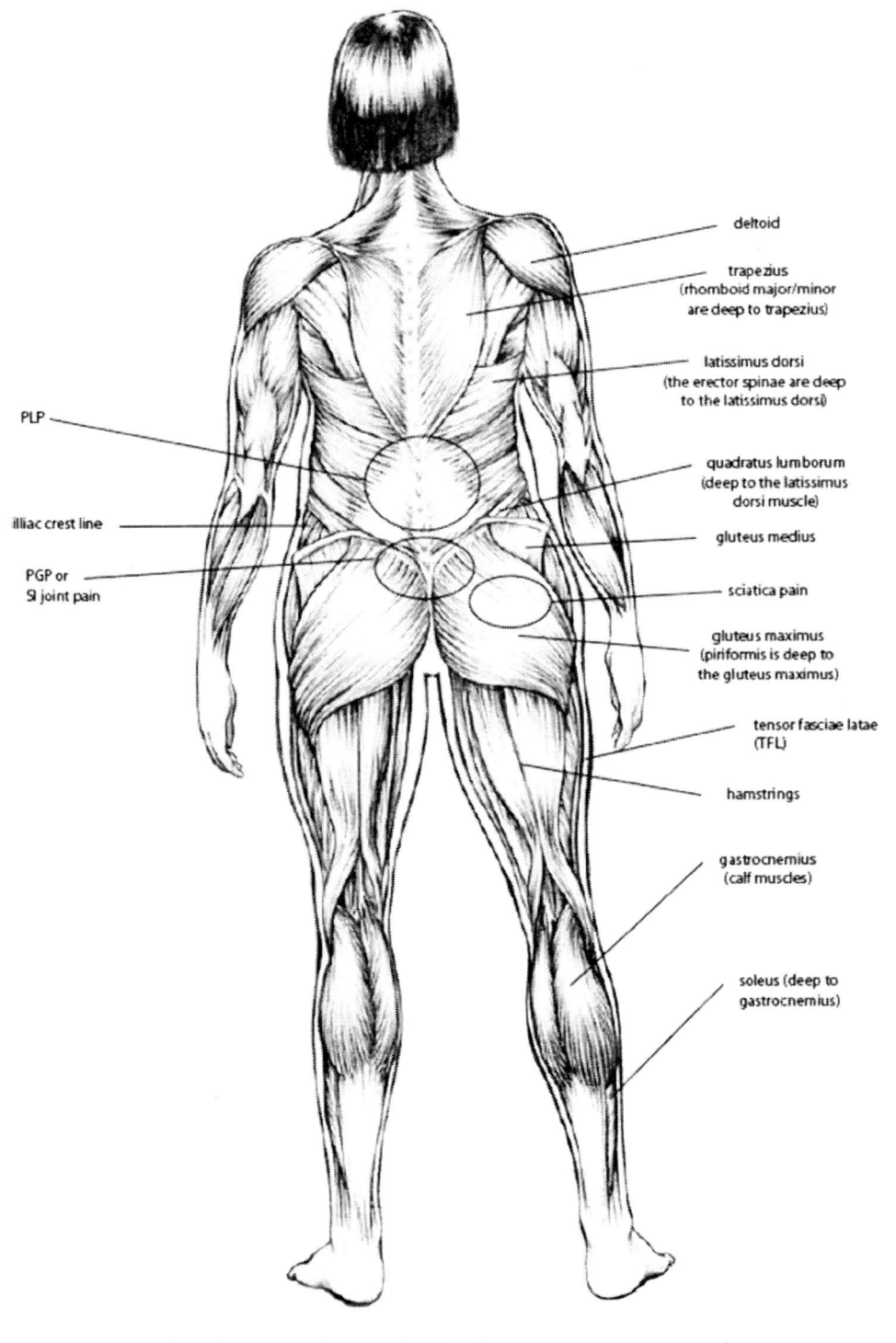

deltoid

trapezius
(rhomboid major/minor
are deep to trapezius)

latissimus dorsi
(the erector spinae are deep
to the latissimus dorsi)

PLP

quadratus lumborum
(deep to the latissimus
dorsi muscle)

illiac crest line

gluteus medius

PGP or
SI joint pain

sciatica pain

gluteus maximus
(piriformis is deep to
the gluteus maximus)

tensor fasciae latae
(TFL)

hamstrings

gastrocnemius
(calf muscles)

soleus (deep to
gastrocnemius)

Description: Circles indicate type of pain and possible location. Source: WInston Johnson.

Pregnancy-Related Lumbar Pain

Definition and Causes

Pregnancy-related lumbar pain is defined as pain found in the lumbar region with or without radiation to the leg. Individuals with lumbar pain sometimes respond to repeated motion testing, where a specific direction of movement is identified which peripheralizes or centralizes the pain. Pain is said to peripheralize if symptoms go down into the leg, while centralization occurs if the symptoms come out of the leg and into the low back region, or sometimes dissipate completely. Repeated motion testing should be carried out by a trained physical therapist to determine your peripheralization or centralization pattern.

PLP can be the result of mechanical, chemical, hormonal, metabolic, and psychosocial factors. For example, postural changes, ligament laxity due to hormonal shifts, lumbar or pelvic malalignment, muscle spasms and poor ergonomic setup combined with the stress of work-related activities can all cause PLP. Approximately one in 10,000 pregnant women will experience PLP due to disc herniation.

Common Symptoms and Activity Limitations

1. Throbbing or aching pain in the area between the lower ribs and hip bones in the posterior aspect of the thorax.

2. Pain with standing, sitting, or walking for prolonged periods in the low back region.

3. Difficulty with bending forward to pick up objects due to pain in the low back region.

4. Inability to lift objects due to pain in the low back region.

5. Shooting pain down the posterior aspect of the legs which is aggravated with repeated movements, bending forward, lifting objects, prolonged standing, sitting or walking, or positional changes. Also known as peripheralized PLP.

Prevalence

Statistics vary amongst different studies and populations concerning prevalence rates of PLP. However, most would agree that approximately half of pregnant women will experience PLP. Again, although common, this condition is not normal and there are many ways to get yourself out of pain. Please reference the "Treatment" section below to learn ways to combat your PLP.

Relevant Treatment: Watch Your Movements and Know What Motions Increase Your Pain

A general rule of thumb is to avoid directions of movement which aggravate your pain, and stick to the direction of movement which relieves your pain. Contrary to the popular saying, "no pain no gain," individuals with PLP should not try to work through their pain, but rather should seek out directions of movement or positions which centralize or alleviate the pain to keep from exacerbating their condition. In addition to modifying activities to avoid movement patterns which worsen symptoms, there are several simple exercises that will help combat PLP by improving flexibility, strength, and enhancing core stability. Usually with PLP spinal flexion (bending forward) increases pain and spinal extension (leaning back) decreases pain. But the opposite can hold true also. So monitor your pain and listen to your body: it will signal to you loud and clear what it doesn't like.

Pelvic Girdle Pain Also Known as Sacroiliac Pain

Definition and Causes

Pelvic girdle pain (PGP), also known as sacroiliac joint pain, is defined as having pain distal to L5 in the vicinity of the sacroiliac joint with or without radiation to the thigh. In other words, the pain is located below the level of the hip bones, or iliac crests, posteriorly and above the level of the gluteal folds, or folds of the buttocks. Pregnancy can predispose women to PGP for multiple reasons including weight gain, postural changes, hormone-induced ligamentous relaxation, and pelvic trauma associated with birth. Malalignment of the pelvic girdle including sacral torsions, ilium rotations, and pubic symphysis dysfunction can be the cause of PGP. Refer to Chapter 5 to learn how to evaluate your pelvic alignment and correct any malalignment that may be present to help combat PGP. Dysfunction at the pubic symphysis on the anterior aspect of the body near the groin can also be a cause of PGP and is discussed further in Chapter 7.

Prevalence

Approximately 45 percent of pregnant women experience PGP; this common complaint can cause severe pain and disability.

Common Symptoms and Activity Limitations

1. Sharp, achy, or throbbing pain in the region of the sacroiliac joint between the posterior superior iliac spine (PSIS) and gluteal folds.

2. Pain that radiates into the groin or anterior/lateral thigh.

3. Difficulty with dressing or bathing due to pain exacerbated by standing on one leg.

4. Difficulty with positional changes, such as rolling over in bed, due to pain in the sacroiliac joint region.

5. Difficulty with ambulation and/or stair negotiation due to pain and/or instability in the sacroiliac joint region.

Treatment: Simple Exercises to Alleviate Your Pain

Pelvic alignment can have a significant impact on the way a woman feels and functions during pregnancy. At our healing center in New York City, we often find that if the pelvic alignment is not corrected first, women with PGP may have difficulty performing these exercises without pain. If you attempt any of the following exercises and experience pain, stop and listen to your body. Then, read Chapter 5 to learn how to correct your pelvic alignment and try again. If you continue to have difficulty, seek the care of a physical therapist.

Other Strategies for Managing PGP

Pelvic girdle pain can be effectively managed during pregnancy using the proper tools and strategies to create stability in a largely unstable environment. We often find that using a combination of physical therapy techniques can provide great pain relief to women experiencing PGP, while using only one or two strategies can leave you in pain, unstable, and ultimately unhappy. These techniques typically include manual therapy, pelvic alignment, sound ergonomic advice, biomechanics training, stabilizing exercises, and prescription of sacroiliac joint belts for additional external pelvic support. To find out more information about belting advice for PGP, see Chapter 8.

Pain-Relieving Exercises for Pregnancy Related Lumbar Pain (PLP) and Pelvic Girdle Pain (PGP)

We call this group of pain-busting exercises the Magical 8. The beauty of these exercises is that we created them for both PLP and PGP. There is some overlap in the exercises and that makes it easier for you just in case you cannot pinpoint your pain. Many times pregnant women have combination pain that consists of PLP plus PGP, so we have created exercises to treat both. If you do them you will be very successful in combating pregnancy pain. The only treatment difference between PLP and PGP is that PLP requires more hip stability. To address this we added the clam exercise. PLP also requires that the nerve and the nerve roots have more space in the spine and for that we included a side stretch. (We will consider sciatica on its own but there is overlap there also.)

We will describe the exercises and show you what to watch out for so you don't hurt yourself. You must refer to Tables 6.1 and 6.2 for the correct groups of exercises to relieve PLP and/or PGP. Seated neutral spine is very important for any exercise so we will start with that and then get into the Magical 8.

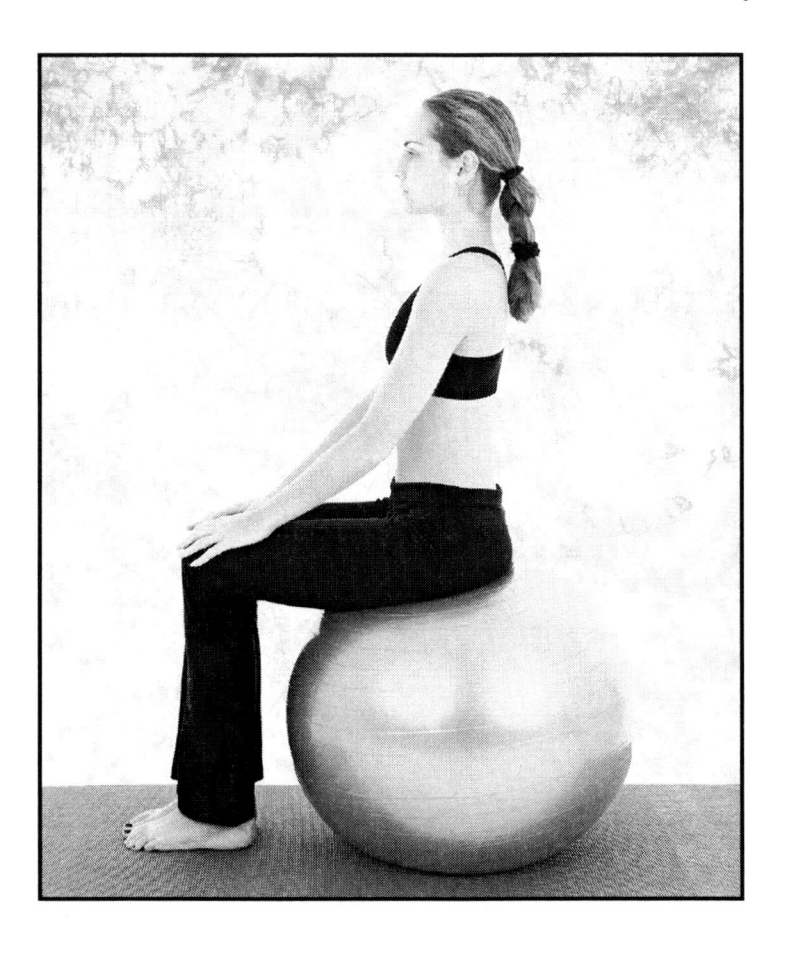

How to Find Seated Neutral Spine

WHAT TO DO:

1. Lie on your back or sit on a stable surface with your feet flat on the floor. Make sure your legs are hip-width apart and in great alignment. Imagine there is one continuous line from your hips to your knees to your feet. To accomplish this make sure your feet are parallel and not out to the side.

2. Keep your arms at your side and keep the body relaxed.

3. Exhale and use your abdominal muscles to round your lower back performing a posterior pelvic tilt (PPT). Inhale and release the PPT through your nose into your belly and release the PPT.

4. Exhale and pull your lower spine into arched position creating an anterior pelvic tilt (ANT). Inhale and relax; release the ANT.

5. Neutral spine is the place in between these two extreme positions. You must practice this until you get a sense of what it means to be in neutral spine. Practice NS and know how to do it before advancing to the Magical 8.

The Magical 8

Trade Secret: Magical Exercise #1 Transverse Belly Holds

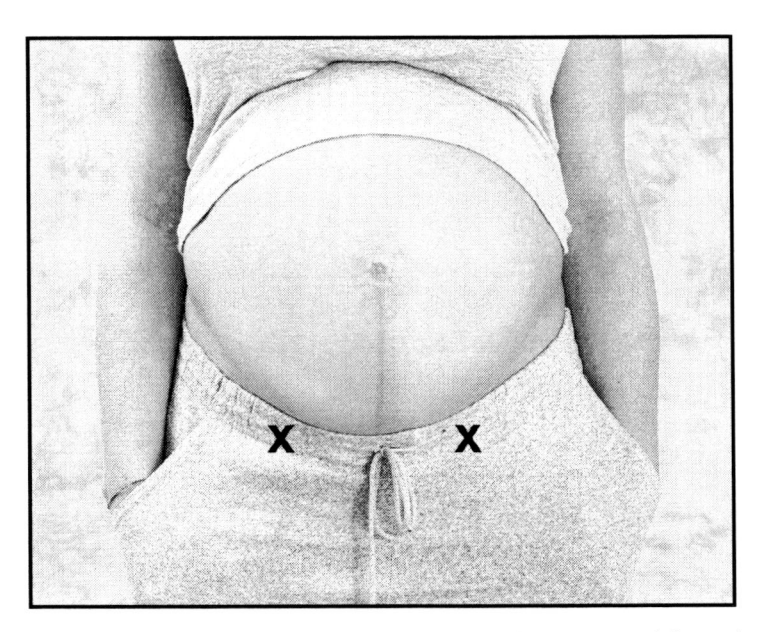

Description: The X's represent the location where you can feel the transverse abdominal muscle when it is properly activated.

Transverse belly holds are the foundation upon which all exercise regimens should be built. You will notice this exercise is included in the treatment for all three conditions discussed in this chapter.

WHAT TO DO:

1. This exercise may be done sitting, supine, or standing. Keep a neutral spine as you take a full belly breath. As you exhale, do a gentle Kegel and draw your belly closer and more firmly toward the spine. As you pull in the abdominals try to imagine that you are trying to squeeze into an old pair of jeans that don't fit.

2. If your belly is showing, you should be able to see the belly rise up toward your nose as you contract the abdominals. The power of your abdominals is actually lifting your baby up!

3. One you establish the above movement, hold for five seconds and repeat ten times. Do one to three sets per day.

WHAT TO WATCH OUT FOR:

1. Holding the breath, which can increase abdominal pressure and cause leaking, pain, and pressure.

2. Over-contracting the abdominals, which engages the more superficial abdominals such as the rectus abdominis and external obliques.

BENEFITS:

1. Activates the deepest core muscle, the transverse abdominis, which keeps your low back and pelvis stable and supported.

2. Can help prevent diastasis recti, or separation of the abdominals, which can lead to increased back pain, incontinence, and weakness.

3. Strengthens the deep abdominal muscles and provides the foundation to build a safe and effective core stabilization exercise regimen.

Trade Secret: Magical Exercise #2 Bridging with Chop

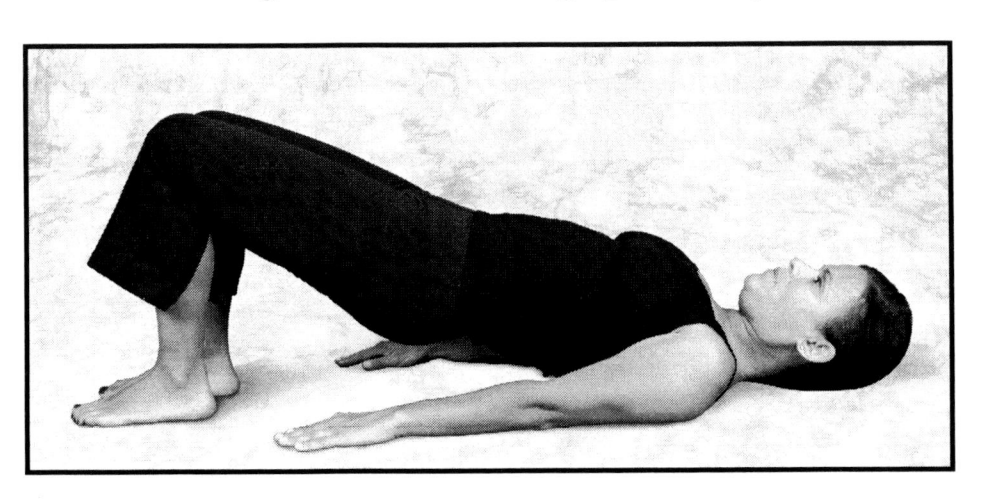

WHAT TO DO:

1. Lie on your back with your knees bent and feet flat on the surface.

2. Your arms should be down by your sides, elbows locked straight, and palms facing down.

3. Contract your transverse abdominis muscle first.

4. Push down into the floor with your feet so your buttocks lift up off of the floor. At the same time, push your hands down into the floor and open the chest up. Envision that you are putting your shoulder blades down and back into your back pockets as you do this. This activates your latissimus dorsi muscle, which plays a very important role in sacroiliac joint stability through the thoracodorsal fascia.

5. Only bridge up as far as you can without losing your TrA contraction. Hold at the top for five seconds. Repeat ten times and do one to three sets per day.

WHAT TO WATCH OUT FOR:

1. Holding the breath, which can increase abdominal pressure and cause leaking, pain, and pressure.

2. Dizziness while lying supine may occur in the second and third trimesters. Monitor how your body responds to lying flat and discontinue if you feel dizzy or faint. This may indicate compression of the vena cava, a blood vessel that allows blood to return back to the heart.

3. Lifting the buttocks too high off of the surface. This may cause you to place too much stress on the spine. Less is more.

BENEFITS:

1. Strengthens core and pelvic floor muscles in addition to the gluteal, hamstrings, and inner thighs.

2. Helps improve lower back spinal alignment and improves lumbar and pelvic stability.

3. Tenses and strengthens the latissimus dorsi muscle and its fascial extension, the thoracodorsal fascia, which provides support and stability to the sacroiliac joint and lumbar spine.

Trade Secret: Magical Exercise #3 Seated Side Stretch

WHAT TO DO:

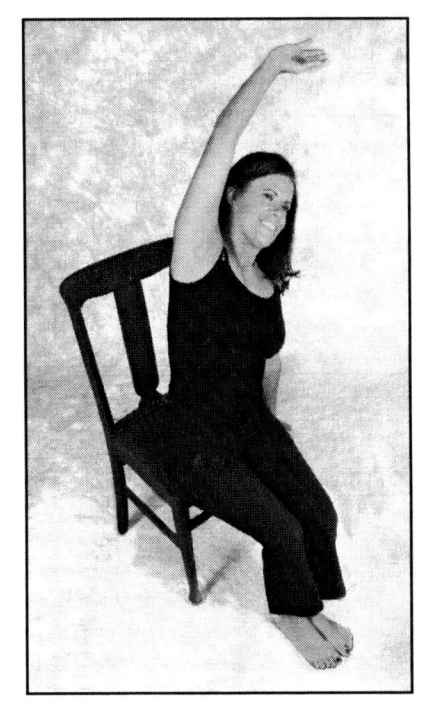

1. Start in a seated position at the front of your chair, using good posture as outlined earlier in this book.

2. Raise your right arm up toward the ceiling and place your left arm at your hips.

3. Bend your upper body to the left while reaching up and over with your right arm.

4. Bring your body back to the center and repeat the pose on the other side.

WHAT TO WATCH OUT FOR:

1. Avoid compressing into the left side. Think tall as you bend sideways.

2. Avoid overstretching and forcing the side-bend as this can cause pain to the intercostals or side muscles.

BENEFITS:

1. Helps increase the flexibility of your spine, arms, and rib cage.

2. Helps to realign pelvic bones and maintains lumbar spine and sacral alignment.

3. Enhances nerve function and releases pain from the side muscles.

4. Facilitates rib expansion, which will help get more oxygen into your lungs and promote better breathing.

Trade Secret: Magical Exercise #4 Seated Abduction

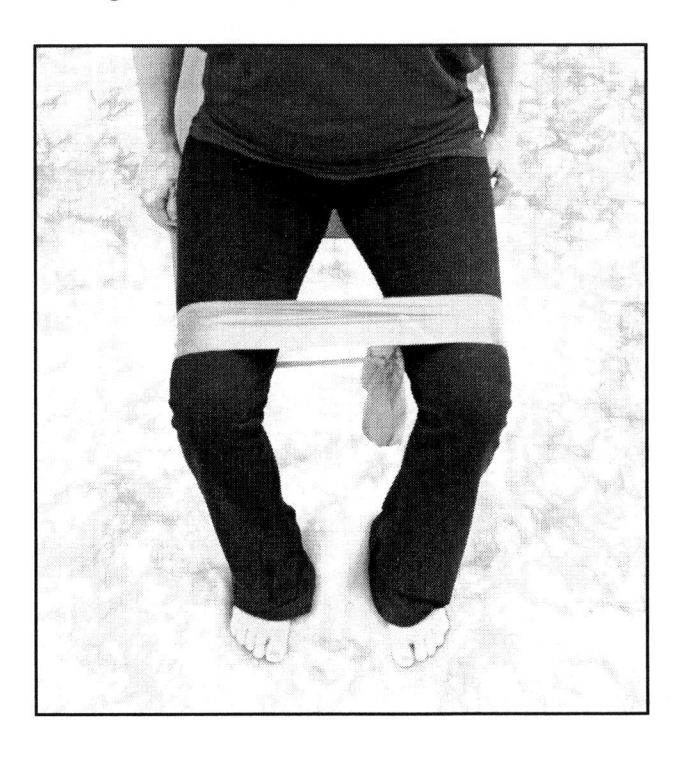

WHAT TO DO:

1. Sit on a stable surface with your feet flat on the floor, hip-width apart, in neutral spine.

2. Place your hands on the outside of your thighs just above your knees. Or if you have a Dyna-Band, you can place the Dyna-Band around both thighs just above the knees.

3. Do a transverse belly hold and simultaneously push both legs out into your hands. This should be an isometric contraction, meaning the legs should not move as you push them into your hands.

4. Hold for five seconds and repeat ten times. Do one to three times per day.

WHAT TO WATCH OUT FOR:

1. Holding the breath, which can increase abdominal pressure and cause leaking, pain, and pressure.

2. Rounding your back when you place your hands next to your knees. You must maintain neutral spine to protect your back.

3. Pushing your legs out with too much force. Ensure your legs stay stable as you push them into your hands. If you are working with a Dyna-Band move your thighs against the band.

BENEFITS:

1. Strengthens the core, glutes, and pelvic floor muscles.

2. Helps to realign pelvic bones and maintains lumbar and sacral alignment.

Trade Secret: Magical Exercise #5 Seated Adduction

WHAT TO DO:

1. Sit on a stable surface with your feet flat on the floor, hip-width apart, in neutral spine.

2. Make a fist with one or both hands, and place them between your knees. You may also use a pillow or yoga block placed between the knees if you have difficulty maintaining neutral spine while reaching forward.

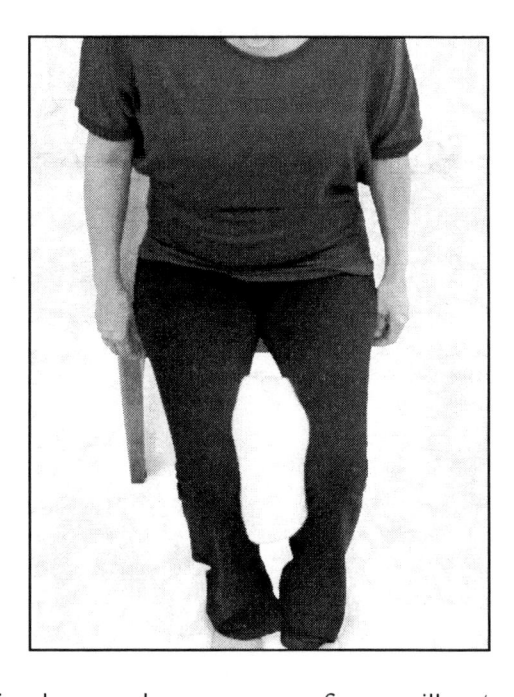

3. Do a transverse belly hold and simultaneously squeeze your fists or pillow/block. This should be an isometric contraction, meaning the legs should not move while you're squeezing.

4. Hold for five seconds and repeat ten times. Do one to three times per day.

WHAT TO WATCH OUT FOR:

1. Holding the breath, which can increase abdominal pressure and cause leaking, pain, and pressure.

2. Rounding your back when you place your hands inside your knees. You must maintain neutral spine to protect your back.

BENEFITS:

1. Strengthens the core, glutes, and pelvic floor muscles.

2. Helps to realign pelvic bones, including the pubic bone, and maintains lumbar and sacral alignment.

Trade Secret: Magical Exercise #6 Straight Arm Lat Pull-Down

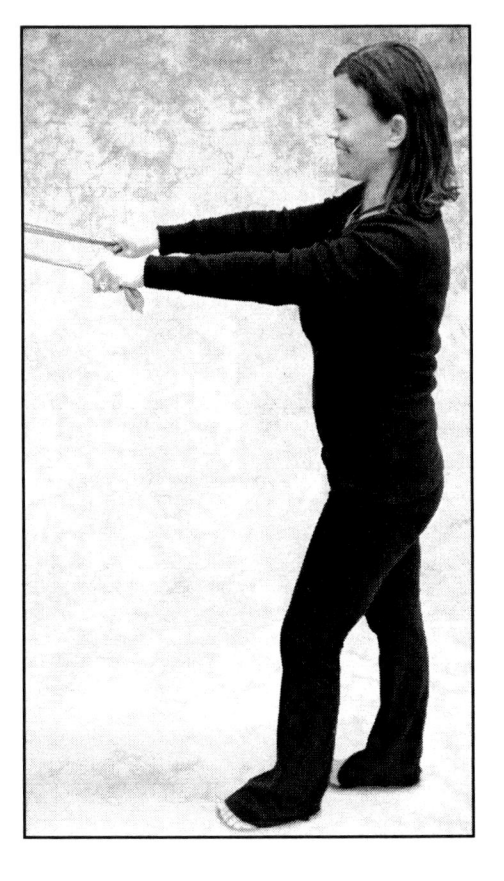 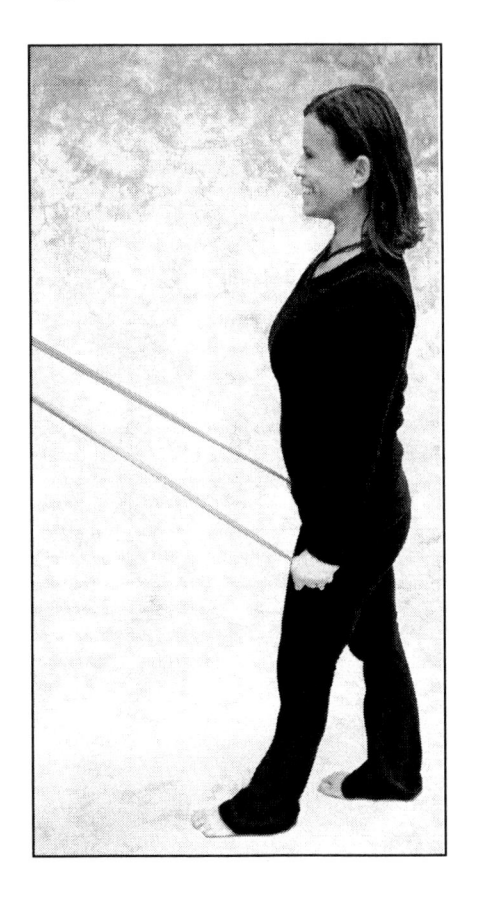

WHAT TO DO:

1. This exercise can be performed standing or sitting. Attach a Dyna-Band high on a doorway so that you have two ends of the band to grasp.

2. Your arms should be slightly in front of your body, elbows locked straight, and hands grasping the Dyna-Bands.

3. Contract your transverse abdominis muscle first (see Transverse Belly Holds).

4. Keeping your arms straight, pull your arms down and back just until they are at the side of your waist.

5. Hold three to five seconds and envision you are keeping your shoulder blades down and back as if you were going to put them in your back pockets. Repeat ten times; do one to three sets per day.

WHAT TO WATCH OUT FOR:

1. Holding the breath, which can increase abdominal pressure and cause leaking, pain, and pressure.

2. Keeping your shoulders rounded or hunched in front which places the cervical spine and upper back in a compromised position. Your chest should be up and shoulders back in excellent posture.

BENEFITS:

1. Tenses and strengthens the latissimus dorsi muscle and its fascial extension, the thoracodorsal fascia, which provides support and stability to the sacroiliac joint and lumbar spine.

2. Can be used to facilitate proper posture and body awareness.

3. Assists in balancing and increasing strength in the posterior aspect of the body. As the baby grows and shifts the center of mass anteriorly, strengthening the posterior column muscles is extremely important to keep your back stable and supported.

Trade Secret: Magical Exercise #7 Lean Backs

WHAT TO DO:

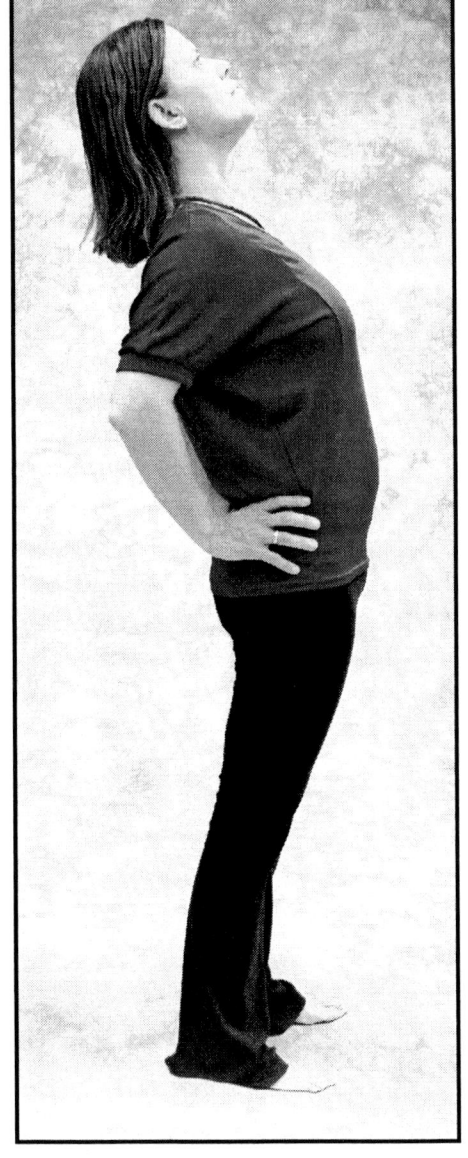

1. This exercise can be performed standing or sitting. Start in neutral spine position.

2. Place your palms on your low back with your fingers pointing forward. This will help support your low back.

3. Gently begin to make an arch in the low back by leaning backward. Initiate the lean back from the head first, then shoulders back, chest out, and finally the pelvis comes forward into an anterior pelvic tilt to create a nice curve in the lumbar spine.

4. You should maintain a slight transverse belly hold while doing the lean back in order to support the lumbar spine.

5. Hold for five to ten seconds and repeat ten times. Do one to three times a day, or as needed for pain control.

WHAT TO WATCH OUT FOR:

1. Holding the breath, which can increase abdominal pressure and cause leaking, pain, and pressure.

2. Arching too vigorously. Be gentle and start with a very small range of motion.

3. Increased pain! If this motion aggravates your lumbar pain or makes your pain travel down the leg, do *not* continue. Your directional preference may not be extending the low back, but rather a neutral spine or flexed position.

BENEFITS:

1. Assists in neutralizing the intervertebral disc. The majority of individuals who have disc herniations occur in the posterior, or backward, direction. A lean back is a gentle way to encourage proper lumbar and disc alignment.

2. Can be used to facilitate proper posture and body awareness.

3. Opens the chest and heart to improve postural alignment and prevent cervical, thoracic, and lumbar spine pain.

Trade Secret: Magical Exercise #8 Clams

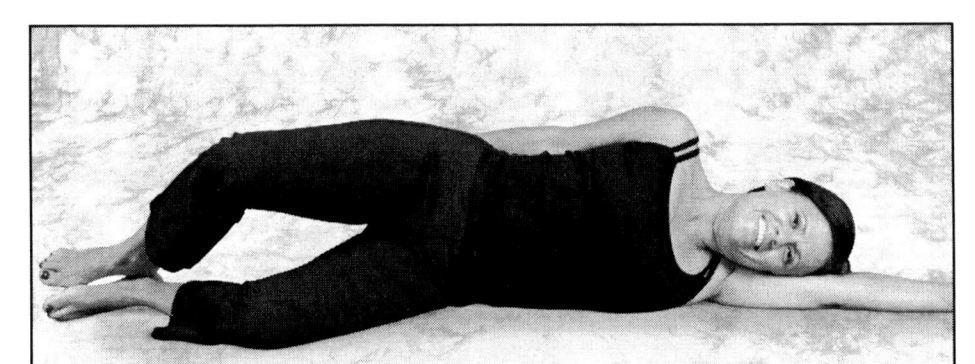

WHAT TO DO:

1. Lie on your side with your knees and hips bent at ninety degrees each.

2. Gently draw in the abdominal muscles to engage your transverse abdominis.

3. Keeping the ankles together and hips stable, lift the top knee away from the bottom knee, mimicking the motion of a clamshell opening and closing.

4. This motion should be done slowly without any movement in the hips. Usually, less range of motion is "more" with this exercise.

5. Gently return back to the starting position. Repeat ten times for one to three sets on each side.

WHAT TO WATCH OUT FOR:

1. Holding the breath, which can increase abdominal pressure and cause leaking, pain, and pressure.

2. Rotating the hips backward as you lift the top leg. This can cause instability, pain, and does not allow the gluteus medius muscle, one of the major hip stabilizers, to contract and strengthen properly.

3. Pain in the pubic bone or groin. If you are experiencing pain in your groin with this exercise, this may not be appropriate for your exercise regimen.

BENEFITS:

1. Activates and strengthens the gluteus medius muscle, a major hip stabilizing muscle that is important for standing and walking tolerance, as well as balance.

2. Assists in achieving and maintaining optimal sacroiliac joint alignment.

SCIATICA

Definition and Causes

Sciatica is defined as pain, numbness, and/or tingling in the gluteal region which may or may not radiate down the posterior or lateral thigh. Common causes of sciatica pain in pregnancy include tightness in the piriformis muscle causing entrapment of the sciatic nerve as it travels through the gluteal region, pressure on the neural structures in the pelvis from the growing uterus and fetus during pregnancy, and hormone-induced ligament laxity causing instability and weakness in the gluteal muscles and resultant compression of the sciatic nerve. One in 10,000 pregnant women may experience sciatica due to intervertebral disc herniation, which compresses the nerves in the lumbar spine that travel down the posterior leg. Although rare, fracture of the sacrum has also been reported as a cause of sciatica pain in pregnancy.

Prevalence

The literature oftentimes does not distinguish between PLP and sciatica when discussing prevalence and incidence rates. Therefore, very few studies exist that discuss rates of true sciatica in pregnancy. Values have been reported ranging from 1 percent to 45 percent of women experiencing sciatica pain in pregnancy. Regardless of the prevalence rate, it is important to recognize the signs and symptoms of sciatica so it can be properly diagnosed and treated.

Common Symptoms and Activity Limitations

1. Pain in the low back region may be present, but is not as severe as pain in the buttock or leg.

2. Pain described as "sharp" or "shooting" or tenderness in the gluteal region, typically on one side more than the other, which is exacerbated by prolonged walking or standing.

3. Pain when the lower extremity is placed in flexion, adduction, and internal rotation. This position stretches the piriformis muscle and can compress the sciatic nerve as it travels through the gluteal region.

4. Inability to sit for prolonged periods due to pain in the buttocks which may or may not radiate into the posterior thigh.

5. Burning, tingling, weakness, or numbness in the buttock region or down the posterior leg.

Table 6.3: Exercises for the Treatment of Sciatica

EXERCISE	POSITION	REPS AND SETS	PURPOSE
Transverse Abdominis Holds	Seated, Standing, Supine, Semi-Recumbent	Beginner: five-second hold: ten reps/one to two sets Advanced: fifteen to twenty reps/two to three sets	Increases pelvic hip and spinal stability and strengthens the core. Protects the organs against adverse pressure.
Tennis Ball Release	Standing or Seated	Press into painful spots for sixty to ninety seconds. Repeat as needed until pain in spot is reduced by at least 50%	Helps to get rid of painful gluteal trigger points that can be contributing to your sciatica.
Figure Four Stretch	Seated	Beginner: ten to thirty second hold: one to two sets Advanced: ten to thirty second hold: two to three sets	Stretches the piriformis muscle and relieves sciatica symptoms.
Seated Adduction	Seated	Beginner: five-second hold: ten reps/one to two sets Advanced: five second hold: ten reps/two to three sets	Helps strengthen the inner thigh and helps to maintain hip alignment.

Table 6.3 continues on following page

Table 6.3 (cont.): Exercises for the Treatment of Sciatica

EXERCISE	POSITION	REPS AND SETS	PURPOSE
Seated Abduction	Seated	Beginner: five-second hold: ten reps/one to two sets Advanced: five second hold:ten reps/two to three sets	Increases pelvic hip and spinal stability and strengthens the core. Protects the organs against adverse pressure.
Lean Backs	Supine or Standing	Beginner: five to ten second hold: ten reps/one to two sets Advanced: five to ten second hold: ten reps/two to three sets	Helps to centralize pain and helps to relieve pain associated with sciatica.
Sciatica Nerve Stretch	Seated	Five-second holds in the stretched position and five seconds in the relaxed phase. Repeat ten times	Helps to centralize pain and helps to relieve pain associated with sciatica.

Transverse Belly Holds

Please refer to page 128 to learn how to perform a transverse belly hold.

Tennis Ball Release

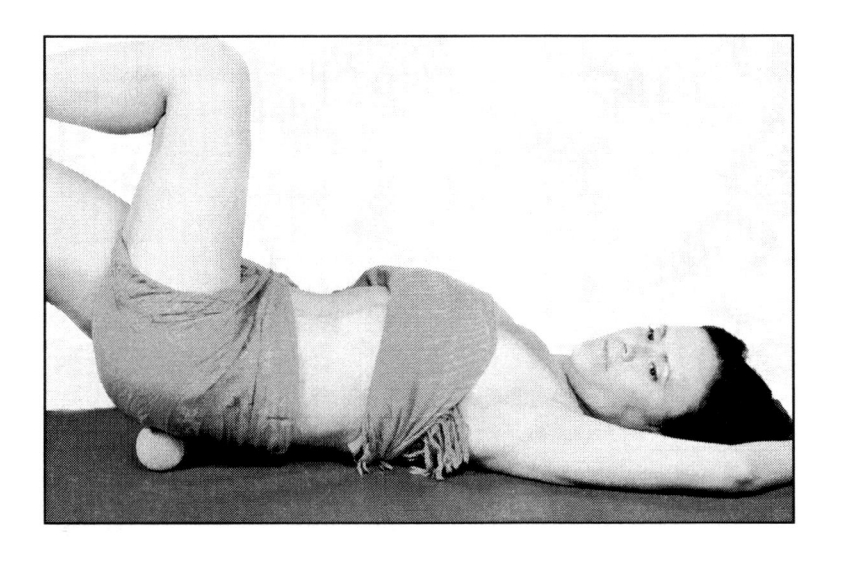

WHAT TO DO:

1. This exercise may be done standing next to a wall, or supine.

2. If standing, place the tennis ball between the wall and your gluteal muscles. If you are lying down, you will place the tennis ball underneath your gluteal muscles and sit on top of the ball.

3. Roll the ball around the gluteal muscles until you find a tender spot. The muscles you are targeting here include the piriformis muscle, gluteus maximus, and gluteus medius muscles.

4. Stop on the tender spot and ask yourself: "What is my pain level on a scale of 0 to 10 (0 is no pain, 10 is the worst pain imaginable)?"

5. Stay on that spot for sixty to ninety seconds, or until your pain reduces by at least 50 percent. Repeat several times until tender spots are relieved. Do this one to three times a day for pain relief. This type of pressure to a tender spot is called trigger point therapy.

WHAT TO WATCH OUT FOR:

1. Avoid pressing too hard into the muscle, which can cause it to spasm more. Try to keep your pain level less than 5 on the 0 to 10 pain scale.

2. Avoid sitting on the tennis ball on the inside of your sit bones close to the anus. This spot can be very sensitive and a tennis ball should not be used to release this muscle.

3. Ensure you are holding each tender spot long enough for your pain to reduce by 50 percent. The trigger point you are targeting will not be shut down if you fail to do this. If you encounter a stubborn spot, you may need to do this trigger point release multiple times before it lets go.

BENEFITS:

1. Reduces muscle spasm in the gluteal muscles, which can help decompress the sciatic nerve as it travels through the posterior gluteal region.

2. Helps facilitate and maintain proper sacroiliac joint alignment by reducing muscle tension, improving flexibility, and allowing pelvic bones to sustain alignment corrections longer.

3. Improves blood flow to the hip and pelvic muscles enhancing vitality and sexual function.

4. Reduces pain by decreasing trigger points that originate from tight posterior gluteal muscles. For more information about trigger point therapy, see Chapter 7.

Figure Four Stretch

WHAT TO DO:

1. While seated in good posture at the edge of your seat,
place the left ankle lightly
on the thigh of the right leg
making a figure four. Keep
your hips square, your shoulders down and back as you
sit straight.

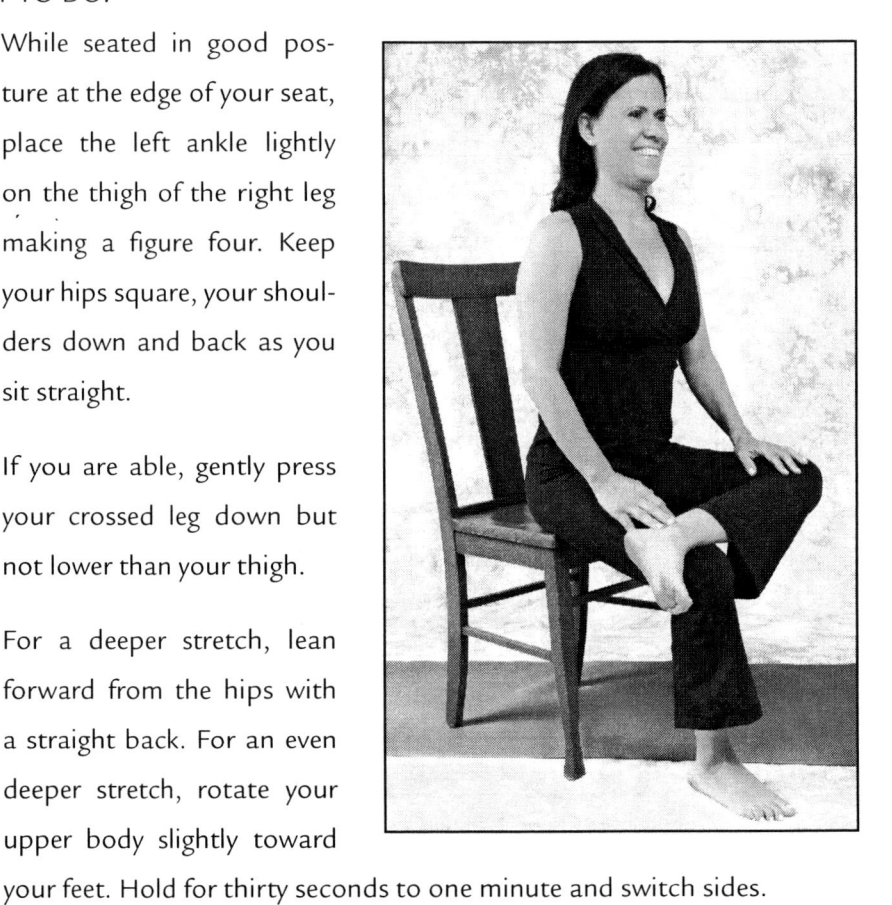

2. If you are able, gently press
your crossed leg down but
not lower than your thigh.

3. For a deeper stretch, lean
forward from the hips with
a straight back. For an even
deeper stretch, rotate your
upper body slightly toward
your feet. Hold for thirty seconds to one minute and switch sides.

4. Bring your body back to center and repeat the pose on the other side. Do
two to three repetitions of the stretch.

WHAT TO WATCH OUT FOR:

1. Don't torque the ankle bone. Remember to keep the anklebone slightly off
the resting thigh to avoid stressing it.

2. Avoid slouching in this posture to prevent stress on the lumbar spinal
nerves and to make this stretch more effective.

3. If your pain increases and/or radiates into your thigh or lower leg/foot, or persists for thirty minutes or longer, discontinue this stretch and consult your healthcare professional.

BENEFITS:

1. Helps to stretch the piriformis muscle and maintain pelvic alignment.

2. Helps increase the mobility and function of the major nerve roots of the lumbar and sacral spine, which innervate the pelvic floor muscles and internal pelvic organs.

3. Improves blood flow to the hip and pelvic muscles enhancing vitality and sexual function.

Seated Adduction

Please refer to page 135 to learn how to do the seated adduction exercise.

Seated Abduction

Please refer to page 133 to learn how to do the seated abduction exercise.

Lean Backs

Please refer to page 138 to learn how to perform a lean back.

Sciatic Nerve Stretch

1. Sit in NS and in great posture.

2. Straighten out the leg of the painful side. Hold this position and then look up. This stretches the nerve. Hold this position for five seconds. Lower the leg and lower the head then look down in this relaxed position. Hold for five seconds. Return to start position. Repeat 10 times.

3. This exercise stretches the sciatic nerve and can give you symptoms that travel down the leg. This is normal. You must do this exercise with caution and don't overdo it. Do one set of ten repetitions and see how you feel afterward. This sciatic stretch may not be appropriate for all pregnant women. Consult with your physical therapist before performing this stretch.

CONCLUSION

The good news: the majority of women who experience pregnancy-related lumbar pain, sciatica, or pelvic girdle pain during pregnancy will have a full recovery within three months of giving birth. However, the literature suggests that one in three women who are three months postpartum have persistent lumbo-pelvic pain causing moderate to severe disability. A substantial number of women thus carry the burden of pregnancy-related pain in the postpartum period. In our clinical experience treating thousands of women both during pregnancy and in the postpartum period, we find that providing proactive care during pregnancy can significantly reduce pain, improve strength and stability, and prevent pain and dysfunction from persisting beyond the birth of the baby. It is essential to address and combat your pregnancy-related pains early on so that you can regain your power and care for your baby without limitation. Pregnancy-related pain may be common but that does not mean it is normal, nor does it mean you have to suffer for the nine-month journey ahead. Use this book or seek out the help of a women's health physical therapist to guide you so that you can learn to stop your pain and reclaim your power.

In the next chapter, we'll discuss a common type of pelvic pain called pubic symphysis dysfunction. Read on and we will show you how to manage this pain with our programs, tools and behavior modifications.

CHAPTER SEVEN

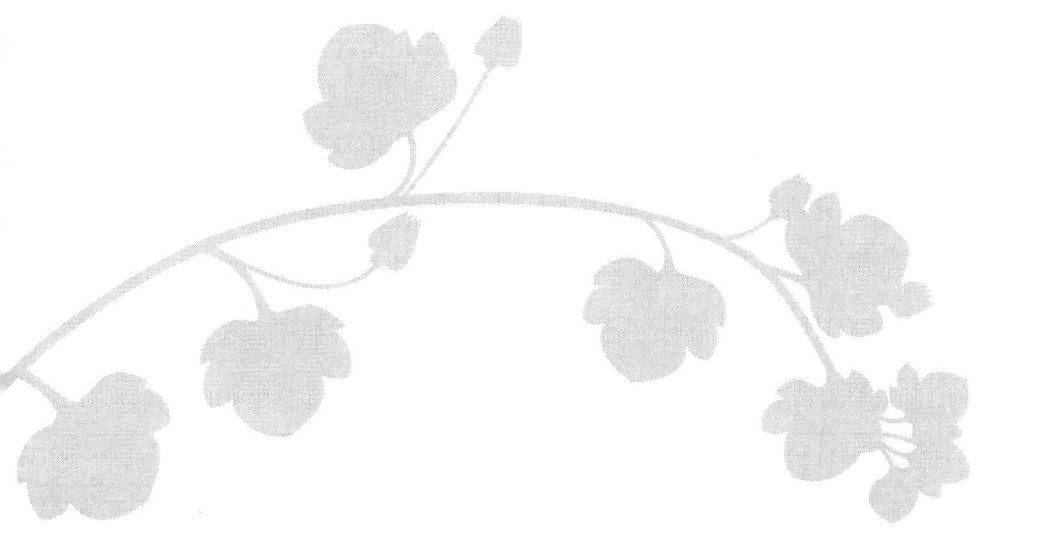

*"Our greatest weakness lies in giving up.
The most certain way to succeed is always
to try just one more time."*

—*Thomas A. Edison*

Chapter 7

SYMPHYSIS PUBIC DYSFUNCTION: TRADE SECRETS THAT REDUCE PAIN

While symphysis pubic dysfunction (SPD) or pubic bone pain (diastasis) is common during pregnancy, it is not a normal part of the pregnancy journey. Yes, something can be *common* yet not be *normal*. Pregnant women suffer in silence with SPD and seek no help or—worse yet—are not advised to try physical therapy. Unfortunately, many OB/GYNs and midwives believe that certain types of aches and pains are a routine part of pregnancy and are unaware that pregnant women can be helped with conservative physical therapy. This is the belief culture here in the United States. But I will prove to you that there is much you can do—not only with a physical therapist but on your own—to alleviate your pain and symptoms. In this chapter you will learn massage therapy, trigger point releases, protection and injury prevention strategies. You will also learn how to align your pubic symphysis joint, an extraordinary pain-relief tool. Since women with SPD tend to suffer from pelvic instability, you will also learn how to belt yourself for optimization and maintenance of alignment and enhancement of stability.

Let's start with a brief anatomy overview (see also Chapter 5). The two pubic bones are connected together by cartilage and ligaments; this connection is called the pubic symphysis. SPD results when the pubic symphysis moves excessively, separates or misaligns creating instability and contributing to high levels of pain. It is normal for the pubic bones to separate during pregnancy to make room for the baby, but if the separation is too great or there is excessive movement the end result can be pain of great magnitude. SPD can start as early as the first trimester when relaxin hormone is at its highest or can begin later on in the pregnancy as the hips begin to widen to allow the baby to position itself for labor and delivery. Pubic bone pain can have debilitating effects on the lives of pregnant women, causing them to resort to medication to deal with the day-to-day pain. I see pregnant women using canes and wheelchairs because they simply cannot walk due to severe SPD pain. By the time a pregnant woman suffering from pubic bone pain comes to my healing center, she is often at her wits' end.

Up to 45 percent of pregnant women suffer from some sort of SPD (also known as pelvic girdle pain), but in my experience, this suffering can be alleviated. Conservative physical therapy can have dramatic pain-relieving effects. (It is important to note here that pregnant women who suffer from SPD pain might need to rest more than usual to allow for the bone to heal.) In the next section I will explain some precautions you can take to help minimize pain and maximize your day-to-day function. I will also explore the top exercises that create stability within the pelvis to give you a simple exercise program that you can follow while you are pregnant. You will also learn how to correct your misaligned pubic bone using a simple pubic bone muscle energy technique. To succeed you will have to adhere strictly to the recommendations and precautions and perform your therapeutic and massage exercises daily. SPD does not miraculously disappear after you have a baby and you may have to continue these exercises and tools well into the postpartum period. Also note that women who suffer from SPD must be careful in the position of labor and delivery. I have seen women get worse and leave the hospital in wheelchairs after having their babies. I advise you to discuss your labor position with your caregiver; I do not recommend any labor position that requires the legs to spread wider than hip-width apart. Make sure to read Chapter 10 which details how to avoid obstetrical trauma in the labor and delivery process.

Diagram 7.1: Pubic Symphysis Joint and Related Structures

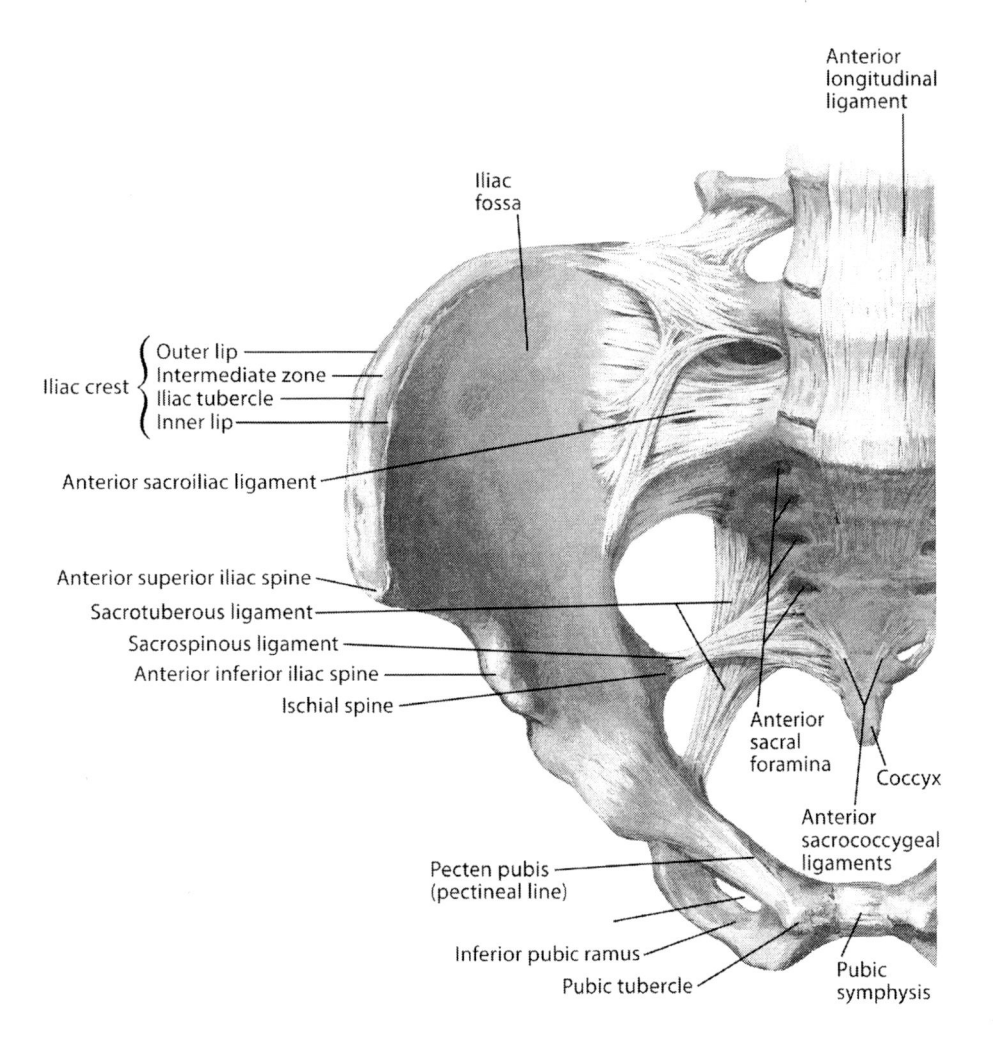

Diagram Description: Notice the pubic symphysis and the cartilage that holds the two pubic bones together. When there is a separation it occurs at the pubic symphysis. Source: Netter Images.

Advice for Pregnant Women Suffering from Pubic Symphysis Pain

Dysfunction at the pubic symphysis can alter the way you walk, contributing to pain in the groin, inner thighs or abdominal muscles. To keep pain in check women who suffer from SPD must make serious modifications to their activity and exercise programs.

At first you must be very strict and diligent with monitoring of activities and exercises, but as you improve and get stronger and the pelvis stabilizes you will be able to do more. So don't panic. I find that many pregnant women get angry because they simply cannot do what they used to do. But it is important to note that SPD is a serious condition not to be ignored. You must listen to your body when choosing and performing activities, chores or exercises. Your body will tell you what it needs. Never override a pain signal; pay attention because if you further injure this joint it is very difficult to manage. Listen to your "Body Talk" and review this chapter carefully so you know how to heal yourself with proper execution of the tools and exercises. Don't despair; instead take the necessary action so that you can continue to stay active while you are pregnant.

SPD Risk Factors

Pregnant women constantly tell me: "I didn't know I was at risk for SPD," and "No one ever told me and I wish someone had." The following list is provided for educational purposes and to increase your awareness of factors that can contribute to the development of SPD. Read carefully and take note of those factors that are within your control; these should be monitored to reduce your risk of SPD.

Table 7.1: SPD Risk Factors

1. Gaining excessive body weight during pregnancy especially in the first and third trimester.
2. Elevated Basal Metabolic Rate (BMI).
3. Multiple pregnancies.
4. History of SPD with previous pregnancy.
5. Expecting a large baby or twins.
6. Poor standing posture, strenuous activities such as running, spinning or other exercises that put excessive strain on the pubic symphysis.
7. Baby's in utero position.
8. Connective tissue health and laxity of the connective tissue.
9. A history of a fracture or trauma to the pelvis.
10. Exercises, posture or activities that bring the legs far apart or wider than hip-width apart.
11. Previous history of performing repetitive motions that increase pain at the pubic symphysis.
12. Laboring on your back with your legs spread wide apart.
13. Pelvic malalignment issues.

Childbirth Positions to Avoid

Women suffering from SPD have to take extra precautions during labor and delivery to avoid further separation of the pubic sympysis joint. Listed below are some of the positions that you should avoid.

Low Squat Birth Position

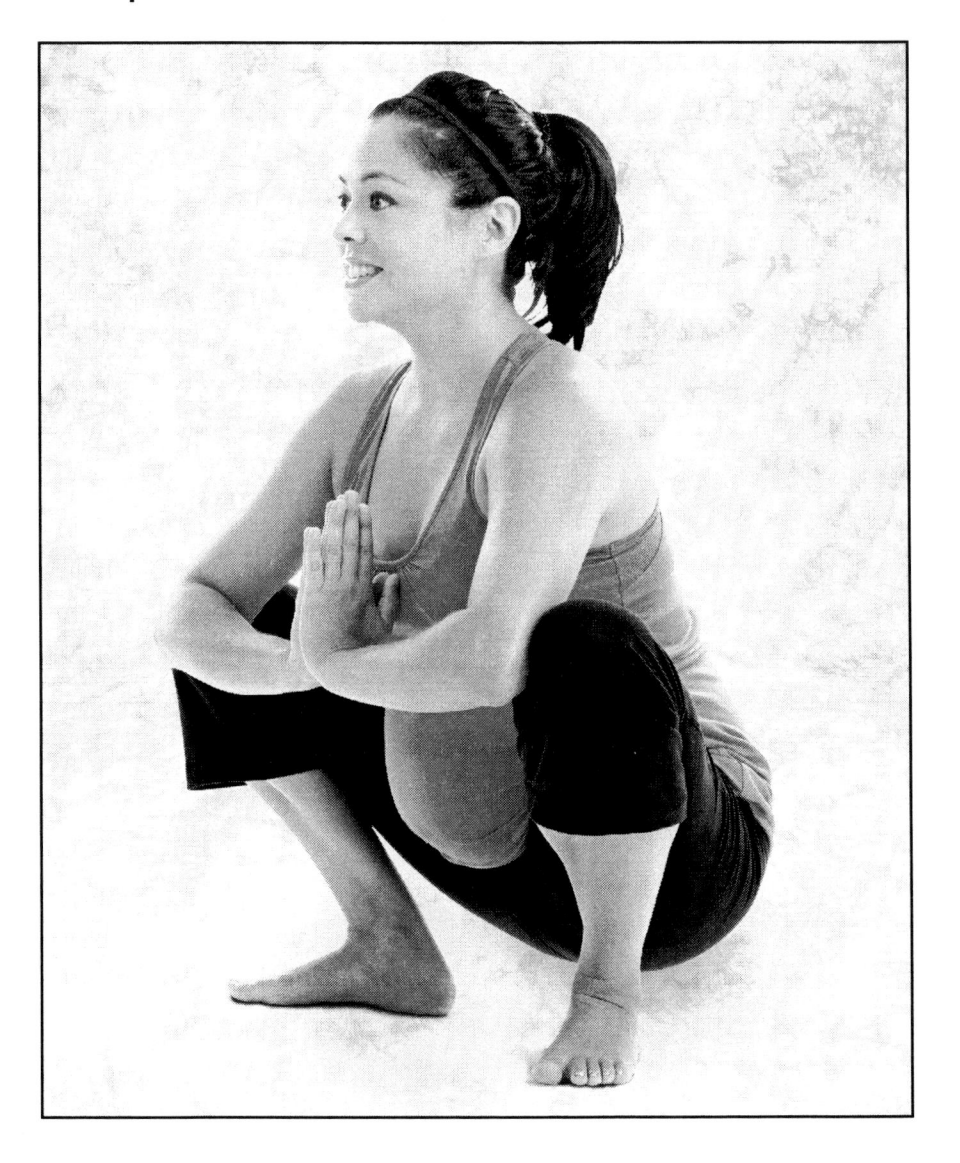

Description: Low squat birthing position not recommended for SPD.

Partner Birth Squat

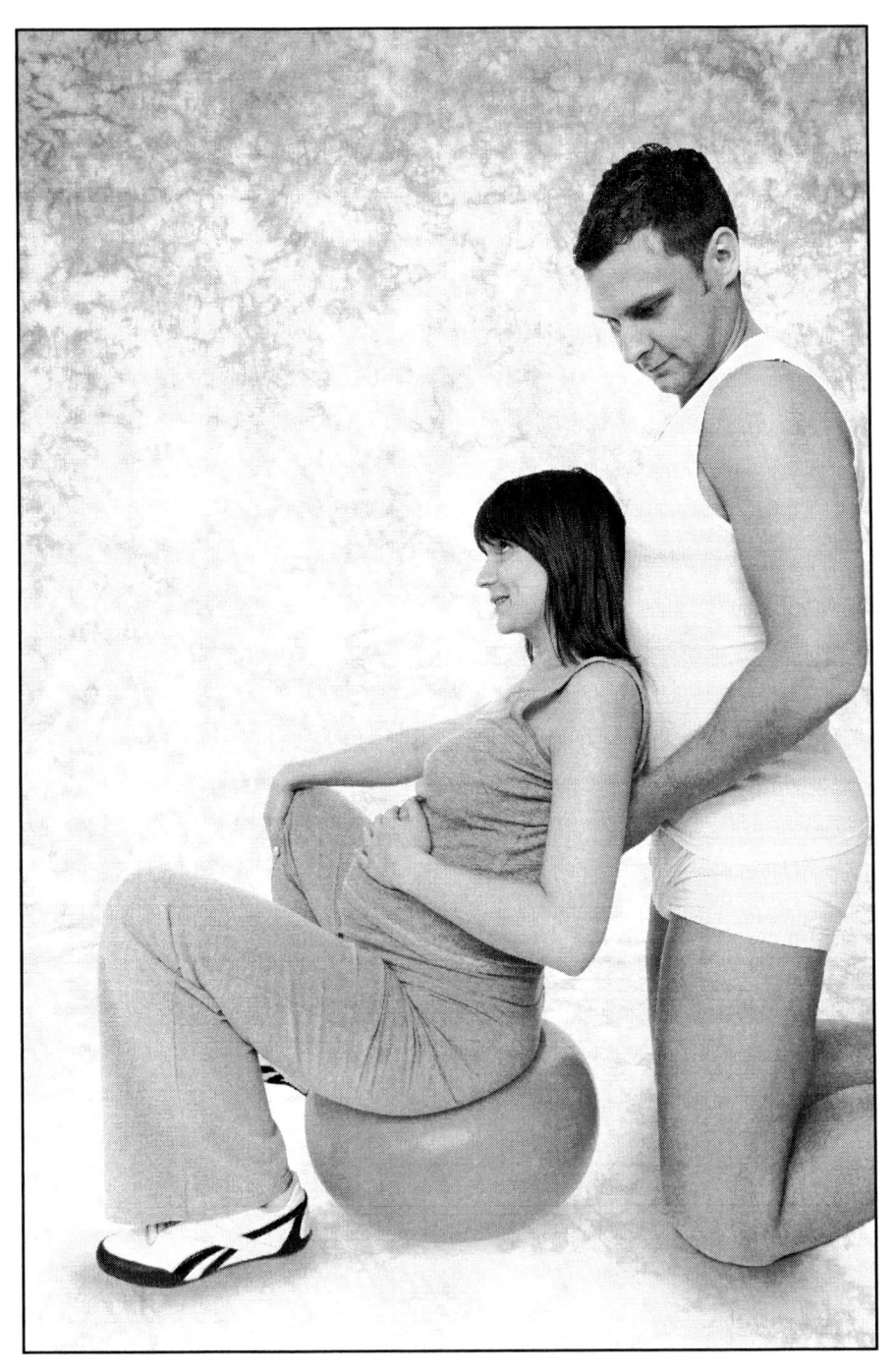

Description: Supported partner low squat birthing position not recommended for SPD.

Recommended Birth Positions for SPD

The best position to deliver in if you are suffering from SPD is the side-lying position. Don't forget to discuss this option with your doctor or midwife.

Side-Lying Birth Position

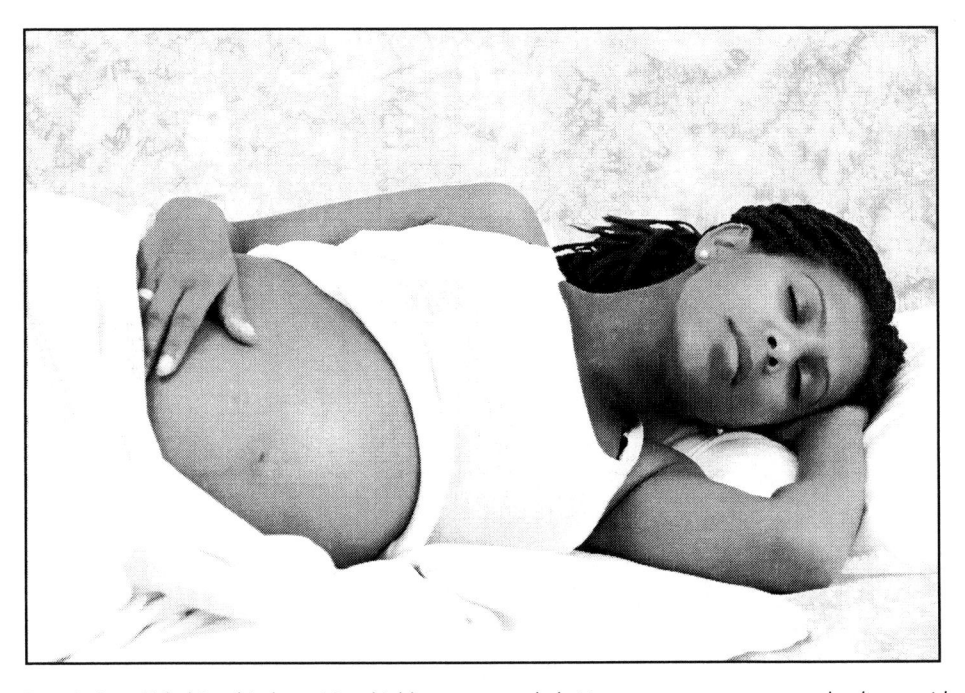

Description: Side-lying birth position highly recommended. Have partner support top leg but avoid bringing the legs too far apart. See Chapter 10 for more details.

SPD Symptoms

SPD has many faces and many symptoms can arise when there is a dysfunction, malalignment, separation or laxity in this joint. Many times women complain about groin/pubic bone pain and lower abdominal pain, usually greater on one side than the other. As discussed in Chapter 5, the rectus abdominis muscle that forms your "six-pack" attaches into the pubic symphysis. With SPD there may be increased tension on these muscles and lower abdominal pain may result. All abdominal pain during pregnancy must be evaluated by your physician or midwife to rule out more serious causes of abdominal pain. Don't assume that your pain is related to SPD. Always consult your MD or midwife. Apart from the lower abdomen and pubic pain and discomfort, SPD may also contribute to the symptoms listed in the table below.

Table 7.2: Symptoms Associated with SPD

1. Pain can get worse when you lift your legs or stand on one foot.
2. Inability to stand on one foot while dressing, bathing and/or exercising.
3. Trouble moving the legs when you wake up in the morning.
4. Pain in the pubic joint, groin and/or inner thigh with turning over in bed, moving sit-to-stand, walking and going up and down stairs.
5. Pain that gets worse when you lie flat on your back.
6. Pain that increases when you try to turn over in bed.
7. Decreased range of movement of the hip bones, causing difficulty and pain with walking.
8. Pain shooting down your buttocks and legs (sciatica).
9. A clicking or popping sound near the pubic bone area when you walk or move your legs.
10. Stress or urge incontinence.

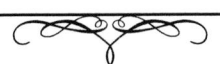

Table 7.2 (cont.): Symptoms Associated with SPD

11. Pelvic pressure or pressure in the vagina as if something is about to fall out.
12. PFM muscle spasms.
13. Sexual dysfunction.
14. Pelvic floor muscle weakness.
15. Lower abdominal pain. Must be checked out immediately as this can be very serious.
16. Diastasis recti separation of the abdominals.
17. Sexual pain or pain with deep thrusting.
18. Low back pain or sacroiliac joint pain.
19. Walking backward is less painful than walking forward.

Reducing SPD with Proven Trade Secrets

When you suffer from SPD you are more vulnerable to injury and you must take extra care to avoid exacerbating your SPD. I have found over the years that certain behavioral changes, body positioning and activities can help to reduce SPD-related pain. Below you will find some of the best techniques/exercises to help manage your pain and keep it in check. Make sure to review this part very carefully and follow as many of these strategies as possible. Also, review Chapter 4 so that you are simultaneously acting to stop destructive forces.

How to Transition from One Position to Another without Excruciating Pain

Perform a pelvic brace (PB) to move around and to get in and out of positions. A pelvic brace will help to stabilize pubic symphysis and greatly reduce pain. This is your go-to exercise when you are moving and the movement is triggering pain. A PB is a combination exercise that incorporates a TrA abdominal muscle hold and a low-level Kegel contraction. This brace will help reduce pain when you move from sitting to standing, in and out of the car, and when changing positions in bed. The pelvic brace is explained in Chapter 4. Take some time to re-read this section. In addition to the PB you will find that keeping the legs together as much as possible will help you control your pain. Sleeping can be challenging. Sleep with a pillow between your knees if you are sleeping in side-lying position. This will help maintain your pubic bone alignment. You may have to try different sleeping positions to see which one works for you.

How to Switch Positions in Bed with Less Pain

Most pregnant women sleep on their sides so I will cover this position specifically, but this process can be performed with any sleeping position. When switching from one side to the other side in bed, first squeeze the pillow between your knees, perform a PB then roll onto your back, re-squeeze the pillow, perform a PB and then roll to the other side. This re-squeezing of the pillow and performing a PB every time you change sides in bed will help to keep your pain in check and prevent the pubic bone from coming out of proper alignment. To sit up in bed from a side-lying position you will do a similar process. First squeeze the pillow between your knees, then perform the PB, then push yourself up to a sitting position as you maintain the PB and pillow squeeze. You can try your positional changes with just the PB if it's too difficult to squeeze the pillow. Try both and see which one works better for you.

Reduce Your Pain by Using a Belt

A sacroiliac (SI) belt will provide the stability your pelvis needs and can be a pain-reducing life saver. (See Chapter 8 for the specifics on how to wear belts.) Many women have pain that keeps them up at night. Sleep with your belt if needed; you will find that you might get a better night's sleep. If you are suffering from severe pain, get two belts: one for everyday use and one that you can use while showering. Don't take the belt off if you are in a lot of pain. Wear it as much as possible—at all times if necessary. Remember to first correct your pelvis using the shotgun technique.

Correct Your Pubic Bone: Shotgun

This is an important and pain-relieving tool that should not be overlooked. The "shotgun" correction is a pelvic muscle energy technique that aligns the joint of the pubic symphysis. (See Chapter 5 for information on how to find your pubic bone and perform the shotgun correction.) The shotgun correction is appropriate for pregnant women who are experiencing symptoms of pubic bone pain or sacroiliac joint pain. This is the best correction for women experiencing SPD and this may be the only correction that you will need but please review Chapter 5 for an overview of all corrections.

Avoid Going Wider Than Hip-Width Apart with Exercise and Everyday Activity

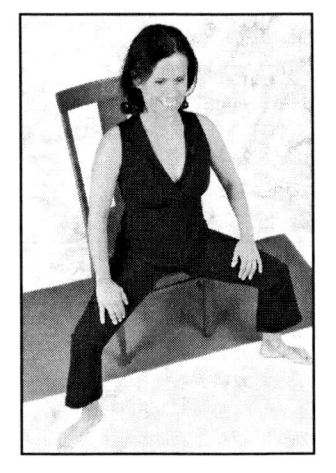

Any exercise or activity that requires the legs to be wide apart or wider than hip-width will either cause you a lot of pain or increase the risk of separating the pubic symphysis further. Avoid excessive stretching of the inner thigh muscles and widening your stance with day-to-day movements or with exercise.

Description: Avoid bringing your legs too far apart if you are suffering from SPD.

Avoid Crossing Your Legs

The inner thigh muscles take a beating with SPD because all the inner thigh muscles attach to this bone. Since the bone is dysfunctional, the neighboring inner thigh muscles get into a tizzy and develop trigger points, muscles spasms and myofascial restrictions. Crossing the legs causes the inner thigh muscles to shorten thereby contributing to all of the above. Do not cross the legs while sitting. Keep your feet planted on the ground and sit in good sitting posture.

Do Not Stand on One Leg to Put on Your Clothes or Shoes or to Exercise

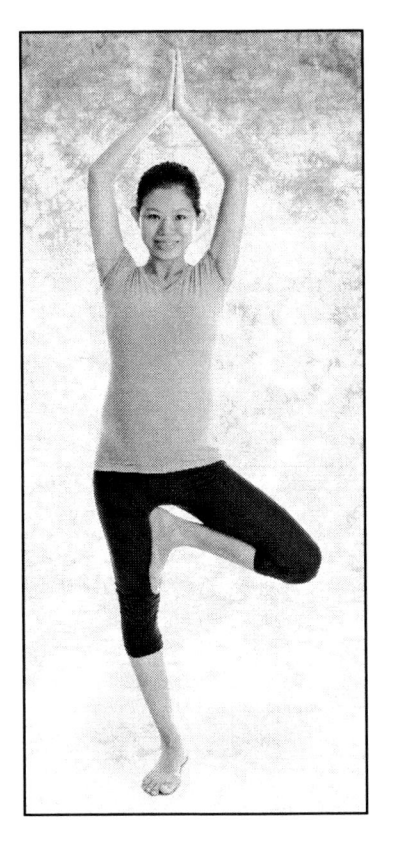

Description: SPD is exacerbated by any action that has you standing on one foot. Avoid standing on one foot and avoid exercises that require you to stand on one foot. Sit down to put on underwear and pants.

Monitor Your Yoga, Pilates and Other Exercise Programs

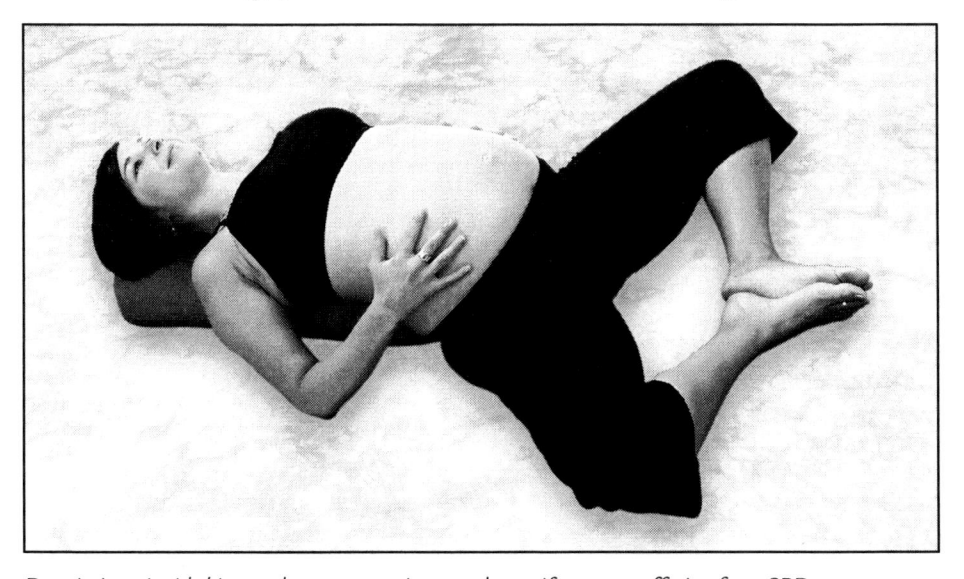

Description: Avoid this popular yoga pose in yoga classes if you are suffering from SPD.

Warrior Pose

Description: Avoid all variations of warrior poses in yoga, or poses that bring the legs wider than hip-width apart if you are suffering from SPD.

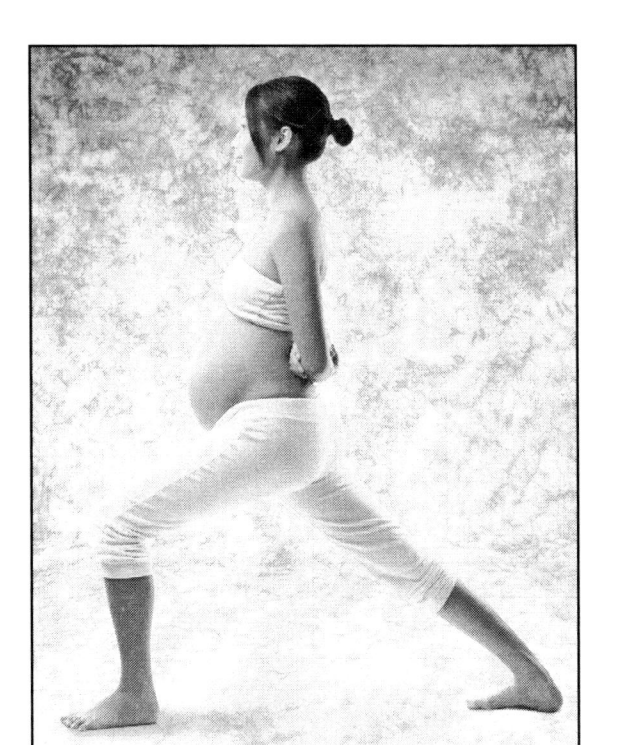

Avoid exercises that increase your pain such as certain yoga poses that bring the legs wide apart. Even certain prenatal poses need to be modified. Monitor Pilates exercises that require unilateral leg swings or exercises that require you to bring the legs far apart. Avoid running or biking because they put too much stress on the pubic bone. Avoid swimming strokes that bring the legs far apart. Keep exercise pain free. Any exercise that increases your pain is not a good idea. It is recommended that you wear your SI belt when exercising.

Sex and SPD

The side-lying position for sexual intercourse is a great position to use to avoid exacerbating your SPD. If that doesn't work try all fours but keep the legs no further than hip-width apart. Although this might seem strange, consider wearing your belt for sexual activity. Don't forget to correct your alignment after sex and then put the belt back on again. Read Appendix 1: Sex during Pregnancy for different sexual positions.

Natural Pain Relief: Ice and Heat

Ice the pubic bone for ten to fifteen minutes one to three times a day as needed for pain. Avoid putting the ice on the uterus. Keep the ice on the bone and remember to wrap the ice pack so you don't burn your skin. Apply heat or a hot water bottle to your inner thighs to keep these muscles supple and less tight.

Walk Like a Geisha Woman

Walking will pose its challenges and can be so painful that many women who suffer from SPD complain their pain with walking is the worst pain they have ever experienced. Move as a unit when changing positions and keep the legs symmetrical and parallel as if wearing a tight pencil skirt. Avoid taking long strides and walking too fast, which will pull on the pubic bone contributing to more pain.

Women with Young Children and Dealing with SPD

If you are a pregnant mom, avoid carrying your young child as much as possible and avoid carrying your young child on one hip. If you have to lift your child, make sure he/she is very close to your body so you are not over-reaching to lift your child. Bend from the knees and use proper body mechanics.

Move as a Unit: Getting In and Out of Cars

Getting in and out of the car will pose some challenges. Move as a whole unit and try to keep a pillow or small yoga block handy. To get in the car sit facing the window of the car with legs close together and a yoga block between the knees. Activate your PB, lift both legs together and pivot the whole body until your legs are facing the front window.

Avoid Stairs

Stair climbing is one of the worst things to do when you suffer from SPD. If necessary, set up a bedroom in the downstairs part of your home.

More Trade Secrets: Six Exercises That Enhance Stability and Help to Reduce SPD Pain

In this next section we start to discover what exercises work for SPD. Pregnant women with SPD need stability in the pubic symphysis bone. Stabilizing exercises for SPD involve working the muscles around the pubic bone several times a day. Exercising this frequently helps to keep the pubic bone stabilized and helps to keep the muscles that surround the pubic bone activated. Pain can often shut down the effectiveness with which muscles do their work. With SPD you need to stay on top of the muscles to prevent shut down and maintain a stabilizing force on the pubic and pelvic areas. Although these exercises seem simple, their effectiveness is profound and their pain-relieving capacity miraculous. The upcoming exercises should be performed five times a day throughout the day with long rest periods between sets. These restorative and stabilizing exercises are isometric holds, static holds that require no movement or change in the muscle length. They are simply holding exercises in certain form. They can be performed in any position but if you are sitting or standing these exercises must be performed in optimal posture.

Table 7.3: Stabilizing and Pain-Relieving Exercises for Women Suffering from SPD

1. Transverse Belly Abdominal Holds
2. Pelvic Floor Muscle Squeezes (Kegel)
3. Butt Squeezes
4. Latissimus Dorsi (LATS) Activation
5. Inner Thigh Squeezes
6. Leg Press

Transverse Belly Abdominal Holds

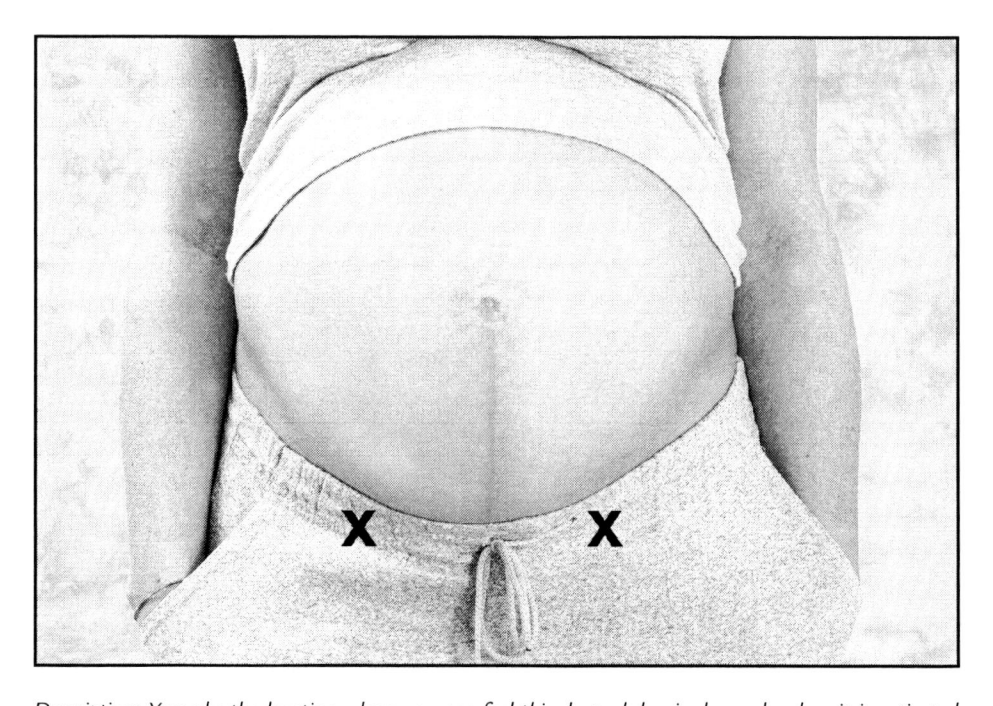

Description: X marks the location where you can feel this deep abdominal muscle when it is activated properly. You will also notice that when this exercise is executed properly you can lift your belly and baby upward. We call this the baby lift.

WHAT TO DO:

1. As you exhale, do a Kegel, or squeeze your pelvic floor muscles as if you are trying to stop the flow of urine. This is a low-level gentle Kegel. Only do 20 percent effort with this Kegel.

2. Draw your belly closer and more firmly toward the spine. As you pull in your abdominals try to imagine that you are trying to squeeze into an old pair of jeans that don't fit. You can also pull in your lower abdominal muscles as if you were hugging your baby.

3. Your belly should actually lift upward toward your nose if you perform the exercise correctly and the belly should move up and inward.

4. Hold TrA for five seconds, repeat five times. Breathe normally as you perform your TrA holds and avoid holding the breath or over-activating the abdominals. This is very subtle work and requires monitoring.

BENEFITS:

1. Strengthens the deep abdominal muscle and provides pelvic and spinal stability.

2. The TrA can also help pregnant women deliver their babies.

Pelvic Floor Muscle Squeezes (Kegel)

WHAT TO DO:

1. Sitting tall in good posture, do a Kegel contraction.

2. Perform the Kegel for five seconds and repeat five times.

BENEFIT:

The pubococcygeus (PC) muscle inserts into the pubic bone and will help to create stability to the pubic bone.

Butt Squeezes

WHAT TO DO:

1. Squeeze your butt cheeks together for five seconds and repeat five times.

2. You can do this exercise in good sitting or standing posture.

3. Perform the Kegel for five seconds and repeat five times.

BENEFIT:

The gluteal muscles provide posterior stability to the pelvis, hip, low back and sacroiliac joint.

Latissimus Dorsi (LATS) Activation

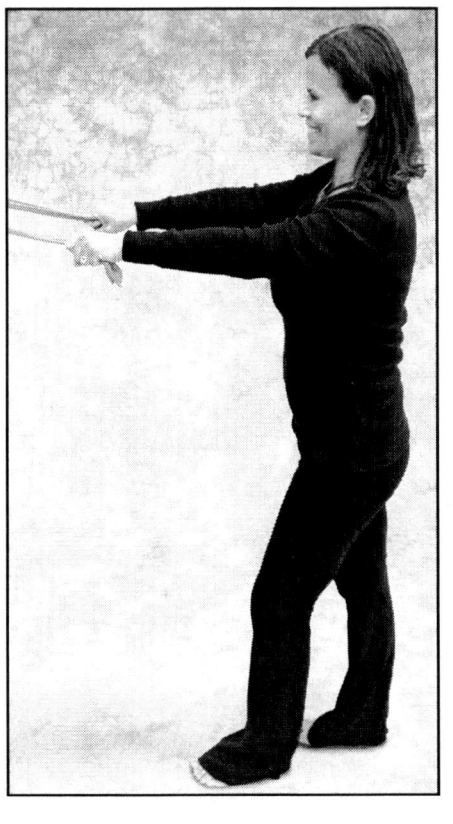 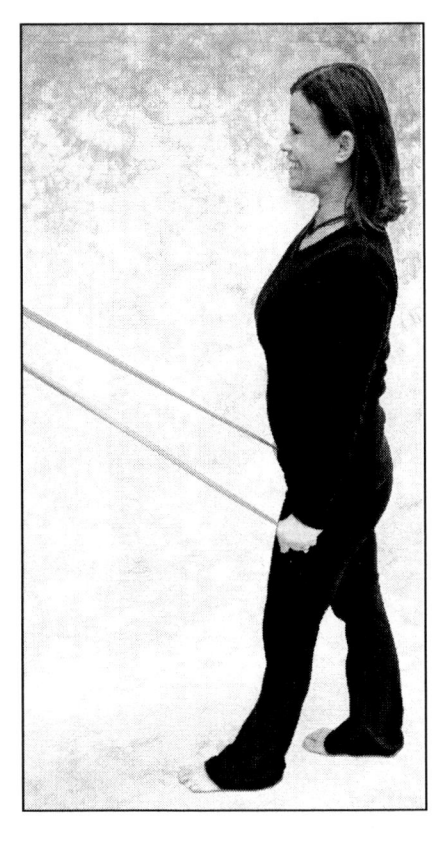

WHAT TO DO:

1. This exercise can be performed standing or sitting. Attach a Dyna-Band high on a doorway so that you have two ends of the band to grasp.

2. Your arms should be slightly in front of your body, elbows locked straight, and hands grasping the Dyna-Bands.

3. Contract your transverse abdominis muscle first (see Transverse Belly Holds).

4. Keeping your arms straight, pull your arms down and back just until they are at the side of your waist.

5. Hold three to five seconds and envision you are keeping your shoulder blades down and back as if you were going to put them in your back pockets. Repeat five to ten times; do one to three to five sets per day.

BENEFIT:

This is one of the largest muscles in the body and has several functions. It connects to the shoulder, spine and pelvis. The LATS help maintain pelvic alignment and help to stabilize the posterior pelvic region.

Inner Thigh Squeezes

WHAT TO DO:

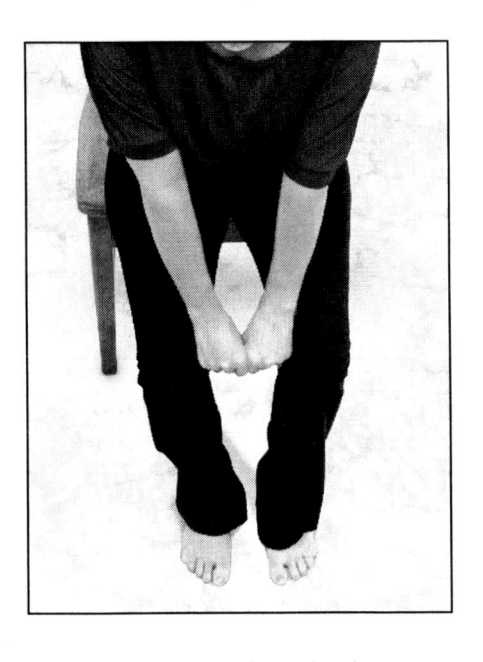

1. Sit down in excellent posture.

2. Put your fist or a rolled towel between your knees; squeeze knees together. This may hurt a little so monitor how much force you are putting into the inner thigh squeezes. Avoid causing yourself too much pain. It is okay to do these squeezes gently until you can tolerate more force.

Description: Instead of your hands you can use a yoga block or a pillow to squeeze between the knees.

3. Hold this inner thigh contraction for five seconds and repeat five times.

BENEFITS:

1. The inner thigh muscles provide a tremendous amount of stability to the pubic bone region.

2. A woman with SPD will tend to develop trigger points and spasms in these muscles which causes weakness in the inner thigh muscles. These squeezes allow the inner thigh muscles to remain strong so they can participate in the stability and thereby reduce SPD. Inner thigh muscles are also used to correct the pubic bone when it is out of alignment.

Leg Press

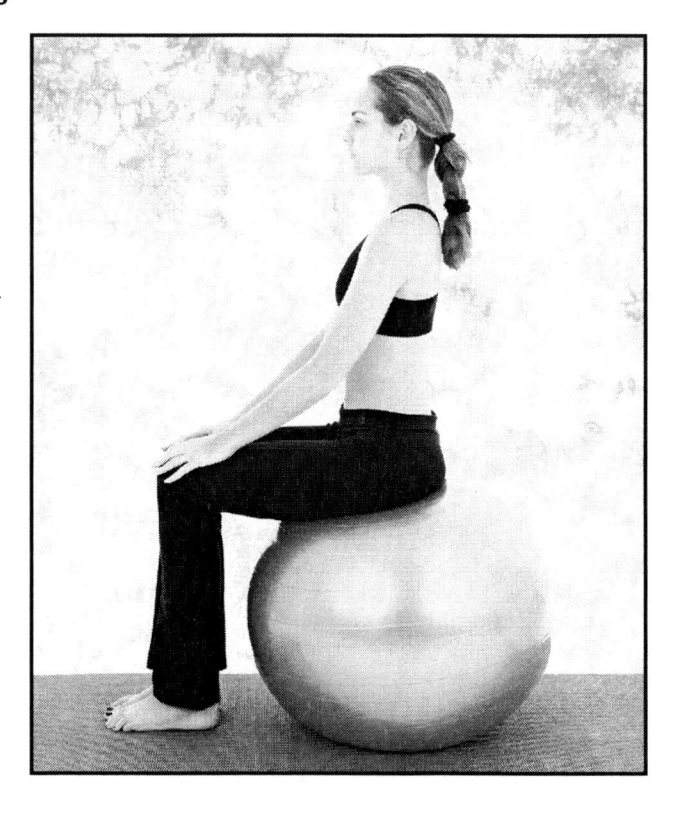

Description: For women suffering from SPD it is best to do the leg press while sitting on a sturdy chair. Once you have your pain under control you can try to progress to the physio-ball.

WHAT TO DO:

1. Sit in good posture placing your palms on your thighs.

2. Bring belly button toward your spine by doing a TrA hold and simultaneously press your hands into your thighs without moving your legs.

3. Hold five seconds and repeat five times.

BENEFIT:

This exercise strengthens the TrA while simultaneously strengthening the deep back muscles.

Listen to your body when performing the above exercise program. If the exercises start to increase your pain check to make sure you are performing them in excellent posture and not overdoing the contractions.

In this next section we will explore how to massage pain away with hands-on techniques and tools. It is a great idea to first do all your exercises and then massage the pain away.

Massaging Your Pain Away: Inner Thigh Trigger Point Release, Inner Thigh Positional Release and Inner Thigh Massage

The following techniques are all for the inner thigh muscles. As previously mentioned the inner thighs are deeply affected by SPD. The tools discussed here should be incorporated into your overall SPD program. You will learn how to massage the inner thigh, how to roll the muscles and how to get rid of trigger points. The goal with these massaging tools is to get rid of your pain. Start by taking note of your current pain level (0= no pain and 10= worst pain ever). After you have performed your massages check your pain level again. Assessing and keeping track of your pain before and after your exercises or massage is a great way to monitor your progress and evaluate what exercises or tools work best for you.

Inner Thigh Massage, Skin Rolling and Trigger Point Release

GETTING STARTED:

The inner thigh muscles require special attention because of their close proximity to the pelvis, pubic bone and PFMs. The inner thigh muscles can develop spasms, trigger points and adhesions as a response to what is happening in the pubic area. These tissue abnormalities can make sitting, walking and positional changes even more painful. The trigger points in the inner thigh can refer pain to the pubic bone, groin or bladder. To restore proper function, muscle length, and flexibility to the inner thigh muscles, use the three techniques described below. Having your inner thighs in optimal health will help you maintain better pubic bone alignment. Perform these techniques up to five minutes a day on both legs. Even if you do less you will gain the benefits. Avoid pressing too hard into the inner thigh muscles as this may cause a flare-up.

Long Deep Inner Thigh Strokes

WHAT TO DO:

1. Massage the inner thigh muscles from the knee to the upper groin, using long deep strokes for five to ten minutes.

2. If performing the massage without oil is too painful, you can use a small drop of oil or massage cream to make the gliding less painful or use aromatherapy oils such as my *Pain Be Gone* available at *RenewPT.com* or Young Living lavender oil.

Inner Thigh Skin Rolling

WHAT TO DO:

1. Gently roll your inner thigh muscles from the knee to the groin using your index fingers and thumbs. Try not to use an oil and stay superficially on the skin so you target the inner thigh fascia.

2. Roll the inner thigh for five to ten minutes or as tolerated.

Inner Thigh Trigger Point Release

WHAT TO DO:

1. The inner thigh muscles can develop trigger points in them as a response to pelvic pain. Search for these trigger points by running your hands slowly along your inner thigh muscles. A trigger point will feel like a hard, small ball and will produce pain when touched.

2. Once you find them, press into the trigger points for ninety seconds until the pain has diminished or gone away. You may have to do several cycles of ninety seconds to accomplish this.

3. Complete normalization of the inner thigh is necessary because this muscle is a major culprit in creating dysfunction and pain in the PFMs and it also contributes to bladder symptoms such as urgency and pain.

You can combine these three massage techniques and do all of them in one session or break them up into different days. The most important thing is to get pain relief and to work within a pain level that is tolerable. Stay between a three or four pain level (0= no pain and 10= worst pain ever).

SPD is a serious condition that requires active surveillance and monitoring—and lifestyle changes. Some women have a lot of pain and others have little pain and dysfunction. The spectrum for SPD is wide but no matter where you are it is important to follow the guidelines put forth in this chapter to make sure you keep your SPD from getting worse and negatively impacting your life. Pregnancy has many challenges; be aware of what can be done so that you can enjoy a pain-free pregnancy journey.

In the next chapter we explore the different types of belts that can help relieve pain for women suffering from SPD. Belts can also help relieve low back pain, sacroiliac pain and pelvic pressure. Don't skip the next chapter; a belt can sometimes make a world of difference.

CHAPTER EIGHT

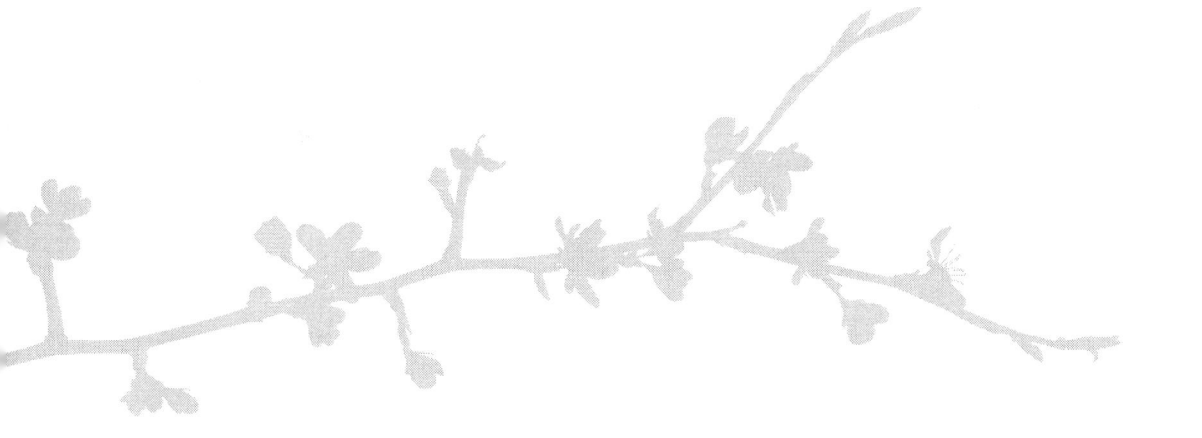

"Making a decision to have a child—it's momentous. It is to decide forever to have your heart go walking around outside your body."

— Elizabeth Stone

Chapter 8

SO MANY BELTS SO LITTLE TIME: HOW BELTING CAN HELP YOU

At Renew Physical Therapy we believe that belts are a key tool in a woman's healing program. Wearing a belt during pregnancy can make a positive difference for a woman suffering from low back pain, pelvic pressure, vulvar varicosities/swelling, diastasis recti separation, sacroiliac joint pain, symphysis pubic dysfunction, pelvic instability and incontinence. Women who use belts can have immediate pain relief, experience better day-to-day functioning and can carry out their days with less pain. When I was pregnant with my child I was the poster child for belts. I used many different types including the sacroiliac joint belt and the prenatal support belt. I am convinced that I was able to treat my patients and stay active during pregnancy because these belts helped me to have a stable pelvis.

We frequently hear: "I used a belt and it didn't help me." But we find that most women who are not getting results with a belt are either not using the correct type or are wearing it incorrectly. This chapter reviews the different types of belts and how to use them. The importance of exploring belts in general and working with the ones that give you the most pain relief, support and stability cannot be overstressed. We have seen over and over again that women are much better able to deal with the demands of pregnancy and postpartum recovery when they add a belt to the toolbox.

Table 8.1: Belt Types and Benefits

TYPE OF BELT	BENEFITS
Prenatal Support Belt	• Helps support the abdominal muscles, pelvic floor muscles, low back, hips, pelvis and upper back. • Can provide pain relief for the neck because these belts typically improve postural alignment. • For upper back stability and neck pain relief use a belt that has the shoulder straps and mid-back support.
Postnatal Support Belt	• Helps support and stabilize the abdominal muscles, low back, and pelvis and helps to reduce the effects of a diastasis recti separation by bringing the abdominal muscles together.
Sacroiliac Joint Belt	• Helps to reduce pain associated with sacroiliac dysfunction and symphysis pubic dysfunction. • Helps to stabilize the sacroiliac and pubic bone when they are unstable. Allows for better walking and day-to-day functioning.
Belly Bands	• Gives light abdominal support in pregnancy and also helps to extend the wear of clothes because you are able to keep the zipper or buttons open and put the belly band on top of the clothes.
Vaginal/Vulvar Support Strap	• To be used during pregnancy for support and compression of the pelvic floor to prevent varicosities, lymphedema, swelling, incontinence, organ prolapse, pain.

Belts for the Prenatal and Postpartum Periods: Belt Types and Indications

Prenatal Support Belt

Many women experience pelvic pressure when pregnant, and wearing a prenatal support belt will help alleviate this pressure by supporting the abdominal area. This pelvic pressure can be caused by the growing baby, weak pelvic floor muscles, weak abdominal muscles, poor posture and generalized body weakness. (Using a prenatal support belt will help, but please refer to chapters in *EPP* for abdominal training, pelvic floor training and full body training so that you can address these fundamental issues. The faster you get yourself on a proper program, the less symptomatic you will become and you will be able to wean yourself off the belt.) Prenatal belts help to reduce back pain by supporting the upper and lower back. Sometimes these pregnancy support belts also help pregnant women who are experiencing neck pain.

Postpartum Support Belt

Women who have just had a baby can benefit from wearing a postpartum support belt and at Renew Physical Therapy we recommend every woman bring her postnatal support belt to the hospital. There are many types of these belts on the market today and many celebrities either endorse a belt or have one of their own. We like belts that are fairly wide and cover not only the abdominal muscles but also support the bladder and uterus. The belt that you buy should be adjustable so that it can provide different levels of support and compression. Postpartum belts can be used immediately after delivery to support the abdominal muscles, low back and/or pelvic muscles. Those who have Cesarean births will find that these belts help to lessen pain and improve function and movement. If you had a Cesarean birth you will have to wait until the staples are out to use the belt. Make sure to ask your MD about belting after Cesarean birth. Some doctors will let you use them in the hospital and some will not. In New

York City there are many doctors now giving women who have had Cesarean births a belt because they realize how important they are for pain relief and support. If you have a diastasis recti abdominis and abdominal muscle weakness you will find a postpartum belt very helpful because the belt helps the muscles to approximate and it also helps to support them. In Latin and other cultures postpartum women are belting immediately after birth; the belts are recognized as a tool that will give them back their bodies and flatten their abdominals. At Renew Physical Therapy, we have seen countless women transform their bodies with the help of postpartum belts.

Sacroiliac Joint/Symphysis Pubic Dysfunction Support Belt

This belt works extraordinarily well for women who suffer from symphysis pubic dysfunction (SPD) or sacroiliac joint dysfunction. It can approximate the pubic bones providing stability and tremendous pain relief. For women with SPD this belt can be a lifesaver. Our recommendation is to use the belt all the time—including sleeping and showering— for acute and very painful SPD. Please remember that first you must correct your public bone alignment using the shotgun technique highlighted in Chapter 5 before putting on the belt. Additionally, you must perform the exercises highlighted in Chapter 7 to get your muscles strong so that over time you become less and less dependent on the belt.

The sacroiliac joint can become highly unstable during pregnancy, the postpartum period or during a woman's cycle. If you suffer from sacroiliac joint pain, this belt will provide you with profound pain relief and stability. This belt should be put on after you have corrected your pelvic alignment (see Chapter 5) and should wrap around your hip bones at the widest part of your pelvis. First find your hip bones and then wrap the belt around your lower hip bones (called the greater trochanter). The placement of this belt around the hips can vary several inches up or down. Make sure you are getting pain relief and you are not experiencing any numbness or tingling down the legs. If you do, you are wearing the belt to high or too low and it's too tight. Adjust the belt and then walk around to see if it makes you feel better. If you don't feel relief and the belly does not feel right, you may be out of alignment. Go back and check your alignment and belt placement.

Belly Band Support Belt

Belly bands offer the least amount of support yet many women love them and use them routinely during the pregnancy and postpartum period. These belts are large and elastic and many women use them to get their clothes to fit right. Belly bands ease the transition from one clothing size to another and help to make the wardrobe last. When I was pregnant I frequently used the belly band over clothes that did not fit and on top of that I would wear my sacroiliac belt and/or pregnancy belt. Belly bands come in many different fabrics and they can easily be disguised under the clothes.

Vaginal-Vulvar Support "V" Belt

The V belt is very similar to a man's jock strap. It is a woman's secret weapon during pregnancy and during the early postpartum period. The V belt provides pelvic floor support and compression by using a perineal strap or underpad. The V belt also helps to compress the perineal area thereby preventing vulvar varicosities, perineal swelling, pain, incontinence and organ prolapse and pressure. If you currently have vulvar varicosities ask your doctor or midwife about this belt. Patients in our center have amazing relief of vulvar varicosities/swelling and pelvic pressure with the V belt. Many women experience a "falling out" feeling in the pelvis and the V strap can help minimize this and support the perineum and the pelvic organs. The V belt fits comfortably over undergarments and can also help women who are experiencing incontinence during their pregnancy. In the postpartum period ask your midwife or doctor about the V belt; it may or may not be appropriate if you have experienced a perineal tear.

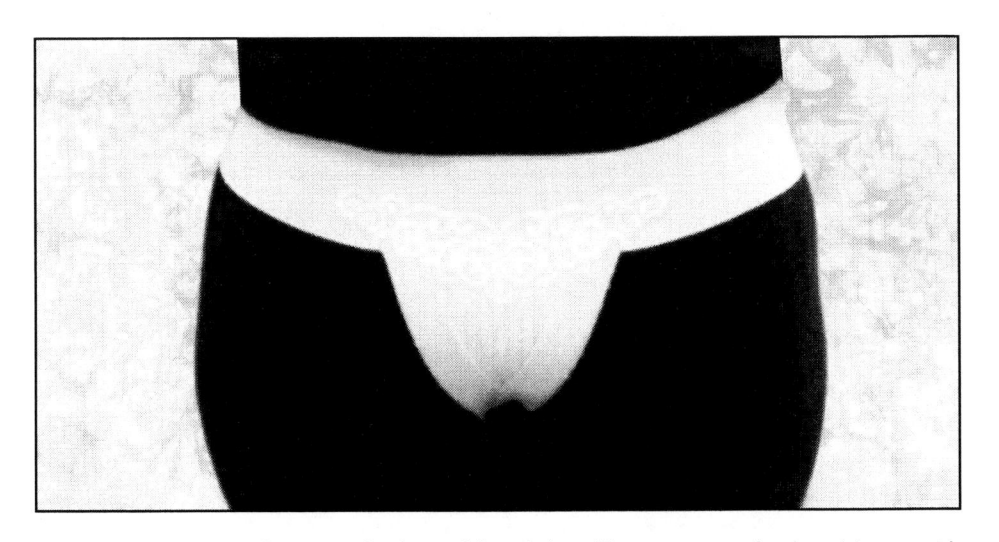

Description: **V Strap Belt.** *Notice the shape of the V belt and how it wraps under the pelvis to provide support and relief of pre- and postnatal symptoms.*

Belts can be the missing link during the pregnancy or postpartum period and should not be overlooked and treated as purely cosmetic. Belts are medical devices that can help to reduce symptoms and pain associated with pelvic and abdominal muscles weakness, scar pain and pelvic pressure. They help to increase pelvic stability and reduce stress to the pubic bone. Belts can provide so much relief that we believe every woman should explore them and add them to her healing journey.

In the next chapter we cover the ins and outs of Kegels. We will review the anatomy and function of the pelvic floor muscles (PFMs) and we will explore three types of perineal massage. After reading this upcoming chapter you will be able to test your own pelvic floor muscles and put yourself on a Kegel and/or reverse Kegel program. All your questions about your muscles "down there" will finally be resolved and answered.

PART THREE:

SURVIVING LABOR AND DELIVERY WITH AN INTACT PERINEUM AND NO INJURIES

"I am determined to be cheerful and happy in whatever situation I may find myself. For I have learned that the greater part of our misery or unhappiness is determined not by our circumstance but by our disposition."

— Martha Washington

Chapter 9

KEGELS THAT WORK: PREVENTING PERINEAL TEARS, INCONTINENCE AND PELVIC PRESSURE DURING PREGNANCY

The pelvic floor muscles (PFMs) are among the primary supportive muscles during pregnancy. They have to perform optimally for your nine-month journey and postpartum recovery to go smoothly— without dysfunction of incontinence, organ prolapse, sexual problems and pelvic instability. The PFMs not only support your baby, which on the average weighs seven to nine pounds, but also support the uterus which is about two pounds of pure muscle. Next add the placenta and the amniotic fluid which weigh about two pounds each. By the end of your pregnancy your PFMs will support approximately an extra eleven to thirteen pounds, in addition to the weight of your internal organs and your pregnancy weight gain.

The PFMs need special attention and care during the nine months of pregnancy to avoid problems in the present and the future. There is conflicting information out there and many pregnant women are left confused and don't know how to train their PFMs. This chapter will provide clarity and a sensible training program. Review the core training chapter also; the PFMs and the abdominal muscles have a synergistic relationship and prefer to be in harmony.

The term Kegel is used to describe a set of exercises, developed by gynecologist Dr. Arnold Kegel, designed to improve the function of the pelvic floor muscles (PFMs). (There are subtle nuances to Kegels that if not taken into account, can actually produce worse results for pregnant women with pelvic pain, low back pain and/or continence issues.) Typically, Kegels are prescribed for women suffering from incontinence or organ prolapse, and are designed to help strengthen and improve PFMs endurance, continence and sexual function by reducing laxity and decreasing weakness. Pregnancy and childbirth are major causes of weakness and disorders of the pelvic floor in women. Women at the highest risk for weakness in the PFMs have had multiple pregnancies, prolonged second-stage labor, episiotomy, forceps delivery, perineal tearing and/or large babies. Many of my pregnant patients complain to me about leaking urine, pressure inside the vagina, sexual problems, and frequent trips to the bathroom. Pregnant patients often tell me: "My doctor does not want me to do Kegels because I will get too tight down there" or "I don't want to overtrain my PFMs because I will have a difficult time getting the baby out." Others have said their doctors don't care whether they do Kegels because there is not much strengthening or conditioning you can do with these muscles while you are pregnant. These perceptions are incorrect. You absolutely need to train PFMs during pregnancy and you must rehabilitate them after the baby comes. The pelvic floor muscles serve a key purpose and special care during pregnancy will prevent further complications in the postpartum period. In this chapter I will give you an intelligent and progressive pelvic floor program. With it you will achieve pregnancy pelvic power and recover more quickly in the postpartum period.

Pelvic Floor Muscle Anatomy and Function

Before we get into the pregnancy pelvic power program you must first understand your body on an anatomical level, a physiological level, and an energy level. Your pelvic floor is a complex set of muscles, nerves, and connective tissues that can accurately be called the cradle or basket of your being. The PFMs are shaped like a basin and they are the size of a small salad bowl. On an energy level, the pelvic floor contains the first chakra, or energy center, and supports the other chakras. If the foundation is experiencing stress and trauma, then naturally all of your energy will be affected. Major nerves that innervate your entire lower extremity pass through the pelvic region, and a complex web of muscles and fascia support your uterus, bladder, vagina, rectum, and other abdominal organs. If the muscles in your pelvic floor are in spasm, weak or are filled with trigger points or scar adhesions, your pain can be both excruciating and debilitating and your weakness compounded.

If your pelvic floor muscles are weak, you can experience sexual dysfunction and a slew of bladder issues including incontinence, urgency and frequency of urination. Many times pregnant women will feel as if they cannot completely empty either their bowels or bladder and they push to get the urine or feces out. Pushing with bowel and bladder is a big no-no as this action strains the PFMs and contributes to spasms, trigger points and more weakness.

To understand this area of your body better, we'll take a look at the various constructs of your pelvic floor muscles, also called the levator ani muscles. This is a lot to cover, so remember to consult the extensive glossary as well as to familiarize yourself with key concepts and terms found in this book. By getting to know your own anatomy and its particular nuances, you will find that you can open the door to your own healing and maintain long-term results. You hold the key to getting on the road to recovery. Now let's look at the PFMs anatomy.

Diagram 9.1: Pelvic Floor Muscles Internal View

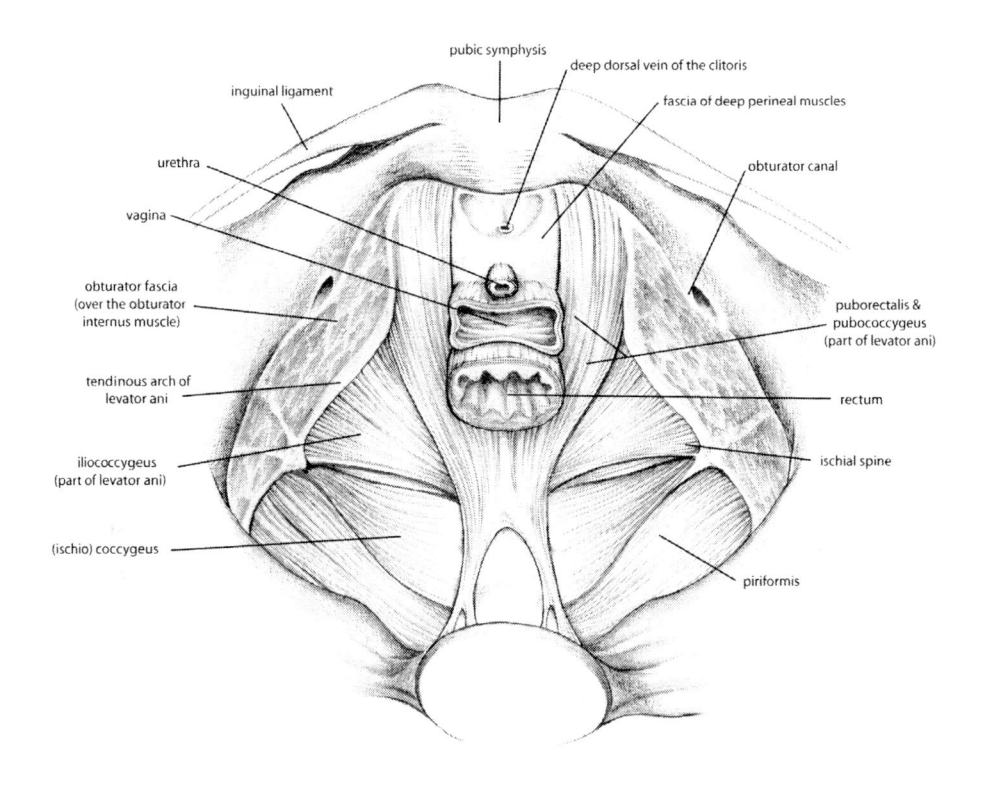

pubic symphysis

deep dorsal vein of the clitoris

inguinal ligament

fascia of deep perineal muscles

urethra

obturator canal

vagina

obturator fascia
(over the obturator
internus muscle)

puborectalis &
pubococcygeus
(part of levator ani)

tendinous arch of
levator ani

rectum

iliococcygeus
(part of levator ani)

ischial spine

(ischio) coccygeus

piriformis

Diagram Description: Top-down view of the pelvic floor. Your body is cut in half at the waist and you are peering down into the third layer of the pelvic floor basket with organs removed. To stretch and work on this layer you would need medical clearance from your OB/GYN or midwife. Many times dysfunctions in this third layer cause a deep ache in the vagina, pain with sexual intercourse and pain in the pelvic hip region. Source: Netter Images.

PFMs Functions

The overall pelvic floor muscle group has four primary functions. First, these muscles are supportive and hold your organs up and in place. Second, they are sphincteric and help prevent urinary and fecal incontinence. Third, they are sexual, enhancing and making orgasms stronger. Fourth, they help stabilize the lumbar, sacral, pelvic and hip regions.

Diagram 9.2: Pelvic Floor Muscles – An Inferior View Highlighting External Genitalia, Perineum, PFM Layer 1, Gluteal Muscles, Levator Ani (PFM Layer 3)

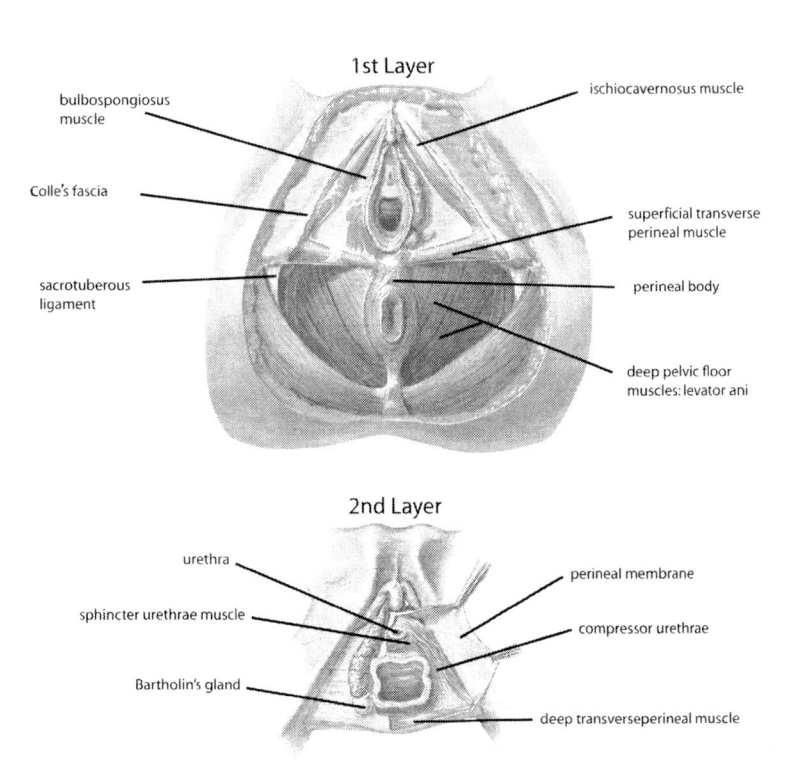

Diagram Description: PFMs first layer appear in the diagram along with some levator ani (third layer PFMs), gluteal muscles. This is the perineal area with the skin removed to reveal the muscles. The first layer is the focal point of stretching during the later part of pregnancy. The first layer is one knuckle deep inside the vagina. This illustration shows the external part of the first PFM layer. Source: Netter Images.

PFMs Innervation

The pelvic floor muscles are highly innervated. PFMs are innervated by the pudendal nerve, perineal nerve, inferior rectal nerve, the sacral spinal and levator ani nerves. These nerves originate in the low back and tailbone region anatomically known as the L4-S4 region.

The muscles of the female pelvic floor can be a source of confusion for many people – even to the trained professional – because they have been given several different names, making it difficult to understand the nomenclature and classification. In this book we will classify the female pelvic muscles into three layers and will describe other structures that must be understood in order to perform pregnancy perineal massages. Please look at Table 9.1 for a description of the main muscles and anatomy of the female pelvic floor. Refer to the accompanying anatomy Diagrams 9.1, 9.2 and 9.3 as you begin to absorb and understand the techniques I have compiled for the stretching of the perineum. Be scientific in your approach to better visualize the musculature of your own body.

PFMs Layer Description and Visualization

The PFMs can be visualized as a tube that has four walls. Think about the walls as an anterior wall, posterior wall and two lateral or side walls. As you move further into the book, keep this visual in mind. The different walls house different muscles, and trigger points in them can reproduce many pelvic, groin or bladder-related symptoms. For instance, if the anterior PFMs are weak and have trigger points and/or muscle spasms and these issues are not resolved, then you can suffer from incontinence, bladder pressure, or urge incontinence. Because the anterior wall of the PFMs houses the uterus and bladder, it is under a lot of stress. In pregnancy we are not allowed to manually stretch this area but you will learn other ways to strengthen and restore function to the PFMs.

Moving a little deeper into the anatomy of the PFMs, we see that the pelvic floor muscles themselves can be divided into three layers, with each layer progressively deeper inside the vagina. Using your index finger as a road map, the first layer corresponds to the first knuckle, the second layer corresponds to the second knuckle and the deeper layer corresponds to the third knuckle. Now let's think about the vaginal opening looking like a clock (see Diagram 9.3). Twelve o'clock is by the pubic bone, six o'clock by the anus, three o'clock to the left side and nine o'clock to the right. Now imagine that each layer is also its own clock, giving you three clocks, one at each level. During pregnancy you will most likely massage and stretch the first layer and not the deeper layers. If you are suffering from a painful PFM condition your MD will have to give a physical therapist a prescription for manual stretching of the deeper layers. (I have performed stretching of the deeper PFMs during pregnancy but only with clearance from an MD.) If you suffer from a PFM condition and you are pregnant I highly recommend that you seek a pelvic floor physical therapist to help you through this transition.

Diagram 9.3: The Clock and Layer Concept

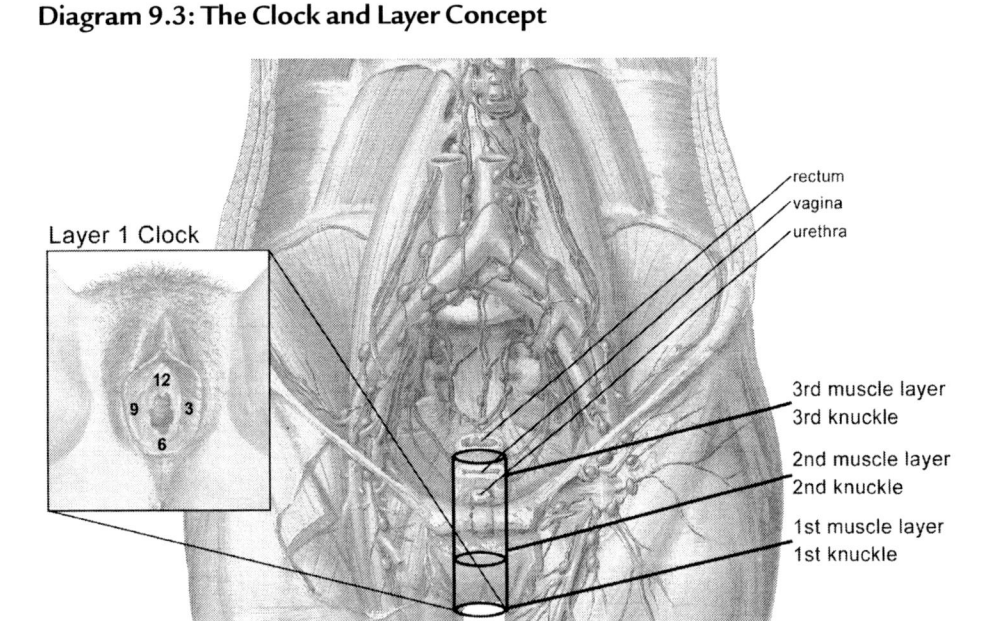

Diagram Description: The PFMs can all be accessed via the vagina. The three pelvic floor muscle layers, each corresponding to a knuckle of the index finger. The inset shows the clock concept of the first layer. In pregnancy most of the stretching if not all occurs in the first layer of the PFMs to allow the baby's head to go through it. Source: Netter Images

Table 9.1: Anatomy of Female Pelvic Floor Muscle Layers

LAYER NAME	MAIN MUSCLES	PFM FUNCTION
• Layer 1 • Located first knuckle of the index finger • Also called urogenital triangle	• Bulbospongiosus • Ischiocavernosus • Superficial transverse perineal muscle • External anal sphincter (EAS) • External genitalia: includes urethra, lower vagina, vulva, mons pubis, labia majora, labia minora, clitoris, vestibular bulb, Bartholin's glands	Sphincteric Sexual
• Layer 2 • Located second knuckle of the index finger • Also called urogenital diaphragm	• Sphincter urethrae • Deep transverse perineal muscle • Compressor urethrae muscle • Internal anal sphincter (IAS)	Sphincteric
• Layer 3 • Located third knuckle of the index finger • Also called pelvic diaphragm	• Levator ani: commonly broken down into pubococcygeus, puborectalis, iliococcygeus • Obturator internus • Coccygeus	Sexual, supportive, sphincteric and stabilization functions

Pregnancy and PFMs: What Is Normal?

When I evaluate a pregnant woman's PFMs, I frequently find that in addition to muscle weakness, the PFMs usually have excessive tone, increased shortness, extreme tension, spasms and multiple trigger points in them, rather than laxity. This can contribute to sexual pain. Why are the PFMs so tight during pregnancy? I believe there are several reasons: pelvic malalignment issues; postural abnormalities; chronic holding of the PFMs; pelvic pressure and scarring from a prior pregnancy. (For more theories see Table 9.2.) I also often find a lack of flexibility in the muscles that attach to the pelvis such as the inner thighs, hip flexors and glutes. The PFMs are normally in a relaxed state, and they respond to what is happening in your body and mind. They can respond to thoughts, past experiences, trauma, visceral problems, abnormal breathing patterns and pain. They also respond to the weight of the baby and the alignment of your pelvis. Usually, their response to any of the above is to become tense and to develop trigger points either in the PFMs or in muscles that are intimately connected to the PFMs such as hips and low back. This tension can go on for the entire pregnancy resulting in shortened muscle fibers filled with spasms, trigger points, and myofascial restrictions. PFMs that are in this state during pregnancy will have a difficult time stretching during labor and delivery.

Once the muscle fibers get shorter and more tense, they are typically weaker. The weakness is not due to looseness, as in the typical incontinence or prolapse patient. Instead, the weakness is caused by muscles which are too tight or hypertonic. The shortened muscle has the ability to contract, but the contractions are weak because there is a decrease in the fiber's ability to move. This type of weakness leads to urinary leaking and urge and frequency of urination, which are typical complaints I hear from my pregnant patients with pelvic, low back and hip pain. To effectively treat these hypertonic muscle fibers, they first need to be lengthened and relaxed before they can be strengthened and toned. So the prescription of regular Kegels—where you are told simply to draw up your muscles to prevent leaking or pain—does not work. In fact it can lead to more pain and weakness as muscle fibers become even shorter, and more hypertonic. As a result, the PFMs often develop more trigger points in them.

Now in pregnancy stretching of these tight muscles cannot be done manually which is the ideal therapy. In order to accomplish the stretching that a tight PFM needs and to get the PFMs more flexible for labor and delivery, I recommend that my pregnant patients do a daily routine of reverse Kegel exercises. First work on getting the muscles more flexible via the reverse Kegel program and then embark on a Kegel contract/relax strengthening program. Having first lengthened the muscles, the fibers can then be better strengthened, leading to reduced pain, improved continence, and enhanced sexual response. The new and improved PFMs can also easily stretch during childbirth preventing the need for an episiotomy and decreasing the risk of perineal tears.

The Kegel programs I have created are to be performed on several levels, beginning with the reverse Kegels to relax and lengthen PFMs, followed by strengthening with the contract/relax, and the quick-flicks Kegels once you have mastered the reverse series. This order is necessary because the release is needed before you can strengthen both slow twitch and fast twitch fibers of the PFMs. Additionally you will have to let go and relax the PFMs during the pushing phase of labor. When it comes to pushing the baby out it is best to keep the muscles relaxed and to avoid tensing them when the pain of the contractions sets in. By better understanding the different types of Kegels, you can achieve success and gain improved control over your PFMS. Before we go into the nuances of pelvic floor training I want to cover several important techniques that can be grouped under perineal massage. These hands-on and internal vaginal massages will help keep your PFMs flexible so they can stretch during labor and delivery with minimal tearing. I will cover three different types of techniques and you can do all three or pick and choose the ones that you feel work the best for you during your pregnancy. It is important to note that the perineal stretching has to be approved by your OB/GYN or midwife and this type of stretching should not start before thirty-four weeks of pregnancy.

Table 9.2: Possible Causes of Pelvic Pain and PFM Tightness and Spasms during Pregnancy

1. Pelvic malalignment
2. Postural abnormalities
3. Chronic holding of the PFMs
4. Pelvic pressure
5. Prolapsed organ: bladder, uterus or rectum
6. Incontinence during this pregnancy or previous pregnancy
7. Perineal tears from previous pregnancy
8. Previous Cesarean birth
9. Previous coccyx injury during birth or new coccyx injury or falling on coccyx (tailbone)
10. Gait deviations during pregnancy
11. Symphysis pubic syndrome (pubic bone pain)
12. Scar tissue from previous pelvic or abdominal surgery
13. Chronic pelvic and sexual pain
14. Herniated disc of the lumbar spine
15. Leg length discrepancy
16. Diastasis recti separation of the abdominal muscles
17. Sacroiliac dysfunction and pain
18. Sciatica
19. Piriformis syndrome and gluteal pain and/or trigger points or spasms in the gluteal muscles
20. Low back pain
21. Emotional pain, stress and fear
22. Chronic yeast infections
23. Urinary tract infections
24. Injury to nerves that innervate the vulva during a previous pregnancy such as a pudendal nerve injury
25. Pelvic floor muscle spasms or trigger points
26. Straining or pushing with defecation and urination
27. Hematoma during previous pregnancy
28. Fibroids

Internal PFM Massaging and Stretching Techniques for Labor Preparation

Perineal massage, PFMs clock stretching and PFMs strumming are internal perineal techniques that stretch, massage and help improve PFM flexibility. Although perineal massage is widely known many pregnant women are confused about how to do this massage. This upcoming section will bring clarity to these techniques. When my patients incorporate these internal massage techniques into their programs they have amazing results. PFM massage and stretching is suggested for healthy and well nourished pregnant women who wish to decrease perineal tearing. Perineal massage has also been shown to reduce the need for an episiotomy. Perineal massage is amazing for women who also suffer from PFMs spasms or sexual pain. You will need medical clearance from your MD or midwife to begin perineal massage. Perineal massage is usually started at week thirty-four and done daily if possible for up to fifteen minutes. You can also perform the perineal massage one to two times a week and still get great results.

These techniques are not that easy to perform on yourself so seek help from your partner. Many pregnant patients come to us specifically because they have difficulty performing the massages on their own. I find that many pregnant women need to try different body positions such as side-lying or sitting back to make the PFMs stretching techniques comfortable. Additionally, you may have to use your right hand to stretch the left side of the PFMs and left hand to stretch the right side of the PFMs. The most important thing is to try and to seek help from a physical therapist if you are having difficulty.

Traditional Perineal Thumb Massage

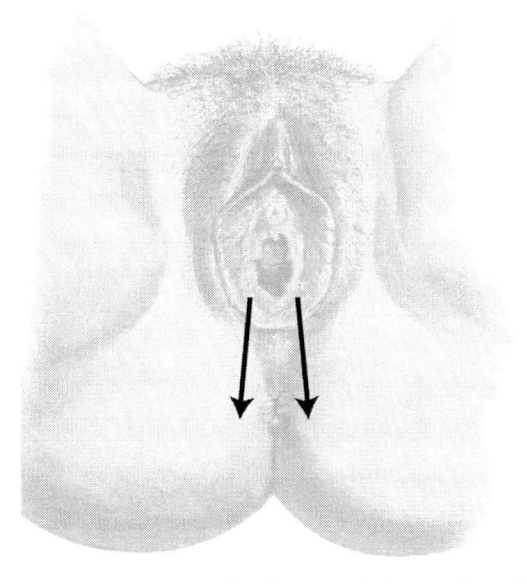

Diagram Description: The arrows represent the direction of the stretching. The stretching pressure is downward toward the rectum. Do this at the first layer only.

GETTING STARTED:

This massage method works great as a preparation for labor and delivery. Pregnant women can start this massage on the thirty-fourth week of pregnancy for three to five minutes.

WHAT TO DO:

1. Lubricate your thumbs, insert them into the vagina up to the first knuckle, and press straight downward toward the rectum for three to five minutes.

2. After three to five minutes, press down to the right for several seconds and then to the left for several seconds.

3. Another technique is to do half-moon strokes with your thumbs. Place your right thumb up to the first knuckle in the inside of your left pelvic floor muscles. Perform half-moon strokes from the top to bottom for about one minute, then change sides and perform the half-moon strokes on the other side. See upcoming pages for details on half-moon massage.

Pelvic Floor Muscle Clock Stretching: First PFM Layer Only

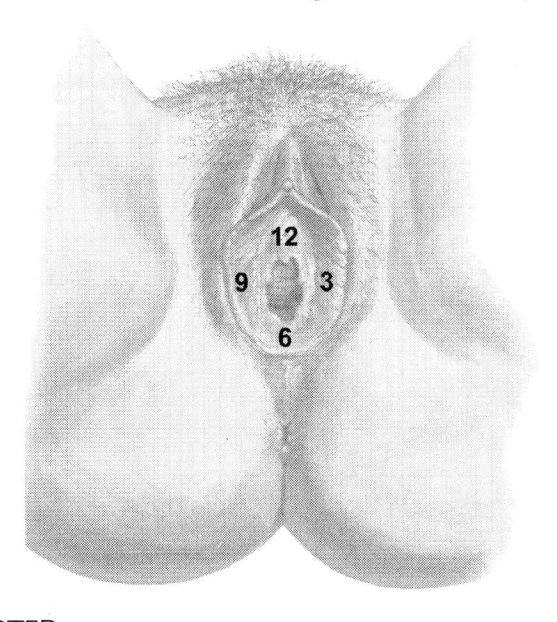

GETTING STARTED:

The pelvic floor muscle clock stretching technique works great for pregnant women who have pain with initial penetration, painful scars, or spasms in their muscles. This PFM clock stretch is more specific and stretches the first layer of the PFMs in a more well-rounded way. With traditional perineal massage the PFMs are stretched at the 6 o'clock spot but with the clock stretch we are focusing on the lower half of the PFMs. For this method, imagine again that your vaginal opening is a clock. To review, 12 o'clock is by the clitoris, 6 o'clock is by the rectum, 3 o'clock is to the left and 9 o'clock is to the right. Using your finger, start stretching your vagina with the clock as visualization. Remember that the PFMs are divided into three layers, each layer corresponding to the knuckles of the finger and progressively deeper inside the vagina. The first PFM layer is knuckle one, the second PFM layer is knuckle two, and the third PFM layer is knuckle three. For this technique you are focusing on PFM layer one ONLY. If you wish to stretch further you must absolutely discuss this with your OB/GYN or midwife.

WHAT TO DO:

1. Focus your stretching from 3 to 9 o'clock positions avoiding 12 o'clock where the bladder is located.

2. Insert your finger into the vagina up to the first knuckle only and stretch PFM layer one only.

3. Press around the clock for thirty to sixty seconds or until you feel a release in the vaginal muscles. You can go around the clock two to three times or you can stay on the same spot for one to three repetitions of thirty to sixty seconds.

4. Only use lubricants that are organic, alcohol free, and parabin free.

Internal Pelvic Floor Muscle Half–Moon Strumming Massage: First PFM Layer Only

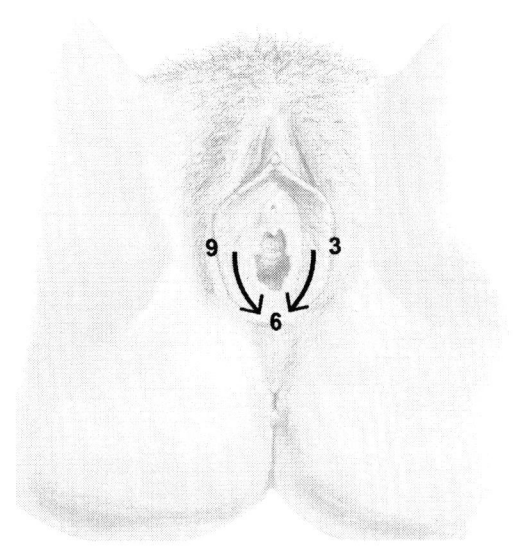

GETTING STARTED:

Strumming is another great way to help prepare the PFMs for labor and delivery. Strumming improves the flexibility of the PFMs so they can maximally stretch during childbirth. This method only involves the first layer of the PFMs.

If you desire to stretch deeper within the PFMs you must get medical clearance from your OB/GYN or midwife.

WHAT TO DO:

1. Strumming massage is a type of massage that is performed in the direction of the pelvic floor muscle fiber. So this massage is from superior to inferior, or top to bottom.

2. Insert your finger (index or thumb) into the vagina up to the first knuckle. First strum the right half of the PFM and then strum the left half, massaging only the first layer of the PFMs.

3. Massage the left half from the 3 to 6 o'clock position for up to one minute. Rest. Switch hands; massage the right half from the 9 to 6 o'clock position for up to one minute.

4. Try different body positions such as side-lying or sitting back to make these techniques comfortable.

Relaxing the PFMs with the Reverse Kegel Relaxation Series

Your ability to have conscious release of the pelvic floor muscles is a critical part of your pregnancy pelvic power. Why? Because the baby will come out more easily if you are able to release the tension in the PFMs while you are in labor. Additionally, a more flexible PFM will stretch more easily reducing the risk for perineal tearing and the need for an episiotomy. The foundation of conscious and mindful release is the mastering of the reverse Kegel relaxation exercises. You must learn to focus on and relax these muscles before they can attain optimal strength. Relaxation and lengthening of the PFMs with reverse Kegels is also called downtraining.

The reverse Kegel downtraining series contains several techniques that will help you gain awareness and control over your pelvic floor. In the beginning, work hard to master the release techniques, and then you can incorporate this focus while practicing the labor positions highlighted in Chapter 10. Practice your relaxation exercises as a way to prep the PFMs for labor and delivery. Do not go through an eight-hour workday without releasing the tension in your muscles especially if you suffer from a PFM condition, PFMs spasms or sexual pain. The following exercises are easy to perform and can be done anywhere or anytime. At first the PFM relaxation exercises will be extremely difficult to visualize and perform. Many of you have had tension and pain in these muscles for a very long time. You will find that the more you practice these exercises, the easier they will become to do and to implement. The reverse Kegel series contains the most effective methods that have brought success to my patients. This series is designed to help you release the tension and then strengthen the PFMs; they are to be used on a daily basis and especially during painful low back, hip and pelvic flare-ups when they could be used every hour until the pain subsides. Since the PFMs are connected to the hip, low back and pelvic areas via fascia you can use the reverse Kegel to release pain from these areas.

The Importance of Breath

To perform the reverse Kegel series more effectively, you must couple the reverse Kegel exercises with proper breathing. When I teach my patients the basics of downtraining, I emphasize diaphragmatic breathing to ensure their success. Diaphragmatic breathing can be defined as a type of breathing that involves the abdominal muscles instead of the ribs, shoulders, and neck muscles. To practice diaphragmatic breathing, place your hand over your belly button. Imagine you are breathing air into your baby. On the inhale, let your belly gently rise out into your hands, and on the exhale, let the belly flatten. Don't let the breath raise your shoulders, and don't bring your belly in on the inhale and out on the exhale, as this is not diaphragmatic breathing. You can also imagine that you are breathing into the PFMs and that they are expanding and lengthening.

The best way to consciously release tension from the PFMs is to try to release the muscles while you inhale. Do not be discouraged if you find this difficult at first. When you inhale properly, your diaphragm actually lowers to make room for the air, so it is natural to also lower and relax the pelvic floor muscles. When you exhale, your diaphragm rises to push the air out, and you can then raise or contract your PFMs. Time your inhalation and exhalation so that they occur simultaneously with a reverse Kegel. For example, inhale for five seconds, and then exhale for five seconds. I usually recommend to my patients that they inhale for a count of five while consciously dropping and relaxing their PFMs downward. This release and letting go is the hardest exercise to do because many women are not even aware of the tension with which they are holding their PFMs. Once the tension is released, the muscle fibers begin to lengthen. Soon you will be able to release on demand, at which point you can begin a regular Kegel strengthening and toning program.

If you have difficulty coordinating the in-breath with the release, don't let that stop you. It's perfectly all right to do a reverse Kegel with exhalation at first until you master the correct techniques. The most important thing is to increase your awareness and focus and to practice reverse Kegels on a daily basis, even an hourly basis, if needed. Also be very careful not to push on your PFMs while you are performing your reverse Kegels. Too many women push on these muscles instead of releasing and letting them go. You may have to insert your finger in your vagina to get the PFMs to communicate with your mind. This is a mind/body connection. Many times women think they are releasing the PFMs but instead they are pushing and/or contracting them as they do the reverse Kegel. Remember that reverse Kegels are critical for labor prep so practice them often and especially in your last trimester.

Test Your Progress

Table 9.3: The Renew Physical Therapy Reverse Kegel Self-Grading System

PROGRESS LEVEL	CURRENT PELVIC FLOOR MUSCLE STATUS	ACTION TO BE TAKEN
Level 1	Not able to release PFM	Continue with PFM Release Exercises. Perform the Release exercise after childbirth if there is a significant perineal tear, episiotomy or pain with Kegel exercise.
Level 2	Able to release PFM a little	Continue with PFM Release Exercises
Level 3	Able to release PFM but not all the way and with some pain	Continue with PFM Release Exercises
Level 4	Able to release PFM completely without pain or with some pain	Start Kegel strengthening contract/relax program but focus on the relaxation part by increasing the ratio of the relaxation part. For example, contract for three seconds; relax for nine seconds.
Level 5	No pain, no urinary incontinence and able to perform a reverse Kegel.	Start Kegel strengthening contract/relax program. Be careful with your ratio and increase if needed. For instance 1:2 or 1:3 ratio which corresponds to the contract/relax ratio.

You should continue practicing your reverse Kegel program until you feel you are gaining control over your PFMs. The only way to tell if you have complete relaxation is to test your PFM by inserting a finger into your vagina and grading the release. I have created a five-level grading system and included it in Table 9.3 so you can evaluate your progress. This is the most accurate way to test because I find many of my patients think they are releasing when in reality they are contracting the muscles and creating more pain and PFM dysfunction. When you test yourself, grade yourself on a scale of one to five. A grade of four or five should be achieved before starting your Kegel strengthening contract/relax program. This is called uptraining.

What will you feel with your finger during your reverse Kegel self-grade test? You should feel the tension or grip around your finger releasing, and the finger should gently slip outward. You can also use a mirror to better visualize the reverse Kegel. When using a mirror, you should see the anal muscles open up and you should also see the perineal body, or area between the vagina and the rectum, drop down toward the mirror. If you see this area lifting up, you are doing the reverse Kegel series incorrectly and instead are contracting your PFMs. Also look at your perineum with the mirror. The perineal body should move outward gently but should not appear to push out, which is a sign of bearing down and straining the PFMs. Again, if you see the anus contract and your perineal body pulls in, you are performing the reverse Kegel incorrectly and are instead performing a Kegel.

Table 9.4: Trade Secrets for the Reverse Kegel Downtraining

TECHNIQUE
1. Rose Petal Flower Release
2. Direct Vaginal Release
3. Child's Pose Release
4. Prayer Squat Release
5. Side-Lying Sit Bones Apart Release
6. Dropping the Panties
7. Body Check Release

Rose Petal Flower Release

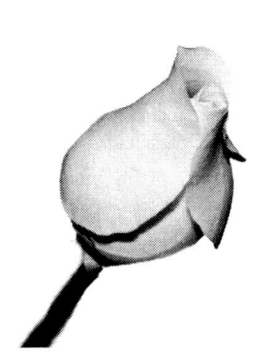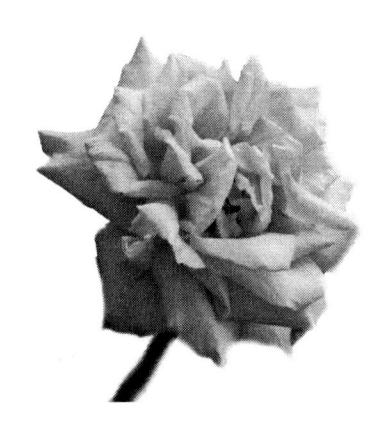

WHAT TO DO:

As you breathe in for five to seven seconds, send your inhalation breath to your vaginal muscles visualizing and imagining them as a large tight rose that is beginning to blossom in the springtime. Imagine the rose opening up petal by petal. You should feel your perineum/PFM relax. Try this exercise for five breaths. Repeat several times throughout the day or as needed to calm down a painful flare-up and prepare the PFMs for childbirth.

Direct Vaginal Release

WHAT TO DO:

1. Place your clean, gloved finger into your vagina. Try to find a position that is comfortable for you to maintain your finger in your vagina for at least five minutes. You can try different positions such as standing, sitting or lying on your side; find the one that works best for you. At times you may be able to do a PFM release in one position but not another. It is important to try all positions to enhance PFM relaxation in any position.

2. As you breathe in, send your in-breath into your perineum/PFM and imagine that the walls of your vagina are expanding away from the finger. The release feels like you are going to pass gas or urinate.

3. If your finger is being pushed out as you do your direct release, then you are forcing the release and putting undue stress and strain on your pelvic muscles. Pushing to get the release is not the same as gently allowing it to happen with your in-breath. Always couple the PFMs relaxation visualization with the inhalation breath.

Child's Pose Release

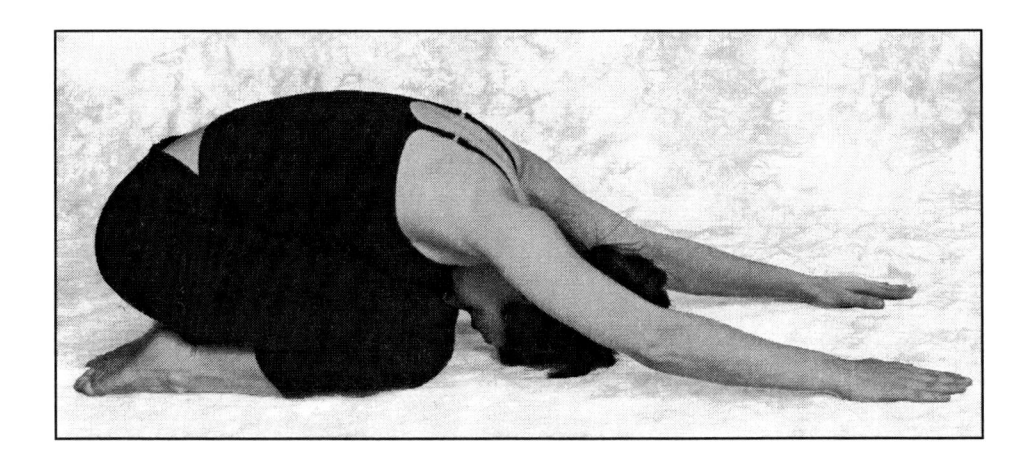

WHAT TO DO:

1. Get on your hands and knees and then bring your body into child's pose as in the above photo. Bring one hand onto each sit bone (not shown) and keep contact with the bones as you perform your PFM relaxation child's pose release (or keep your arms outstretched as in the photo).

2. If your sit bones do not touch your heels, place a pillow under your gluteal muscles and feet. Spread your legs to accommodate the baby. Now imagine as you breathe in for a count of five seconds that your sit bones are moving away from each other. Simultaneously feel your pelvic muscles release and relax. Make sure your in-breath lasts as long as the reverse Kegel (at least five seconds), and then perform for five more breaths.

Prayer Squat Release

WHAT TO DO:

1. Get into the prayer squat position as in the photo. For some women it might be best to hold on to a sturdy object when performing this exercise to facilitate the pelvic floor muscle release and to reduce any undue stress this exercise can put on the thighs, back and calf muscles.

Diagram Description: This is a great position for birth because the pelvic floor muscles are in a naturally relaxed state.

2. If your heels do not touch the floor, place a pillow under your heels to make this exercise more comfortable and less stressful.

3. Send your in-breath into your pelvic floor muscles for a count of five seconds.

4. You can remain in this position for ten releases or you can get up and down within each repetition.

5. Aim to be in this position for five minutes a day especially at the end of your pregnancy.

6. While performing the exercises, focus on inhalation breathing, making sure not to hold your breath.

7. Avoid this position if you have a pudendal nerve condition and pain in this position.

Side-Lying Sit Bones Apart Release

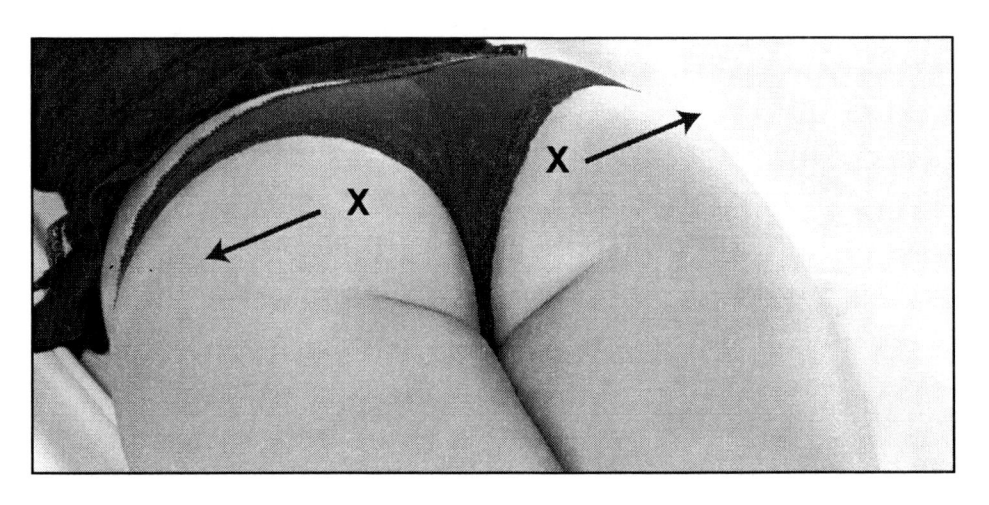

The X's represent the location of the sit bones. This exercise can be done in any position, but is described below in a side-lying position because many pregnant women cannot exercise on their tummies after the first trimester.

WHAT TO DO:

1. Lie down on your left side and place your right hand on your right sit bone.

2. As you breathe in, very gently pull the right sit bone away from the left. Feel and imagine your pelvic floor muscles dropping outward, relaxing and releasing.

3. Hold this release for five seconds and repeat for five breaths. Now try it with the right hand on the right sit bone.

4. Which side gives you the better pelvic floor muscle release?

Dropping the Panties

WHAT TO DO:

1. Sit with good posture with your weight evenly distributed on your sit bones.

2. Practice diaphragmatic breathing for several minutes to center yourself.

3. Breathe in for a count of five and imagine that your underwear and PFM area and vaginal area are dropping into the chair.

4. Make sure to direct your in-breath to your PFM.

5. Repeat this for five repetitions.

Body Check Release

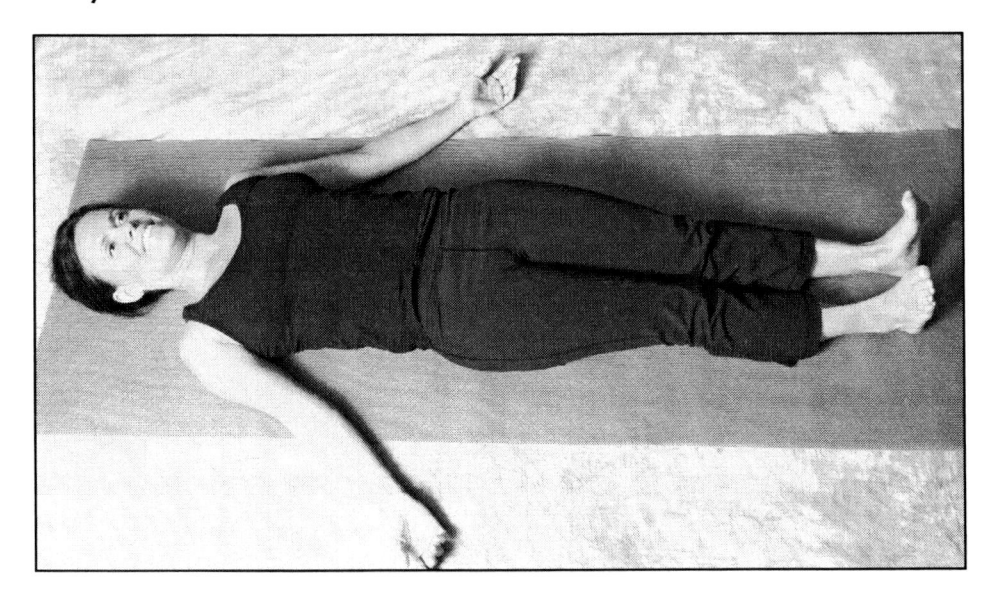

The body check is about focused attention and awareness. The PFMs are smart and respond to what is going on in your life. During flare-ups, stressful and trying times, these muscles increase their muscular tension. Tune in and learn to listen to your PFMs because they are sending you a subtle message and are asking for help. Help them by tuning in to them on an hourly basis. Through this very-focused awareness you will learn when to release these muscles during your day.

WHAT TO DO:

1. Position yourself in any comfortable position. Start with one to two minutes of diaphragmatic breathing to center yourself.

2. Tune in to your PFMs and ask yourself, "Where are my muscles in space? What state are they in?"

3. Practice releasing and relaxing the muscles with the inhalation breath.

4. This technique should be utilized during stressful times such as when you are arguing with someone, and also during periods of painful flare-ups.

Traditional Kegel Contract/Relax Series for Pregnancy Pelvic Power

Congratulations! If you are reading this section and getting ready to move into the contract/relax series, then you are doing really well with the downtraining. Take a conscious moment to congratulate yourself for getting this far. For women in this phase of their pelvic pain recovery, or for women suffering from urinary/urge incontinence, pelvic pressure or organ prolapse I like to begin with a contract/relax program. But I always teach them how to release their PFMs first before doing a contract/relax uptraining program. Please note that contract/relax is the same thing as Kegel/reverse Kegel. This program works really well in establishing and restoring pregnancy pelvic power. This power translates into improved sexual function, less leaking or none at all, better support for your baby and reduced overall pelvic, hip and low back pain.

Contract/Relax Series or Kegel/Reverse Kegel

The contract/relax series is recommended for all women. It creates balance, restores PFMs coordination and strengthens the PFMs and simultaneously lessens bladder issues and improves other symptoms such as pelvic pressure.

This series is great for women who have mastered the reverse Kegel exercise. If you are suffering from pelvic pain and start this series before you are ready, you risk a flare-up and exacerbation of your pain by creating more tension and pain in your PFMs.

Start by examining your PFMs. Perform an internal vaginal examination with your index finger, similar to the self-grading exam for the reverse Kegels. During this self-exam you need to find out how many seconds you can hold a PFM contraction(Kegel) and conversely how many seconds it takes you to release your PFMs completely (reverse Kegel). These two numbers will determine a ratio that you will use as a starting point of your contract/relax program.

How to Determine Your Contract/Relax Program Ratio

1. Please have a mirror and lubrication on hand for your exam.

2. Start off by first looking externally at your perineum area and performing a contract Kegel.

3. For correct Kegel execution look for the following motions: your anus should "wink"; the perineal body, the area between your vagina and anus, should move up and in; and your clitoris should move downward in a nod movement.

4. After looking at your Kegel contraction, look at your reverse Kegel. You should see your perineal body move outward toward the mirror and your anus gently open up or expand.

5. Once you are performing the Kegel and the reverse Kegel correctly, place a well-lubricated index finger into your vagina and contract your PFM around your finger. Count to see how many seconds you can hold the contraction: "*one Mississippi, two Mississippi, three Mississippi,*" etc. Stop counting once you feel the contraction of the Kegel get weaker or release. This is the number of seconds to use for the contract.

6. Start releasing your muscles and see how many counts of Mississippi it takes you to release your PFM completely. From these two numbers, determine your contract/relax ratio. For example, you might start out with a five-second Kegel contraction and a ten-second release so your ratio would be 1:2. Or your ratio could be much bigger such as 1:3.

7. Always err on the side of safety by giving yourself more time to release.

What to Look for in a Correctly Executed Kegel

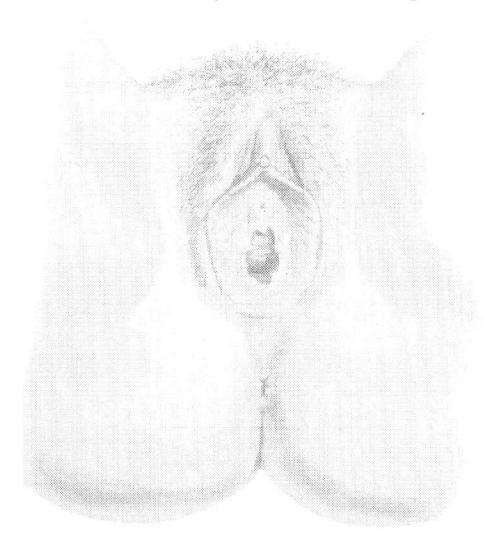

Diagram Description: A proper Kegel has three motions associated with it. The clitoris should nod and move downward. The anus should close or wink and the perineal body (the area between the vaginal opening and anus) should move up and inward. Use a mirror to see if you are performing your Kegels correctly.

Trade Secret: Kegel Strengthening Program—Pregnancy Pelvic Power Program

Body Position Is Everything

Start your Kegel program in a flat-on-your-back position. This is the easiest position for the contract/relax program. After the first trimester, this position is no longer recommended. The semi-reclined seated position requires that you place a couple of pillows behind your back so you are slightly leaning backward. Next comes the upright seated position and then the standing position. Your body will tell you when to move to the next difficult level. You should be able to do three sets of slow and quick Kegels in one position before advancing to the next level.

For pregnant women who have incontinence and/or pelvic pressure you can incorporate the level five Kegel which trains and strengthens the anterior wall of the PFMs. To strengthen the anterior wall sit upright in good posture and slightly arch your back. This arching of the back emphasizes the anterior wall of the PFMs and helps to strengthen the bladder and the supporting function of the PFMs.

Level Five Kegel: Anterior Wall Kegels on Physio-Ball

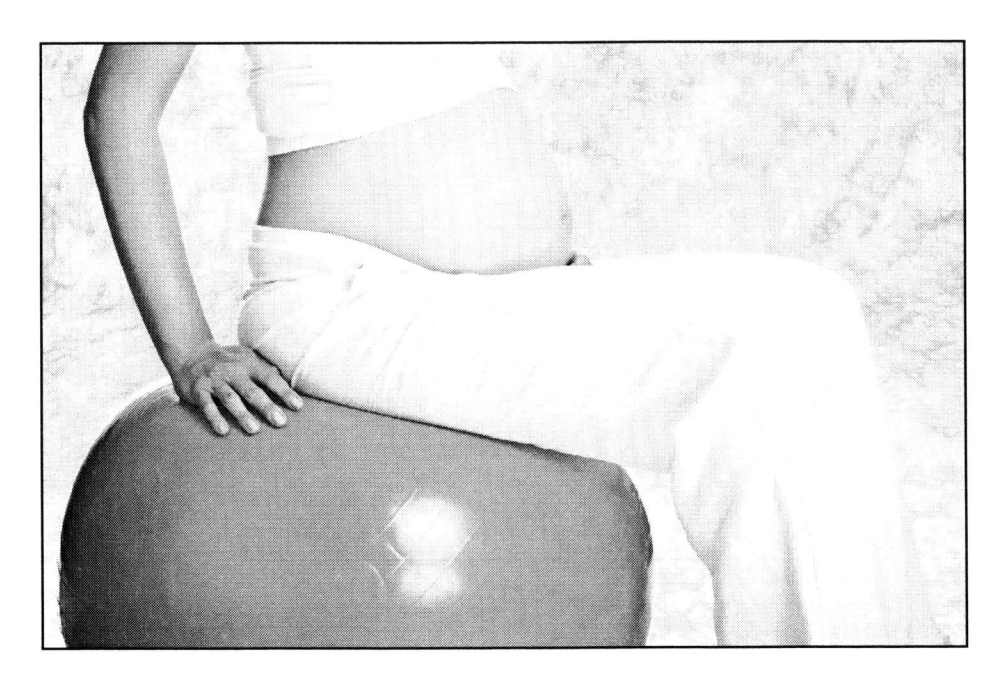

Diagram Description: I love doing Kegels on the physio-ball because you get good feedback from your pelvis. For anterior wall Kegels arch your back slightly so your whole perineum including the clitoris has contact with the ball. You can also do the anterior wall Kegels sitting down in a regular chair.

Trade Secret: Contract/Relax Program: Level of Difficulty and Body Positioning

Level One: Flat on your back—Not recommended after first trimester
Level Two: Semi-reclined: Leaning back on pillows position
Level Three: Seated upright position
Level Four: Standing position
Level Five: Anterior Wall Kegel for incontinence and pelvic pressure

Contract/Relax Pregnancy Pelvic Power Program

The pelvic floor muscles consist of slow and fast twitch muscle fibers. To effectively train the PFMs you can do a combo of slow and quick-flick Kegels.

1. Now that you have determined your ratio, start your strengthening program conservatively by performing ten repetitions of contract/relax three times daily, incorporating your ratio as your guide.

2. Pay close attention to make sure your pelvic pain does not increase with your current strengthening program. If you start to experience more pain, stop the contract/relax exercises immediately and go back to the relaxation exercises.

3. After one to two weeks, if you are doing well with your contract/relax program, start doing your program four to five times daily.

4. After two weeks, retest to see if your PFM contract endurance has improved. If it is longer, then add more seconds to your contraction Kegel. For example, after two weeks of diligently doing your strengthening exercises, you can now hold your slow Kegels for seven seconds. Then start doing your program with seven seconds contract and fourteen seconds release, using the same 1:2 ratio as a guide. You may find your ratio changes over time, and if so, this is acceptable.

Quick-Flick Kegels

In conjunction with your contract/relax Kegel, add the quick-flick Kegel exercises as well. These consist of one to two second contractions followed by one to two second releases, repeated ten to twenty times. These quick Kegels should be performed after resting for one minute after the slow Kegels. This type of Kegel can also be used to suppress the urge to urinate and can help you to regain your pregnancy pelvic power so you don't leak.

For strengthening programs, the goal that I usually set for my pregnant patients is a ten-second slow Kegel contraction with a ten to twenty second release, performed three to five times daily. After one set of the slow Kegels, I recommend waiting one minute and then doing ten to twenty quick Kegels. By performing both types of Kegel strengthening exercises, you will hit the slow twitch and fast twitch muscle fibers of the pelvic floor.

Correct Kegel downtraining followed by Kegel strengthening uptraining is part of the foundation of your pregnancy journey. Master your Kegel program in conjunction with the self-perineal massage. Do not quit if you find yourself feeling frustrated with your breathing and releasing on the inhale. Be content to make small improvements if needed, in the beginning. You will achieve breakthroughs as long as you continue to persevere. If you have difficulty following this program, seek the help of a trained pelvic floor specialist. These specialists can also use external biofeedback technology that will help you to connect to these hard-to-visualize PFMs.

In Chapter 10 we reveal trade secrets that will help you have a safe, successful, and fulfilling labor. You will learn how to choose a birth position that works for your "body type." We will also teach you effective comfort measures and TENS therapy for natural birth pain relief. This information will help you to have an empowered birth experience.

CHAPTER TEN

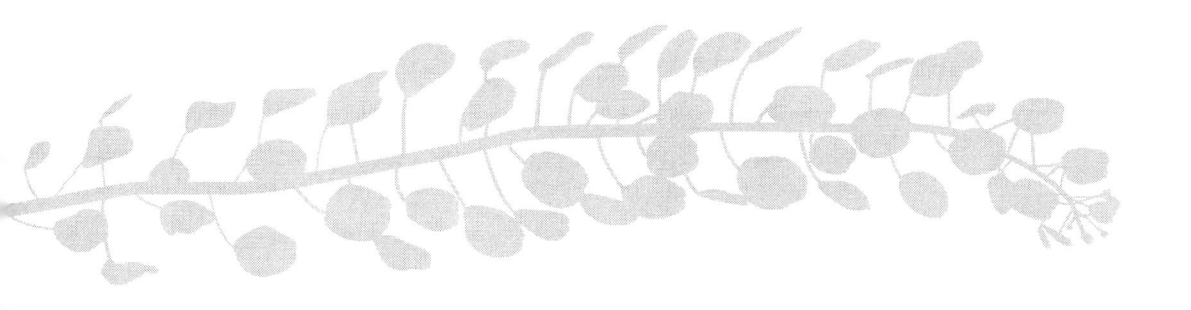

"A mother is she who can take the place of all others, but whose place no one can take."

— *Unknown*

Chapter 10

AVOIDING CHILDBIRTH OBSTETRICAL TRAUMA, RELIEVING PAIN NATURALLY AND LABOR POSITIONS THAT WORK

At Renew Physical Therapy we deal with trauma and injury during labor and delivery on a day-to-day basis. We see women during the postpartum period struggling to take care of their children because the pain that they are experiencing is great and they find it difficult to do their everyday activities without pain. The types of pain that they describe may or may not have been present during the pregnancy, but the labor process has either brought them to the surface or has created a new injury. We treat women suffering from postpartum perineal tears, severe back pain, abdominal separation and herniation, displaced bones, organ prolapses and many other conditions. (Please refer to Chapter 11 so that you can be aware of the things that can happen and what you can do once an injury has occurred.)

We frequently hear from postpartum women: "If only I had known that this could happen..." or " I wasn't prepared for what would happen" or "I didn't know I could choose a birth position that would complement my orthopedic condition and keep my body safe." We find many women suffering from post-traumatic stress disorder as a result of their births and many more suffering from physical pain that could have been prevented or at the very least minimized. In this chapter you will find information on how to protect yourself and how to minimize your exposure to injury during the birthing journey. We have included a very important chart that shows you how to modify labor positions for your orthopedic, spinal and pelvic conditions. This information is based on hard science as well as our clinical experience and uses physical therapy biomechanics principles of injury prevention. The recommended labor positions in Table 10.2 correspond to different orthopedic conditions such as sacroiliac joint pain and lumbar spine herniated disc. Additionally we review several other labor positions that, when used properly for your body type and medical condition, will get you out of labor in one piece and free of injury. Make sure to read the table and show it to your caregivers so we can spread the word and educate as many people as possible. Table 10.2 represents trade secrets we want to share with the world.

Today there is a strong movement toward natural childbirth and women are looking for ways to deal with their labor pain that do not involve drugs. We have included a section on comfort measures for labor that can help you deal better with labor pains. For pain relief we have included detailed information on how to use transcutaneous electrical nerve stimulation (TENS), a natural solution for pain control during labor and delivery. TENS is easy to use and manage during your birth and we recommend adding this to your labor toolbox. We have also included a sample birth plan in this chapter. We recommend that every woman have a birth plan and that you discuss your plan with your birth team. It serves as a blueprint to follow. Read this chapter carefully and show it to your labor partner and medical team. Make sure to keep an open mind: labor is unpredictable and many things happen that are beyond our control. We find many women have a hard time with the emotional journey of recovering as a new mom. The key thing is to move forward, get help and to forgive and to accept your labor as the one you were meant to have. Now let's get started.

In Their Own Words—A Birth Story

"After laboring for fifteen hours at home with my husband and doula, I arrived at the hospital and was told to lie on my back and say goodbye to my support team. Having labored in a semi-squatting position thus far, obviously depending on my doula and husband, I was very angry at these directives. It was enough to make me ask for an epidural, which I received an hour and a half later.

When it was time to push an hour after that, I did as instructed, but it was difficult to know if I was doing it right since I couldn't feel my lower half. After three pushes, my daughter's heart rate was dropping, so the doctor recommended using the vacuum to get her out quickly. I agreed. She was born minutes later and was perfectly healthy. My husband and I instantly fell in love with her.

"I had little physical recovery afterward. I felt bloated, clumsy and a little sore in my vaginal area as I had torn a bit, but these things improved every day until I didn't notice them about two weeks later. What was getting worse was the sharp and throbbing pain in my tailbone. With all the nursing I was doing, I was sitting a lot more than I had in the past. Maybe that was the reason? It didn't really hurt while sitting, but when I would stand up, I'd get a very sharp pain and then throbbing for a while after. It also hurt to squat and to go to the bathroom. By the end of the day, I'd be sore but would find relief when sleeping.

"My tailbone pain was my only complaint when I went for my six-week follow-up appointment with my doctor. He didn't offer a cause, but said that it would probably go away with time. When I went to see him two months later with the same problem, he referred me to an orthopedic surgeon, who sent me for an MRI. The pictures showed that nothing was wrong — no fracture, no tumor, no swelling. That doctor sent me to his mentor, who examined me and the MRI and came to the same conclusion: nothing was wrong. He suggested I see a colorectal specialist to rule out any soft tissue problems. I did so and again was told nothing was wrong. All of these doctors suggested I take over-the-counter pain relievers daily until the pain subsided. Frustrated, I gave up and decided to wait it out — maybe it would heal on its own.

"A little over a year later, I saw a play with my doula. Afterward, I mentioned that I had been struggling with tailbone pain and that it wasn't improving. She explained that this type of pain was common after giving birth, especially when the baby is pulled out quickly. It's possible that my daughter's head or shoulders hit my tailbone and knocked it out of alignment. Getting it back into place was possible with physical therapy. She told me to call Renew PT.

"At my first appointment, I was again reassured that I had a common issue and that it was treatable. After my examination, it was confirmed that my tailbone was out of place. The therapist explained to me how it was positioned and how the muscles attached to it could go into spasm, tighten, and keep it pulled to one side. The therapist mapped out a two-sided plan for my recovery: learn how not to aggravate the injury and work on getting the tailbone back into place.

"Even after my first visit, I had improvement. My therapist taught me how to sit, stand and sleep correctly to not put any pressure on my tailbone. During my visits, 100 percent of my pain was relieved by massage, manual manipulation, cold laser therapy, and stretching. To help me combat pain between visits, I was taught how to release the muscles of my tailbone. I was also taught to use heat therapy, relaxation techniques, manual manipulation, stretching, self-massage and body-strengthening exercises. I was never told I needed to take pills or needed to go buy some gadget to get relief. If something was going to be useful, I was taught how to use a household item (like making a sitting cushion out of a towel, or a massager out of a tennis ball). Being able to understand what was going on with my body and work it out myself was incredibly empowering. It was also a huge relief to be heard, understood and to receive empathy.

"Today, I am almost 100 percent recovered. My therapy has moved into a final phase of maintenance of my tailbone and core strengthening for avoiding injury in the future. It took discipline and patience to make it this far, but I am totally appreciative of the therapists at Renew for their support and confidence in me and the solutions they employ. Thank you!!!" — KR

Labor and Its Stages: A Brief Overview

There are three stages of labor each with its own distinctive characteristics and parameters: first stage, second stage and third stage. Many decisions can and will be made depending on where you are in your labor. I will cover these differences here so that you understand what doctors and midwives are referring to and to give you and your birth partner a timeframe for when to leave for the hospital or birthing center or when to call your homebirth midwife. Knowledge also provides peace of mind.

First Stage of Labor

The first stage of labor is divided into three phases: early phase, active phase, and transition phase. It is highly variable and can last days or hours. During the first stage of labor you want to start timing your contractions. Depending on this timing and how you are feeling you, your caregiver, doula and birth partner will determine when it is time to leave for the hospital. In early labor the contractions can be far apart.

In the first stage, you generally use upright positions instead of squatting positions unless your labor is not progressing. Studies have shown that the first stage of labor is more efficient and less uncomfortable when carried out in an upright position. When you are upright, your baby puts pressure on your cervix, which helps open it up faster. So, listen to your body talk and follow your instincts during the first stage of labor, using any of the upright positions listed in the following chart for the first stage of labor. Try to keep your daily activities as normal as possible until your contractions start demanding all of your attention. Remain upright for as long as you can. Rest when needed, by sitting down. If you find it difficult to remain standing during stage 1 contractions, try neutral positions, on your hands and knees, to relieve your discomfort.

Table 10.1 outlines helpful suggestions on how to make your first stage of labor as comfortable as possible. One of the suggestions is to go for a walk with your partner, which works because moving and remaining upright in the first stage relieves pain and speeds the opening of the cervix. Your contractions are more efficient, stronger, and more regular when you're in an upright position. Being upright also provides many women with a psychological boost. The women in my prenatal class who have labored upright have told me they feel more comfortable, are able to relax easily, and can handle the pain better if they move around or remain upright.

During the contractions it may benefit you to lean forward. This helps your uterus do its work because mechanically, your uterus tilts forward when it contracts. Use your partner and lean against his/her body during your contractions. Psychologically, having your partner's body close to you will comfort you and make you feel safe. As often as possible, change positions and rest by sitting down between contractions. Resting is crucial because it will preserve your energy for later, when you have to push your baby out. Have your partner help you relax, using the relaxation techniques you have worked on in Chapter 9. The more relaxed you are, the less pain you will feel. Make sure to drink water or an electrolyte after every contraction to prevent dehydration, which will slow down your labor. In the early part of your labor, have your partner put warm compresses on your perineum, helping it relax. During your actual labor you should refer to Table 10.2 and, most importantly, listen to your body talk.

Summary Points for the First Stage of Labor

Early Labor:

- Your cervix opens to three to four centimeters.

- Contractions during early labor can be unpredictable and can be short and wide apart.

- Things are still manageable but you can start to use the TENS unit here for pain control if you feel that you can no longer cope with the labor pains.

Active Phase:

- Your cervix dilates even more (up to seven centimeters) and your contractions can last one to five minutes apart. The duration of contractions can be highly variable. The contractions are stronger and more powerful; using the TENS unit here will help you manage the pain.

- This is an intense part and you will need your strength and resolve because you are now almost ready to push your baby out. This phase can last two to six hours but is highly variable.

Transition:

- Your cervix dilates even more (up to ten centimeters) and your contractions can be as little as one minute apart. These contractions are very intense and the TENS unit can help you here. Many women find this part the most difficult; have your comfort measures and birth team there to help you. We always recommend a doula for birthing; doulas are well equipped to help you deal with labor from the beginning to the end and beyond.

Second Stage of Labor

Squatting and remaining upright during the second stage of labor is psychologically the most effective position for delivery. During the second stage, laboring upright includes such positions as squatting, standing, and kneeling. Using them provides numerous benefits. When you squat, the pelvic outlet is 20 to 30 percent wider than when you lie on your back. That's great news if you're having a bigger baby. Remaining upright makes each contraction more efficient and stronger. Gravity is working with you, and the downward pull helps baby get out faster. Birthing in upright positions relaxes the perineal muscles, reducing the likelihood of an episiotomy, and making delivery over an intact perineum possible. Maternal supine hypotension (low blood pressure) is avoided in upright

Table 10.1: Recommended Positions for the First Stage of Labor

1. Hands and Knees (on all fours)
2. Upright , standing, leaning forward on partner or wall
3. Kneeling and leaning forward with support (such as on a chair or birth ball); to avoid back injuries keep your back straight.
4. Standing and holding onto your partner
5. Kneeling on one knee
6. Walking and staying active until your contractions demand your attention
7. Sitting in a rocking chair
8. Side-lying position

and squatting positions. Supine hypotension can occur when a woman labors on her back and the weight of her uterus compresses her inferior vena cava vein. This compression reduces blood flow to your uterus and heart. It also decreases oxygen and blood flow to your baby, which can lead to fetal distress. When back pain is severe, as in back labor, remaining upright or squatting will help relieve the mother of her pain.

There are few disadvantages to laboring upright, but if a woman has a history of precipitous labors (very fast labors), upright positions should be avoided. For fast labors, neutral positions such as kneeling, on the hands and knees or in side-lying position work the best because neutral positions can slow down a very fast labor. The opposite is also true: upright positions during second stage are recommended for women who are not progressing. In other words, if your labor is slow and you want to speed things up a bit, remaining upright can often do the trick.

There are several squatting positions I teach to my students for second stage labor; instructions for each follow. Use any combinations of these positions to enhance comfort, guarantee some progress, and help avoid fetal distress. The birth squats pictured on the following pages should be used when you are fully dilated, when the baby is about to crown, or when you have the urge to push. It is best to use these positions only at the times suggested previously, because using the birth squat too early will fatigue your legs. The second stage can last anywhere from one to two hours or longer, and it's impossible to stay in the same position for that long. So switch positions often, about every thirty minutes if possible. Resting and getting out of the squatting positions after each contraction will preserve your energy and keep your legs from getting too exhausted. Sit back, kneel, or use the child's pose as resting positions.

You may discover that squatting makes your contractions stronger because your baby's head is putting direct pressure on your cervix. If the contractions become too intense for you, switch to another upright labor position or to a neutral position such as hands and knees or side-lying. Listen to your body talk, and labor in whatever position you are the most comfortable in, but try to avoid laboring on your back (lithotomy position). Laboring on your back decreases your pelvic diameter. You work against gravity, your contractions are less efficient, and you increase your chances of tearing the perineum. Talk to your physician about the pros and cons of the various positions, and don't be afraid to raise questions and concerns. It is your birth experience; make sure you make an educated choice.

Summary Points for the Second Stage of Labor

The second stage of labor is where the actual pushing and birth of your baby occurs. Typically you will find the following:

- Your cervix is fully dilated here at ten centimeters.

- This phase can last from fifteen minutes to two hours but we have had patients who have had to push for much longer so don't be surprised if this is the case.

Third Stage of Labor

The third stage of labor is the phase where you deliver the placenta. This can be an intense stage and is worth mentioning here. In this phase abdominal massage can be used to get the placenta out. This can be painful, but it's a short phase and you are now holding your baby so things are looking up and you are in a state of euphoria over your baby. Don't be surprised if your medical team has to manually get the placenta out via the vagina. Many women that we see are not aware that this can happen and experience not only emotional pain but also physical pain when the placenta has to be extracted manually (rather than the body expelling it naturally). Be prepared and know that this extraction can happen as part of the labor and delivery journey.

How to Choose the Best Labor Position

Physical therapists are uniquely equipped to make recommendations for birthing. We understand the pelvic floor muscles, the abdominal muscles and what positions pose a threat to the body. In Table 10.2 we tackle different orthopedic conditions and make birth position recommendations to avoid exacerbating an old injury and to prevent a new injury from occurring. Furthermore you can use this chart to determine among other things which birth position will help you prevent a perineal tear. There are some positions that are considered to be safer than others. As seen in Table 10.2 side-lying position is the go-to position if you have a preexisting condition. Table 10.2 highlights different labor positions that you may want to consider using for your birth. These recommendations are mostly upright labor positions that use gravity to get the baby out and maintain the spine in optimal alignment. Additionally we highlight the side-lying position because we find this position to be the easiest on the pregnant woman's body. Please read them all and practice them with your birth partner before the big day so that everyone is well versed on how to do them.

Table 10.2: Modifying Labor Positions for Pregnant Women with Orthopedic, Spinal and Pelvic Conditions (Excerpt from our Renew Physical Therapy Case Study)

ORTHOPEDIC DYSFUNCTION	MEDICAL DEFINITION	LABOR POSITIONS TO AVOID	RECOMMENDED BIRTH POSITIONS*
Lumbar or Thoracic Disc Herniation or Bulge	Protrusion/Extrusion of discal material out of intervertebral space with possible nerve compression	• Squatting • Semi-reclining with knees to chest • Lithotomy • Hands/knees if nerve root tension is an issue	• Side-lying • Semi-reclined with lumbar support • Hands/knees if nerve root tension is not an issue

Intervertebral Spinal Stenosis	Decrease in joint space between vertebrae due to degenerative changes in spinal column	• Standing	• Positions that open the intervertebral foramen:
			  • Side-lying with side-bending to the opposite side with or without flexion
			• Positions that encourage spinal flexion:
			  • Squatting
			  • Forward bending over a physio ball, bean bag chair or pillows

Spondylolisthesis	Slippage of one vertebrae forward over the vertebrae below	• Standing	• Any position that avoids increased lumbar spine extension (see above)

Table 10.2 (cont.): Modifying Labor Positions for Pregnant Women with Orthopedic, Spinal and Pelvic Conditions (Excerpt from our Renew Physical Therapy Case Study)

ORTHOPEDIC DYSFUNCTION	MEDICAL DEFINITION	LABOR POSITIONS TO AVOID	RECOMMENDED BIRTH POSITIONS*
Sacroiliac Dysfunction	Excessive or inadequate sacral motion	• Walking during first stage • Semi-reclining with the lower extremities unsupported • Lithotomy	• Any position where the lower extremities are symmetrically supported: • Semi-reclining with pillows under both knees • Hands/knees or upright kneel if weight bearing is comfortable • Squatting
Pubic Symphysis Dysfunction	Disturbance or hypermobility of the pubic bone connection	• Positions that abduct the legs wider than hips • Positions where feet are not planted on a surface • Squatting or lithotomy	• Side-lying (lower extremities should not be widely abducted) • Hands/knees or upright kneel if weight bearing is comfortable
Coccyx Dysfunction	Excessive or inadequate motion	• Semi-reclining • Lithotomy	• Any position where the coccyx is free to move: • Side-lying • Squatting • Standing • Hands/knees • Upright kneel
Cervical Disc Herniation or Spondylosis	Decrease in joint space due to disc extrusion/ protrusion or joint degeneration with possible nerve compression	• Lithotomy with unsupported cervical spine/ cervical flexion • Hands/knees if difficulty maintaining neutral cervical spine	• Any position that avoids excessive flexion of the Cervical Spine: • Side-lying • Semi-reclining with pillows under knees • Upright kneel • Squatting • Standing
Pelvic Floor Muscle Dysfunction (including incontinence and pelvic pain)	Pain, spasm, weakness, or in-coordination of the pelvic floor muscles	• Increased Valsalva • Lithotomy position • Episiotomy • Excessive, prolonged pushing	• Side-lying

Table 10.3: Optimal Labor Positions for the Prevention of Obstetrical Trauma and Perineal Tearing

1. Side-lying
2. Hands and Knees
3. Partner Supported Squatting
4. Low Squat
5. Dangling Squat
6. Standing with Partner
7. Half Squat-Half Kneeling Position

Side-Lying Labor Position

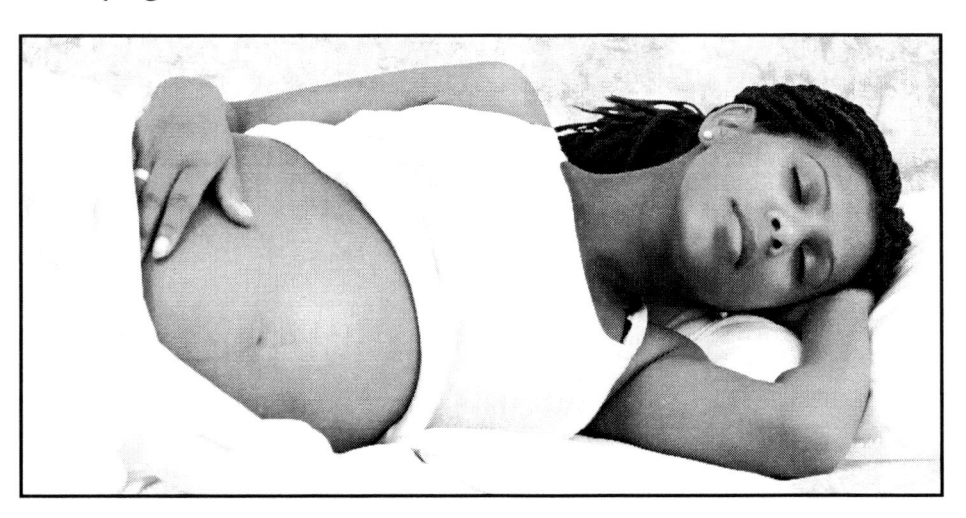

WHAT TO DO:

Partner

- Can hold the top leg when it's time for pushing. Make sure not to spread the top leg too far as it will put the pubic bone at risk for an injury or separation. Your partner will help support the top leg during labor and your doula can massage your back and shoulders or apply warm compresses to the perineum or low back.

Pregnant Woman

- Lie on your side with your knees slightly bent. Get as comfortable as possible and use pillows for your head and belly if needed. You can also place a pillow between your knees which will help keep you in alignment.

WHAT TO WATCH OUT FOR:

- Keep the legs hip-width apart and make sure your birth partner knows not to let anyone pull your leg further than hip-width apart as this can strain the pubic bone and its accompanying ligaments.

BENEFITS:

- Decreases risk of tears and orthopedic injuries and helps decrease the risk of perineal tearing.

- This position also conserves energy and decreases the risk of fatigue and is the go-to position if the labor is progressing too quickly.

Hands and Knees Labor Position

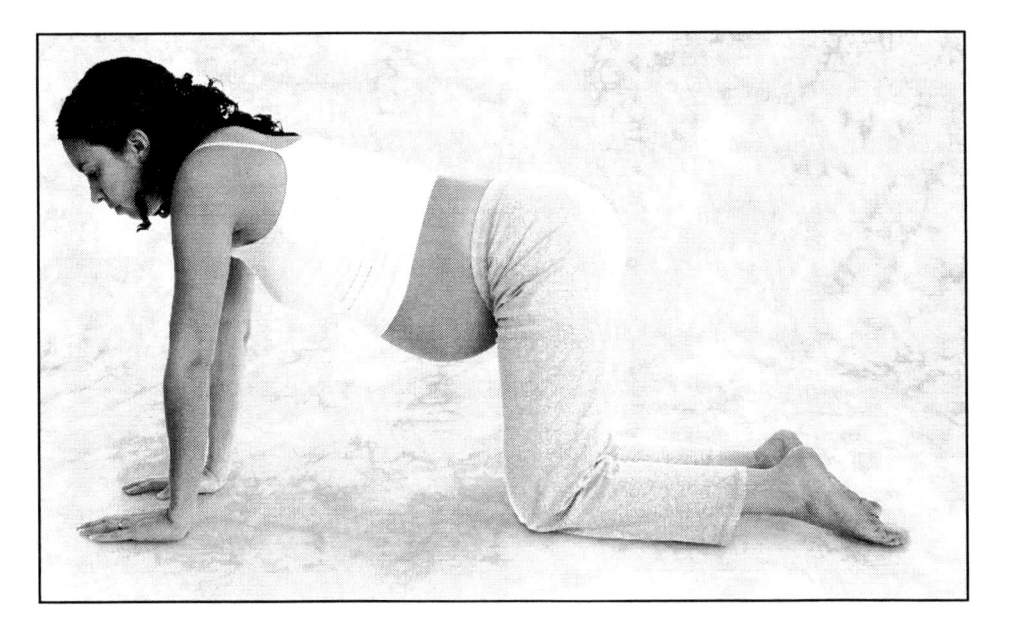

WHAT TO DO:

Partner

The partner can massage the pregnant women here and/or compress the hips to alleviate back pain.

Pregnant Woman

Place weight on the palms of the hands and the knees and keep the upper back relaxed.

WHAT TO WATCH OUT FOR:

- Women who suffer from neck pain, shoulder pain and carpal tunnel pain should use this position with caution.

- Avoid locking out the elbows if possible; this will help minimize pain in the wrist and shoulders.

- You can still use the TENS unit with this position.

Beginner

- Hold this position for one to three minutes, two to three repetitions. Rest thirty to sixty seconds between sets. Don't forget to stretch afterward.

Advanced

- Hold this position for up to five minutes. Rest thirty to sixty seconds between repetitions. Don't forget to stretch afterward.

COMMON MISTAKES:

- Overarching the back. Keep your back in neutral alignment.

- Locking the elbows or hanging the head. Keep elbows slightly bent and neck in neutral alignment.

BENEFITS:

- The hands-and-knees position avoids putting pressure on the coccyx (tailbone), sacroiliac joint and low back muscles and nerves.

- A great position to avoid perineal tearing and the birth partner and doula can still perform the hips squeeze technique if you are suffering from back labor.

- This is the go-to position for a woman suffering from back labor. See Table 10.2 for additional benefits.

Squatting Labor Positions (Three Types – Supported, Low, Dangling)

Partner Supported Squatting Labor Position

WHAT TO DO:

Partner

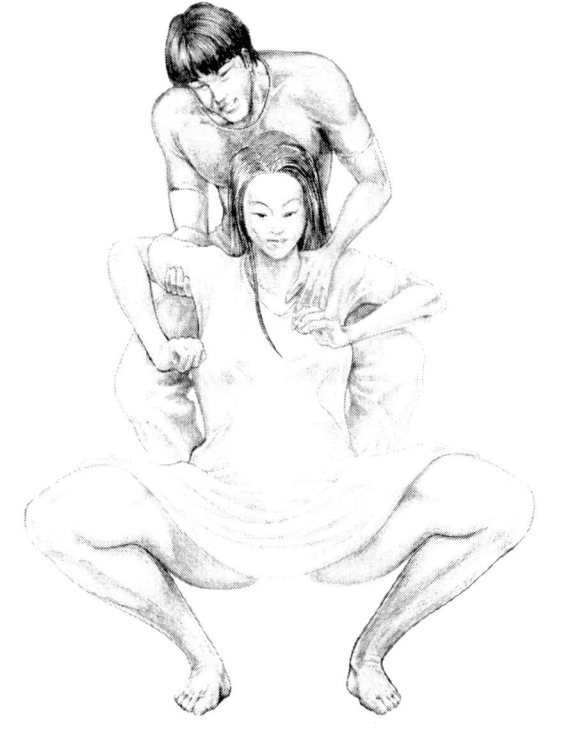

- Sit behind the mother-to-be on a chair or bed. Make sure that you are sitting forward enough so your pregnant partner can lean against your body.

- Hold your pregnant partner under the armpits for extra support, but only if she wants you to.

Pregnant Woman

- Squat all the way down between your partner's inner thighs. Lean your back against your partner's body and place your elbows or inner upper arms on his thighs for extra support.

- Your partner will sit behind you and hold you under the armpits for extra support if needed. You can also lean your body against your partner for emotional and physical comfort

Beginner

- Hold this position for one to three minutes, two to three repetitions. Rest thirty to sixty seconds between sets. Don't forget to stretch afterward.

Advanced

- Hold this position for up to five minutes. Rest thirty to sixty seconds between sets. Don't forget to stretch afterward.

CAUTION:

- Avoid this squatting position, and the one that follows, if you have a cervical stitch, hemorrhoids, vulvar varicosities, or severe varicose veins, or if your baby is in a breech position after thirty-four weeks. This position should also be avoided if you suffer from symphysis pubic dysfunction (SPD). Your pain will tell you if this position is right for you. If you have symphysis pubic dysfunction avoid having the legs wider than hip-width apart.

COMMON MISTAKES:

- Birth partner not sitting forward enough. Your pregnant partner needs to lean against your body, so make sure you are sitting forward.

BENEFITS:

- A great position for partners who suffer from backaches.

- Gravity helps get the baby out.

- Supine hypotension is avoided.

- Pelvic outlet is at its largest diameter.

- The baby has a more direct route because the vagina is wider and smaller.

- A great position to see the baby as it is born, and it's very easy on the back.

- Squatting positions make the contractions more efficient and relax the perineum completely.

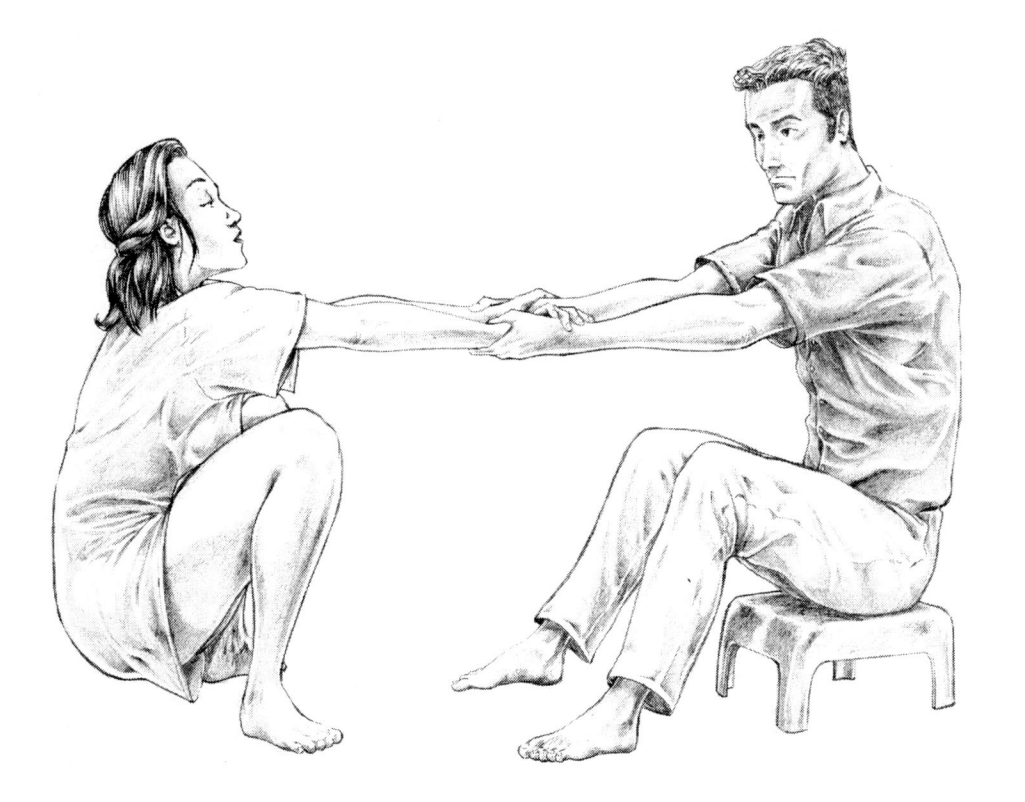

Supported Low Squat

WHAT TO DO:

Partner

- Sit on a low stool or chair. Hold your partner by her wrists, keeping your elbows straight.

- Avoid leaning forward, and keep your back straight.

Pregnant Woman

- Keeping your elbows straight, hold onto your partner's wrists and lower yourself into the low birth squat as explained in the previous exercise.

- Be sure to keep your feet flat on the floor. If it is too difficult, have your partner roll a couple of towels and place them under your heels.

Beginner

- Hold this position for one to three minutes, two to three repetitions. Rest thirty to sixty seconds between sets. Don't forget to stretch afterward.

Advanced

- Hold this position for up to five minutes. Rest thirty to sixty seconds between sets. Don't forget to stretch afterward.

CAUTION:

- Avoid this squatting position, and the one that follows, if you have a cervical stitch, hemorrhoids, vulvar varicosities, or severe varicose veins, or if your baby is in a breech position after thirty-four weeks. This position should also be avoided if you suffer from symphysis pubic dysfunction (SPD). Your pain will tell you if this position is right for you. If you have symphysis pubic dysfunction, avoid having the legs wider than hip-width apart.

COMMON MISTAKES:

- Bending your elbows. Keep your arms straight
- Raising your heels. Keep your heels flat on the floor. Use towels if necessary.
- Letting your knees cave in. Keep your body weight on the outer edges of your feet and your knees in alignment with your toes.
- Leaning forward. Keep your back straight and chest lifted.

BENEFITS:

- A great position for partners who suffer from backaches.
- Gravity helps get the baby out.
- Supine hypotension is avoided.
- Pelvic outlet is at its largest diameter.
- The baby has a more direct route because the vagina is wider and smaller.
- A great position to see the baby as it is born, and it's very easy on the back.
- Squatting positions make the contractions more efficient and relax the perineum completely.

Supported Dangling Squat

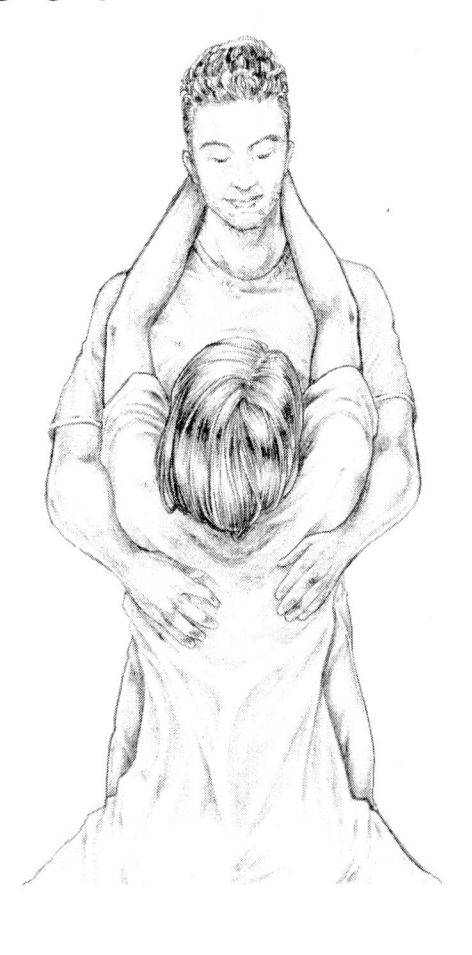

WHAT TO DO:

Partner

- Stand with your feet hip-width apart and your knees bent. While supporting your partner, you should always keep your abdominals tight and your back straight. Bending forward can hurt your lower back.
- It's best not to wear socks and shoes, in order to get good traction. This will prevent you from slipping while holding your partner.
- Keep your shoulders relaxed and down while holding your partner. This position is really hard work, so it needs to be practiced on a regular basis.

Pregnant Woman

- Face your partner and wrap your arms around his neck. Allow yourself to hang from his neck.

- Keep both feet flat on the floor and let go of your mind and your body. Keep your abdominals relaxed.

Beginner

- Hold this position for one to three minutes, two to three repetitions. Rest thirty to sixty seconds between sets. Don't forget to stretch afterward.

Advanced

- Hold this position for up to five minutes. Rest thirty to sixty seconds between repetitions. Don't forget to stretch afterward.

COMMON MISTAKES:

- The birth partner leans forward or arches his back. Keep your back straight and the front of your legs (thighs) and buttocks muscles contracted.

BENEFITS:

- Same as Supported Low Birth Squat

Standing Labor Position

WHAT TO DO:

Partner

- Stand with your feet hip-width apart and knees bent.

- Keeping your abdominals tight and your buttocks contracted, lean back slightly so that you can support your partner's weight against your thighs and pelvis.

- Keep your shoulders relaxed and down while holding your partner.

- Keep your back as straight as possible and avoid leaning forward. Leaning forward will put excess stress on your lower back.

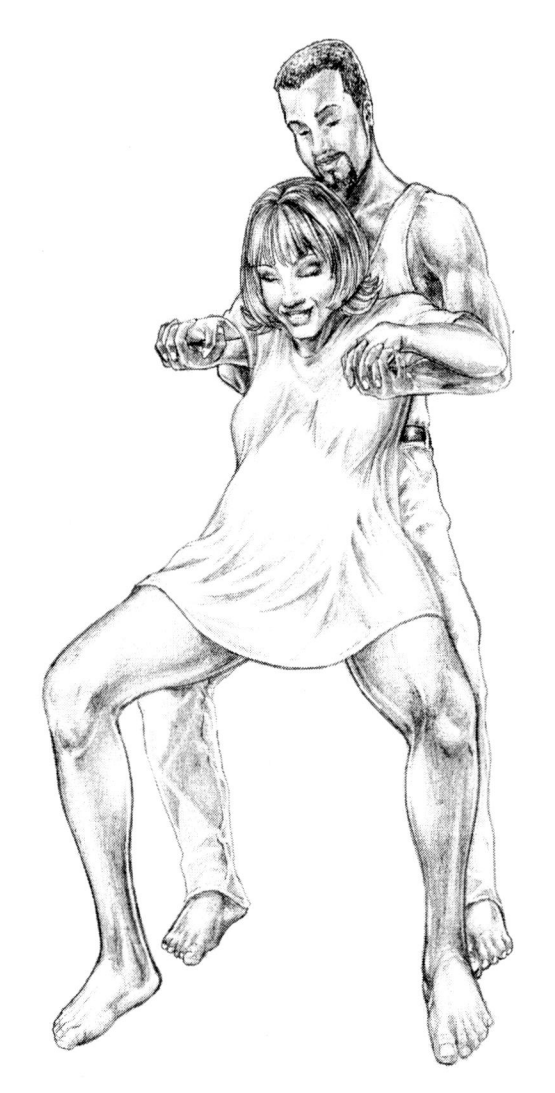

- In order to get good traction, do not wear socks or shoes. This will prevent you from slipping while you hold your partner.

Pregnant Woman

- Let your partner hold you under your arms and lean back against his thighs while you squat about two to four inches.

- Hold onto your partner's hands and forearms for added physical and emotional support.

Beginner

- Hold this position for one to three minutes, two to three repetitions. Rest thirty to sixty seconds between sets. Don't forget to stretch afterward.

Advanced

- Hold this position for up to five minutes. Rest thirty to sixty seconds between repetitions. Don't forget to stretch afterward.

COMMON MISTAKES:

- The birth partner leans forward or arches his back. Keep your back straight and the front of your legs (thighs) and buttocks muscles contracted.

BENEFITS:

- Same as Supported Low Birth Squat.

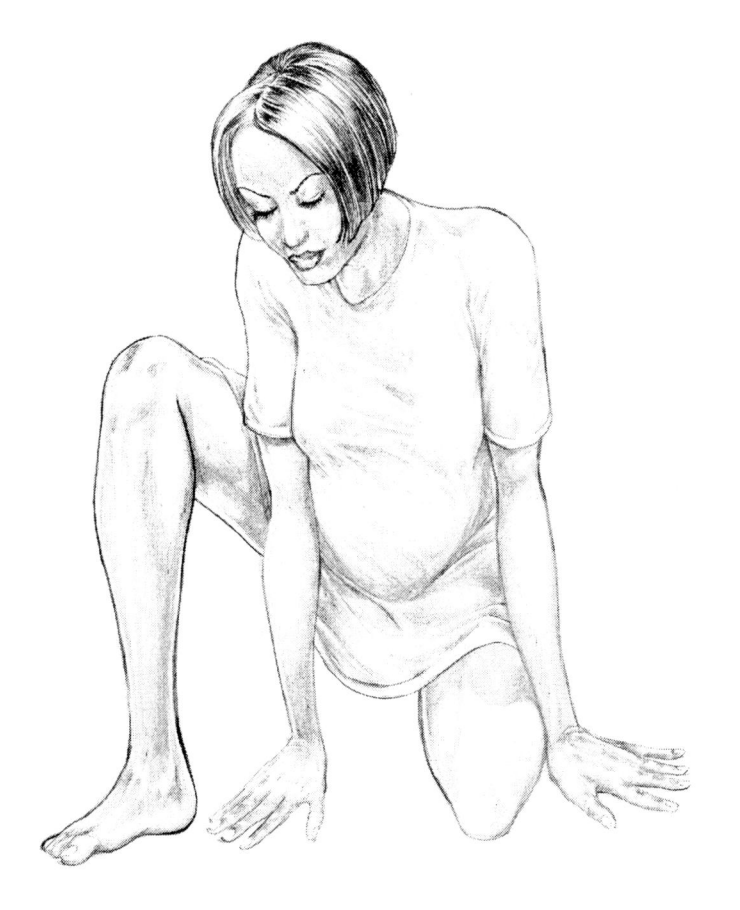

Half Squat-Half Kneeling Position (Solo)

If you become tired or exhausted from the squatting positions during your labor, try the half squat-half kneeling position. This alternative position has the same advantages as the squatting positions, but it's not as difficult. It's also a great position to use if you're experiencing back labor. Try to change legs after each contraction, and rest in between contractions. To rest, lean back on your legs and place your head on a couple of pillows.

WHAT TO DO:

Pregnant Woman

- Kneel down on your left knee and bend your right knee, as in the figure.

Beginner

Hold this position for one to two minutes, two to three repetitions. Rest thirty to sixty seconds between sets. Don't forget to stretch afterward.

Advanced

- Hold this position for up to three minutes. Rest thirty to sixty seconds between sets. Don't forget to stretch afterward.

- Keeps the spine in neutral position and decreases the risk of injuries related to coccyx, low back, hips and sacroiliac joint.

The positions highlighted above are mostly for the pushing part of labor but can be used at any time you feel the need to change positions. Changing positions will help to make your labor more effective and could possibly shorten it. In addition, changing positions and using positions that are right for your body type will help to reduce obstetrical trauma and prevent a long recovery after the baby arrives. Have your birth partner and birth team remind you to change positions often (at least every thirty minutes) during the early phase of labor. Have them also remind you to use the pushing positions you have practiced. It is very easy to get lost in the labor, but practicing beforehand and having a plan will be very beneficial for you and the baby.

Breathing and Different Types of Pushing

Although there are countless types of birthing and pushing techniques and breathing methods, we will cover three that we think you should be aware of; they include directed pushing, spontaneous pushing and Renewal Pelvic and Exhale Pushing™.

Directed pushing involves holding the breath for a certain count (usually to a count of ten) while you push even though you may not have an urge to push. The pushing and breath holding usually occur for the duration of the contraction. Any activity that requires breath holding carries an associated risk. The risk with directed pushing is increased fatigue and it's correlated with a higher rate of perineal tearing and decreased oxygenation for the baby and laboring mother. If there is fetal distress or if the baby is in danger, directed pushing can get the baby out very quickly and is used to protect the baby. But as a rule this type of breathing is not efficient and is not desirable.

Spontaneous pushing is natural and works with the rhythm of labor and with the rhythm of the laboring woman's body. The laboring mom is in control and only pushes when she feels an urge to push and is breathing through the contraction and not holding her breath. Groaning, vocalizing and exhaling are all part of spontaneous pushing. The woman is free and is not subjected to the commands of those in the room. She follows her instincts and is going with the labor and her body signals and she is listening closely to its messages. Her body will signal her when to push. This can be animalistic in nature and many sounds can come out of you when you are deep into your birthing process. This is an ideal method and no training is required. It's based on the deep messages of your body. Additionally, research has shown that women who use spontaneous pushing have shorter births and their babies have higher Apgar scores.

Renewal Pelvic and Exhale Pushing™ requires training and has to be practiced prior to the big day of labor. This technique is based not only on science and normal physiology but it also incorporates the pelvic floor and abdominal muscles. This is the technique we teach to most of our pregnant patients. It's not easy to master because it involves training and working with the abdominal and pelvic muscles and the corresponding breath. Renewal Pelvic and Exhale Pushing involves three things: (1) active exhalation; (2) engaging the transverse abdominis muscle; and (3) a reverse Kegel or relaxed pelvic floor. The catch here is that you have to do all three actions at the same time. These techniques should be practiced at least ten weeks before the due date. A common mistake with this technique is forcing the exhalation and/or over-activating the outer abdominal muscles instead of the deep transverse abdominis. Performing and practicing this pushing technique incorrectly can increase pelvic pressure, incontinence or organ prolapse. Make sure to seek help from a women's health physical thera-pist or a pelvic floor physical therapist to make sure you are performing it cor-rectly. Don't fear. Try it and practice it so you have another technique in your labor toolbox.

Transcutaneous Electrical Nerve Stimulation (TENS): A Natural Solution for Pain Control during Labor and Delivery

TENS for the relief of labor pain has been used for a long time and dates back to the 1970s. The TENS unit works great for natural pain relief because the signals from the TENS unit block the body's labor pain signals from reaching the higher pain centers. The TENS unit is also thought to increase the production of endogenous opiates which are powerful pain-relieving substances. In many countries TENS therapy is commonplace and the TENS units can be bought at local pharmacies. In the United States we are not that lucky; to get a TENS unit you will need to get a prescription from your OB/GYN or midwife. You will also need to get permission from your medical team to use it for your labor and you should also investigate the hospital's TENS unit policy. Policies regarding the usage of TENS vary from hospital to hospital and from birthing center to birth-ing center. Most hospitals and birthing centers, from our experience, have few issues with women using TENS therapy for natural pain relief during labor and delivery. By getting confirmation in advance, you will avoid having issues on the day of your labor with the hospital, the doctor or the midwife.

The TENS unit is convenient to use because it is a small handheld unit that runs on a battery. Many TENS units are equipped with a small clip so that you can put it on your gown allowing your hands to be free. Low-level electrical mes-sages are given off by the TENS. You will feel a slight tingling feeling like tiny little zaps. The signals from the TENS unit are sent up the spine and reach the higher pain centers before the pain signals of your body. The electrical signals coming off the TENS unit travel faster than the nerve signals that produce labor pain. A TENS unit blocks pain by this mechanism, and it's based on the premise of the Gateway Theory of Pain.

The TENS sends its impulses to the skin via four or more surface electrodes of varying sizes. These electrodes have a self-adhesive gel and are easy to use and to stick onto the body. Always make sure to turn off the TENS unit before moving an electrode otherwise you will receive a shock. Care has to be taken not to get the electrodes to stick to anything else such as the hospital gowns or other materials on the labor bed. Electrodes will lose their effectiveness to conduct the signal if they are not taken care of properly so handle them with care. Electrodes can be used many times over again and should last for a very long time. Careful placement of the electrodes is necessary and we have included a photograph to help you place the electrodes correctly on the body. Learn the surface anatomy in the photo below and you will easily be able to place the electrodes on the correct body position. TENS therapy is a very forgiving pain-relieving modality in that you don't have to be exactly on the right spots with the electrodes — just close to them. This is one of the reasons that we recommend you use the larger electrodes because they cover more space and you don't have to be 100 percent correct in your placements.

Nerves play a big part here and we will review where the signals are coming from because they guide you as to where to place the electrodes. The pain felt during the first stage of labor is due to contractions of the uterus and effacement and dilation of the cervix. These pain signals come from uterine nerves and hypogastric nerves, which correlate to T10 to L2 (thoracic spinal nerve number 10 to the lumbar spinal nerve number 1). T10 to L2 would be the ideal area to place the electrode pads for the first stage of labor. See the photograph below to get an idea of these landmarks.

The second stage is more intense and you may have to use several different electrode placements to find pain relief. Pain signals for the second stage of labor come from pudendal nerves and reach S2 to S4 (sacral spinal segment

2 through sacral spinal segment 4). Pain signals for this phase also come from uterine contractions involving T10 to S2 (thoracic spinal nerve number 10 all the way down to sacral spinal nerve number 2).

Setting Up Your TENS Unit Machine

You must have a labor-specific TENS unit with the correct parameters for use during labor. You must have a "constant/continuous" mode which is used for all stages of labor, and this is a continuous stream of sensation. Ideally, you also have a "burst" mode which is a low frequency stimulation between 1 to 4Hz with high frequency trains between 100 to 150Hz. With this burst setting you will see a visible muscle contraction and it looks as if the muscles are twitching.

Some TENS units have an "M" (known as a Modulation mode) and this mode is not used for labor. TENS units have a pulse width setting; make sure to set this at 100 microseconds. The other setting you should pay attention to is the pulse rate, which has to be set at four cycles/second.

Table 10.4: TENS Unit Parameters and Set-Up

TENS UNIT SETTINGS	TENS UNIT PARAMETERS FOR THE SETTINGS
Continuous Setting for Stage 1 and Stage 2 of labor	Frequency: 100 Hz Pulse width: 4 Hz
Burst Mode Setting for when the baby is crowning or at peak of contractions	Frequency: 100-150Hz Pulse width: 1-4Hz
Intensity for continuous setting or burst measured in milliamps	Usually rated at 1 to 10 and you can dial up the intensity as needed. Many times it can take up to one hour before you feel pain relief so don't give up on the TENS therapy.

Table 10.5: TENS UNIT Set-Up for Stage 1 and Stage 2 of Labor

STAGE	TENS MODE SETTING	ELECTRODE PLACEMENT
Labor Stage 1	Continuous sensation	• T10-L2: Between the bra line and the belly button.
Labor Stage 2	Continuous sensation Burst sensation for crowning or at peak of powerful contraction Be sure to shut the TENS off before moving the electrodes	• S2-S4 sacral spinal segments and L4 and L5 lumbar spinal segments. S2 to S4 are located near dimples and L4 and L5 are located on the lower back above the hip crease. • Or you can place the electrodes on multiple areas such as a combination placement that includes T10-L2; S2-S4;L4-L5 (stage one plus stage two electrode placements)

Now that you know the set-up and electrode placement, please review Tables 10.6, 10.7, 10.8, and 10.9 for additional considerations that you must take into account before using your TENS unit for the relief of labor pain. These considerations include benefits, disadvantages, contraindications, and precautions.

Table 10.6: Benefits of Using the TENS Unit for Your Labor and Delivery

1. The woman can be in control of pain relief and in control of the TENS unit. She dials up the intensity as needed to receive maximum pain relief.
2. TENS is a handheld unit or it can be attached to the gown. This small unit allows for freedom to change positions and walk as needed by the laboring woman.
3. There are many other comfort measures that can be used alongside the TENS unit since it doesn't interfere. See Tables 10.10 and 10.11.
4. Certain medications have side effects that can affect emotional states. The TENS unit is natural and does not negatively affect the laboring woman's emotional and mental states.
5. TENS can be used early in labor and there's no wrong time to use it. TENS can help the laboring mother cope with pain in all stages of labor and delivery.

Table 10.7: Disadvantages of Using the TENS Unit for Your Labor and Delivery

1. Back massage may be difficult to perform by labor partner.
2. TENS can be expensive to purchase. Find out if your insurance will cover the cost. Many times to get insurance coverage you will also have to get a prescription from your MD.
3. It is difficult to obtain labor-specific units in the United States.
4. TENS can interfere with electronic fetal monitoring equipment and your hospital might not allow you to use it if you are being monitored.
5. TENS cannot be used in a birthing tub or in the shower or in a regular bath tub.
6. To get a TENS unit in the United States you will need a prescription from your midwife or doctor.

Table 10.8: Contraindications of Using the TENS Unit for Your Labor and Delivery

1. Using the TENS before the thirty-seventh week of pregnancy can bring on premature contractions. Sometimes TENS is used during pregnancy but you must be supervised by an MD or midwife.
2. Never place electrodes on the • Pregnant belly. • Front or side of the neck or throat. • Never place the electrodes on the head or on the eyes. • Never use TENS if you suffer from cardiac arrhythmias. • Never use TENS if you have a cardiac pacemaker. • Never use over carotid sinus. This is the pulse that can be found in the side of the neck and is frequently used to determine heart rate.
3. Women who suffer from epilepsy should not use a TENS unit.
4. Women with undiagnosed pain should not use a TENS unit.

Table 10.9: Precautions with Using the TENS Unit for Your Labor and Delivery

1. Skin irritation because the electrodes stick to the skin.
2. Avoid all water when using the TENS unit.
3. Exercise care when storing your TENS unit. Avoid storing or placing your unit near heat or radiator.
4. Never use the TENS unit where there is flammable gas including oxygen.
5. Always have extra batteries on hand. To maintain your unit remove the batteries when you are not using them.

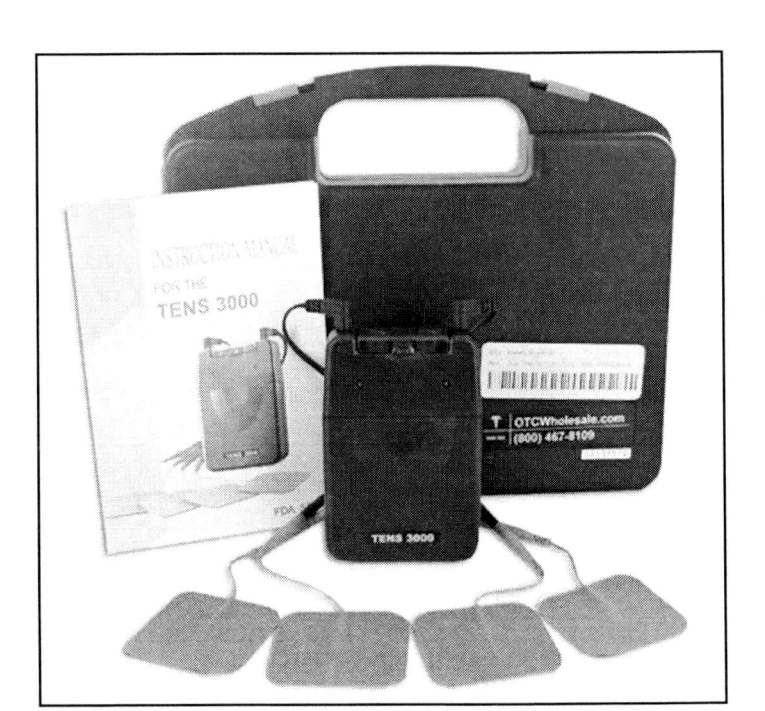

Description: Notice the TENS unit electrode pads. When we use the TENs unit we like to have two different types: a small electrode pad (pictured here) and a larger rectangular one (seen in the photograph on page 254). Try to have both types for your birth.

Diagram 10.1: Electrode Placements and Landmark Anatomy

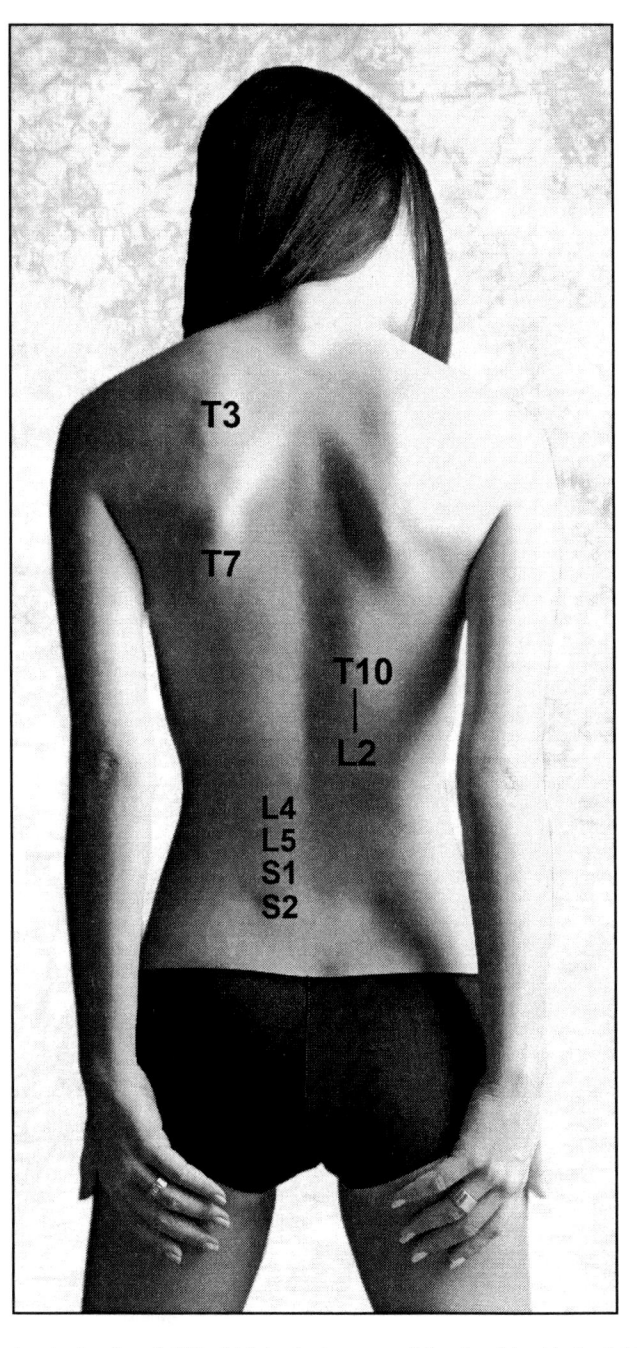

Description: Notice the landmark T7 which is the bottom of the shoulder blade. L4 is located at the top of the iliac crest (hip bone) and S2 is located at the dimples of PSIS.

Diagram 10.2: TENS Unit: Large Pads

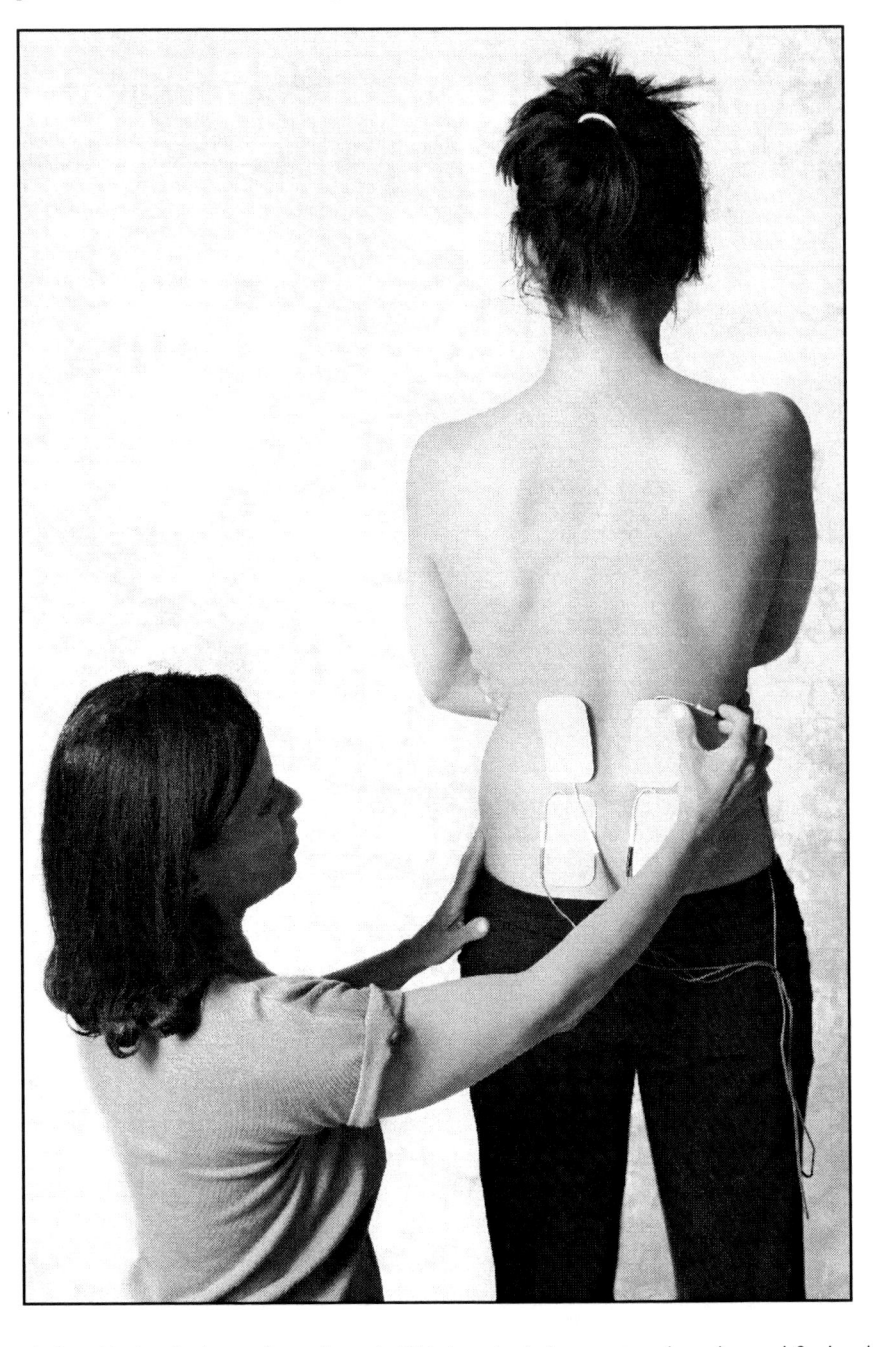

Description: Notice the large electrode pads. This is a dual placement and can be used for low back pain during labor and delivery. The large pads make the placement more forgiving and you don't have to be 100 percent covered as they cover a lot of space and multiple nerves.

Comfort Measures for Labor and Delivery

Comfort measures during labor and delivery can help you cope better with labor pain and with the transitions of labor. In Tables 10.10 and 10.11 you will find common comfort measures that can be used stand-alone or simultaneously with the TENS unit. We advise that you research others as well. We recommend that you also work with a birth doula as doulas are miracle workers in comfort measures. The next table lists comfort measures for the mom-to-be and the table that immediately follows that one provides comfort measures for the birth partner. Read each table carefully.

Table 10.10: Labor and Delivery Comfort Measures for the Mother-to-Be

1. Rest as much as possible during the early stage of labor. You'll need your energy later on.
2. When you first go into labor, try to continue doing your normal daily activities, but rest as much as possible. Your labor could be a very long one and you shouldn't exhaust yourself.
3. Eat whatever and whenever you want.
4. Use hot compresses during the first stage of labor to relieve pain and help relax your perineum.
5. Change positions every thirty minutes if possible: stand, walk, sit semi-reclining, squat, lie on your back, lean on your partner, or lean against a wall.
6. Put a hot water bottle on the lower back, lower abdomen, and between the thighs to relieve pain.
7. Take a warm bath if the membranes have not ruptured. If the membranes are ruptured, take a shower by yourself or with your partner. When your membranes rupture you will feel a gush of liquid seep out through your vagina. If you are in any doubt, call your caregiver and ask if it's okay to take a bath.
8. Take a walk in the park. Walking can shorten and reduce pain.
9. Keep your favorite Popsicle in the freezer or electrolyte drinks in the refrigerator.

Table 10.11: Labor and Delivery Comfort Measures for the Partner

1. Time the contractions on a watch with a second hand. Note when the water breaks and when you think her labor started. To time a contraction:

- Note when the contraction started
- Track the duration of the contraction in seconds
- Time the frequency of the contractions
  (keeping track in minutes from the start of one to the next).

2. Make sure she drinks after every contraction. Keep her as hydrated as possible. Dehydration makes the contraction less effective.

3. For a backache and back labor, use strong counter pressure. Press the fist, heel of your hand, or a firm object such as a tennis ball, or ice pack, on your partner's low back. With your other hand, hold onto the front of her hips as you press (because she may want to have you press hard and this can push her over otherwise). You will need a very strong upper body in order to provide this type of pressure.

4. Very lightly, massage using fingertips only on the mother's abdomen during contractions. Massage other body parts that will help the mother relax, especially the feet. Note that massaging can work during early labor but might be intolerable later on.

5. Hold her hands. Match your emotions to hers and try not to distract her from these contractions. Her labor needs all her attention.

6. The time to ask her a question is not during a contraction. Breathe with her during the contractions and ask her the questions when the contraction is over.

7. Remind her to urinate frequently, every hour.

8. Watch the mother during her contractions and help her to relax her entire body. Don't just say "relax"; be specific as to the body part you want her to relax.

9. Help the mother decide when to call her healthcare provider. Most doctors will determine whether she should go to the hospital by the sound of her voice and by the length and frequency of her contractions.

10. Use the acupressure point Ho-Ku to relieve pain. It is located on the back of the hands, where the bones forming the bases of the thumb and index finger come together. Press steadily during a contraction. Repeat as often as the mother wants.

Sample Birth Plan

Birth plans come in all shapes and sizes and can range from the very specific to the very general. For peace of mind make a plan with your partner and share it with your caregiver, coaching team and/or midwife. Think of it as a blueprint that can be followed during labor and delivery. Sometimes we find patients are very strict with their birth plans and they forget that birthing is an act of divinity and things can happen that are beyond your control. Keep an open mind and surrender to the process. When your coaching team and partner know your wishes, they can help re-enforce them and help you stay focused. Please use the birth plan provided below as a guideline and discuss your wishes with your doctor or midwife before the birth of your child.

Sample Birth Plan

The following are our wishes regarding the birth of our child, our labor experience and our recovery.

During Labor: Procedures/Practices/Options

Pain Relief:

We would like to have a natural birth and avoid medications: for pain relief we prefer emotional support from partner, doula and staff. We would also like to use relaxation breathing and other comfort measures such as bath, acupressure points, whirlpool, shower, essential oils, or TENS. We would like to avoid an epidural.

Presence of Others in Labor Room:

Partner and doula and others at discretion of mother.

Vaginal Exams:

At mother's discretion or by doctor only and only when necessary.

Position for Labor:

Freedom to change positions as necessary and mother would like to walk around.

HEP Lock:

If necessary place it at the forearm not the hands.

Enema:

No enema unless used to stimulate labor.

Onset of Labor:

Spontaneous onset. Would like to avoid using Pitocin.

Enhance Speed of Labor:

Walk, change positions, nipple stimulation, enema, rupture of membranes. No Pitocin unless truly necessary.

To Empty Bladder:

Walk to toilet. No catheterization.

Photographs:

Birth to be photographed by partner and/or doula.

Food/Fluids:

Eat and drink as desired: water, juice, Popsicles, Gatorade.

Monitoring Fetal Heart Rate:

Auscultation with stethoscope or Doppler and/or intermittent external electronic fetal monitoring and only when necessary.

For Birth: Procedure or Practice and Options

Position:

Mother's choice for positions.

Expulsion Techniques:

Spontaneous bearing down, exhalation pushing, avoiding prolonged breath holding and straining as much as possible.

Speed up Birth:

Gravity-enhanced positions and prolonged pushing on command. Avoiding episiotomy.

Bed for Birth:

Mother's choice.

Covering of the perineal area:

Undraped, mother may touch baby during birth.

Care of Perineum:

Try for an intact perineum with massage, support, hot compresses, controlled pushing and positions to promote perineal stretching. Ice packs immediately after birth.

After Birth: Procedures/Practices and Options

Cord Cutting:

Partner will cut cord after it stops pulsating.

Delivery of Placenta:

Spontaneous.

Maintaining Uterine Tone:

Massage by mother or nurse.

Contact Between Mother/Partner/Loved Ones:

Regulated by mother/partner.

Discharge of mother and baby:

One to three days after birth.

Cesarean Birth: Policy and Options

Anesthesia:

Regional anesthesia with little or no pre-medication.

Participation:

Screen lowered at time baby is delivered and doctor explains events as they go on.

Presence of Partner/Others:

Partner and doula present: Partner seated at mother's head; doula photographs event.

Incision:

Bikini cut only; opening and closing of incision by doctor only, NO RESIDENTS.

Discharge:

One to four days.

Baby Care: Procedures/Practices and Options

Circumcision:

None. Absolutely no circumcision.

Airway:

Baby coughs and expels own mucus; suctioned if necessary.

Immediate Care:

None or baby held by parents and suckled by mother in parent's arms for observation. Partner to accompany baby for all care.

Contact between Baby and Mother and Partner:

Twenty-four-hour rooming.

First feeding:

Breastfeeding on demand.

Vitamin K:

Okay.

Eye Care:

Use of nonirritating agent, such as erythromycin or tetracycline.

Hepatitis B immunization:

None. Our pediatrician will take care of it.

Warmth:

Baby skin to skin with mother with blanket covering both.

Sick Infant

Contact between baby and mother/parents:

Parents visit and care for baby as much as possible.

Feeding when baby is able to digest food:

Mother nurses baby.

Contact with support group:

Initiated by parents.

Medical Procedures:

To be approved by parents ahead of time. Doctor must explain all procedures to parents.

This is a sample birth plan. You must determine the plan that is appropriate for you and your partner and review the plan with your caregiver.

It is our hope that you have found this information empowering and helpful for your birthing experience. Pass it along to your doctor, midwife and doulas. Just show them this book and let them know you intend to use the TENS unit and act on other recommendations in *Ending Pain in Pregnancy*. It is important to spread the word to your medical community so that other women can benefit from this information. Education and spreading the word is key.

In Chapter 11 we make you aware of twenty-five things that can happen in birth. So many times we hear from new moms: "I wish I knew. No one told me this could happen." We didn't write this chapter to scare you but to enlighten and empower you. Not only do we cover very important topics but we also provide you with trade secrets that will help you recover if you do experience any of the twenty-five things discussed in Chapter 11.

CHAPTER ELEVEN

"Giving birth and being born brings us into the essence of creation, where the human spirit is courageous and bold and the body, a miracle of wisdom."

– *Harriette Hartigan*

Chapter II

TWENTY-FIVE THINGS YOU MAY NOT WANT TO KNOW ABOUT BIRTH— AND THE TRUTH THAT WILL SET YOU FREE

Birth is an all-encompassing experience filled with ups and downs. Its unpredictable nature can fill both grown women and men with fear. Fear is predominant because so many things can occur. Many times birthing partners are not prepared to handle the unpredictability or simply just don't know that things can happen beyond their control.

When I thought about writing this chapter I wanted it to be an exposé of sorts. As a physical therapist that rehabilitates women with obstetrical trauma I can share what I know in an honest way that is not as scary as what you may see on TV or read in the paper. Not only do I share things you may *not* want to know about birth but I take it a step further and provide you with simple solutions. I always tell my patients if I had had the perfect birth and recovery I probably would not have opened my amazing healing center. Life is like that: it teaches us lessons so we can share and help others along the way.

When you read this chapter, I don't want you to become fearful or scared. Instead I want to give you information so that you can—if needed— seek appropriate help and regain your health more quickly. Knowledge is power and this chapter is filled with knowledge that most girlfriends don't share. Why? Birth is a visceral and animalistic experience and many women are embarrassed by their experience or feel guilty because it didn't go as "planned." Society lays a heavy trip on women. The movies and the media are all filled with picture-perfect births and movie stars that recover in a New York minute. I find this depiction unfair and unjust. Women need to know that no matter what happens with their births they are both strong and resilient and will bounce back.

All recovery has its time frame and the postpartum period is no different. We find that some women bounce back quickly but the majority of women struggle in their recovery phase. Some women can take up to one year to feel like themselves again, even if they didn't have a "complicated" birth. For others this can take longer than a year. *That's right: it can take longer than a year and that's okay.* It is my belief that the more women honestly discuss their birth experiences the better off all women will be. When there is open communication among women and when the media stops misleading us, we will be free of misconceptions and find joy in our births.

Open communication will paint the correct picture of birth. Birthing is messy and imperfect, but it's our experience and we can ultimately accept our births as the ones we were meant to have. Women will understand that unexpected and even unpleasant things may happen in their births but nevertheless their experience can be a satisfying one. Arm yourself with knowledge of the "what if" so you are not taken by surprise. Help is available: This book (and my first book *Ending Female Pain*) will empower you with many of the tools you need to get back on track again after the baby comes. Read on and become the fearless warrior of your own story.

Twenty-Five Things You May Not Want to Know About Birth

1. You can injure the disc material between your vertebrae and/or hurt your back.

A herniation of a spinal disc or an injury to the low back area can occur during the pushing phase of labor especially if you are holding your breath (as in directed pushing) or bending from your waist. The pain in the back can be localized to the injury site or it can present itself as a sciatica-like pain that radiates into the buttock or into the legs or feet.

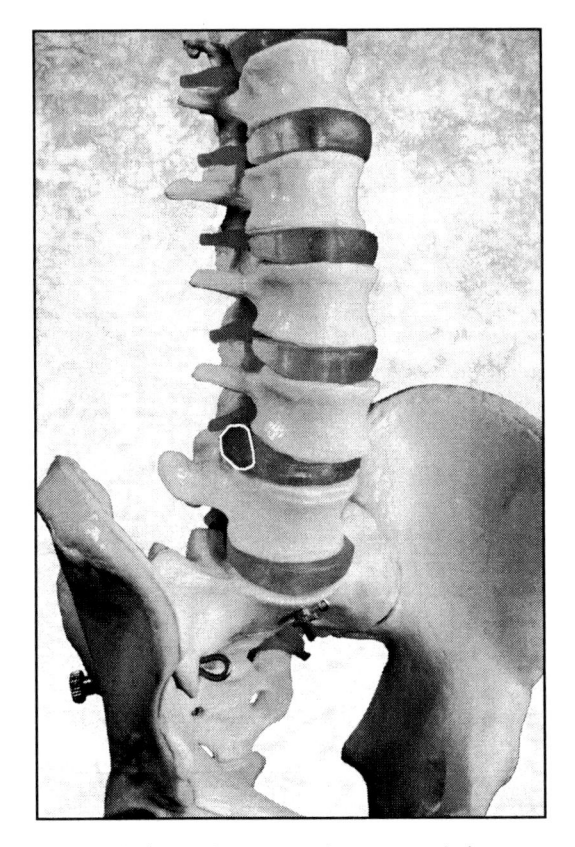

1. See a medical team and report this pain to them; they should refer you to an orthopedic doctor.

2. Work with a women's health physical therapist to receive manual therapy care and pain-relieving exercises.

3. Avoid bending from the waist to reach for items or to put your baby in the crib. Instead bend your knees and use a squatting position to do your day-to-day activities. Keep your back in optimal alignment which is straight and never bend from the waist. Perform a pelvic brace (see Chapter 4, page 79) with all movements that include changing positions, lifting and squatting. Review Chapter 4 and become familiar with correct postural and proper biomechanics.

2. You could separate your pubic symphysis.

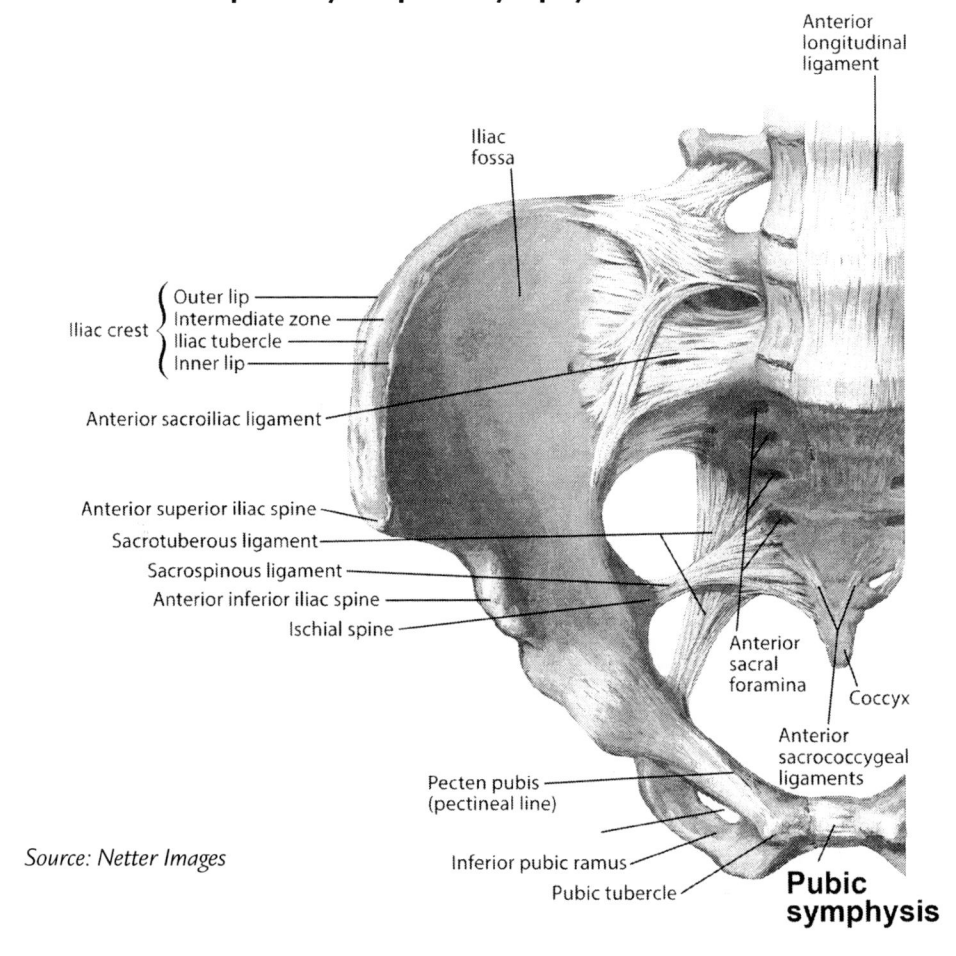

Source: Netter Images

The pubic symphysis (see diagram above) can separate during childbirth. This split can happen when the legs are spread very far apart while you are laboring. Read Chapter 7 for extensive information on symphysis pubic dysfunction.

1. See your doctor or midwife immediately and get a referral to a women's health specialist. The faster you get help and start to get the massage and exercises you need the faster you will recover. Try to find a women's health expert that uses cold laser therapy. This type of therapy can help reduce pubic bone pain.

2. Belt yourself to bring the bones together. Refer to Chapter 5 and Chapter 8 for more information on belting and alignment corrections.

3. Avoid standing on one leg, avoid doing activities that bring your legs far apart and perform the pelvic brace exercise with transitional movements. See Chapters 4, 5 and 7 for more information.

3. You could injure, fracture or have a misaligned tailbone (coccyx).

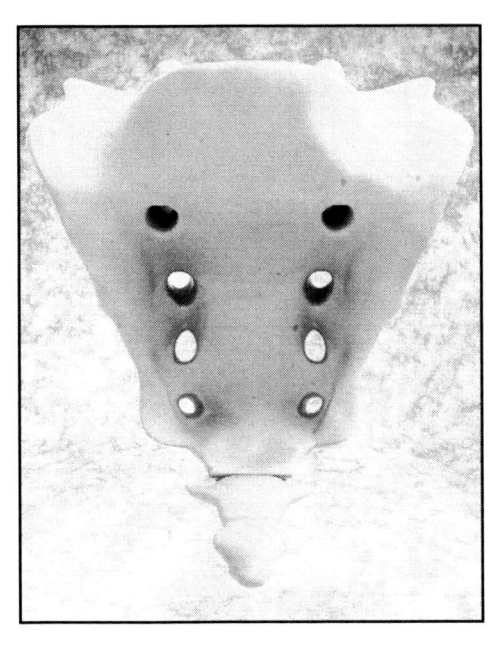

Tailbone injuries are very common and we treat many women who break, strain or misalign their tailbones in childbirth. Tailbone pain is strong pain at the base of your spine; it can be constant and just plain awful. This pain makes it impossible to sit and/or breastfeed and many women may need pain meds to deal with the pain.

1. If you suspect a broken tailbone get an X-ray right away. To detect issues with the coccyx bone it is best to get a seated X-ray.

2. Seek help from a trained women's health expert. Don't wait and go right away.

3. Sit on a donut cushion and avoid slouching, which can put more pressure on the coccyx and result in more pain. Instead sit upright and in good posture and avoid sitting for longer than thirty to forty-five minutes.

4. Your bones will feel out of place.

Labor is a physically-challenging activity and the bones can easily come out of their alignment contributing to localized or full body pain. There are things you can do to get yourself back into alignment and this book will help you.

1. Read Chapter 5, correct your own pelvis and seek the help of a women's health physical therapist.

2. Avoid all destructive forces, avoid standing on one leg, avoid poor posture and use proper body mechanics. Don't despair and seek help immediately.

3. Use the pelvic brace and other relevant exercises and techniques highlighted in Chapters 5, 6, 7 and 8.

5. You will still look pregnant after the baby comes.

It takes eight weeks for the uterus to shrink and go back to the right place. What this means is that you will still look pregnant after the baby arrives. I remember how shocked I was to see my postpartum belly. There are things you can do to make your belly look smaller and to regain your pre-pregnancy shape.

1. Use a postpartum belt immediately after the birth of your child. Try to bring it to the hospital with you.

2. Work with a trained women's health physical therapist so that you can get your core back in shape.

3. Correct your diastasis abdominal separation. Read Chapter 12 and start with the transverse holds and corrective abdominal exercises for the separation.

6. Epidurals can give you a big "spinal headache" or pain at the injection site.

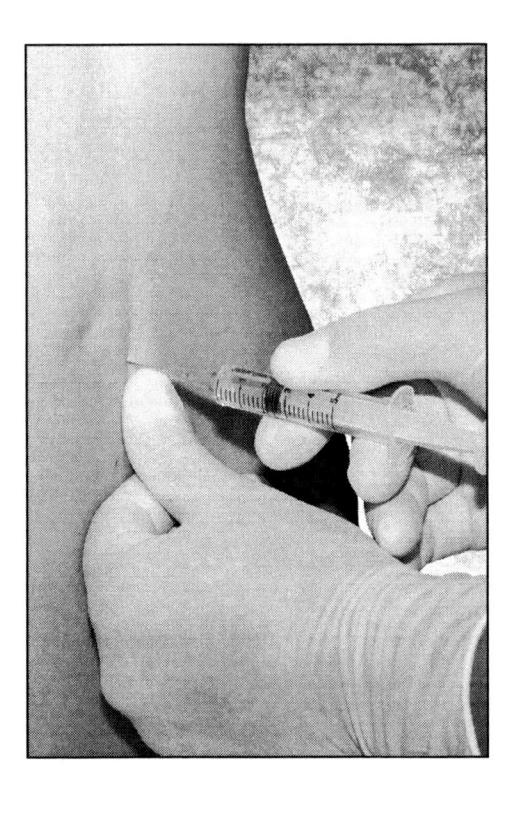

Epidurals can cause local pain at the injection site or lead to severe headache (sometimes known as a "spinal headache") and pain in the low back area.

1. Call your medical team immediately and let them know that you are experiencing this type of headache or lower back pain.

2. You may need a further medical workup and this is best determined by a trained medical team that can include a neurologist, orthopedist and a women's health physical therapist.

7. You may feel as if you just ran a marathon: sore, tired, and achy.

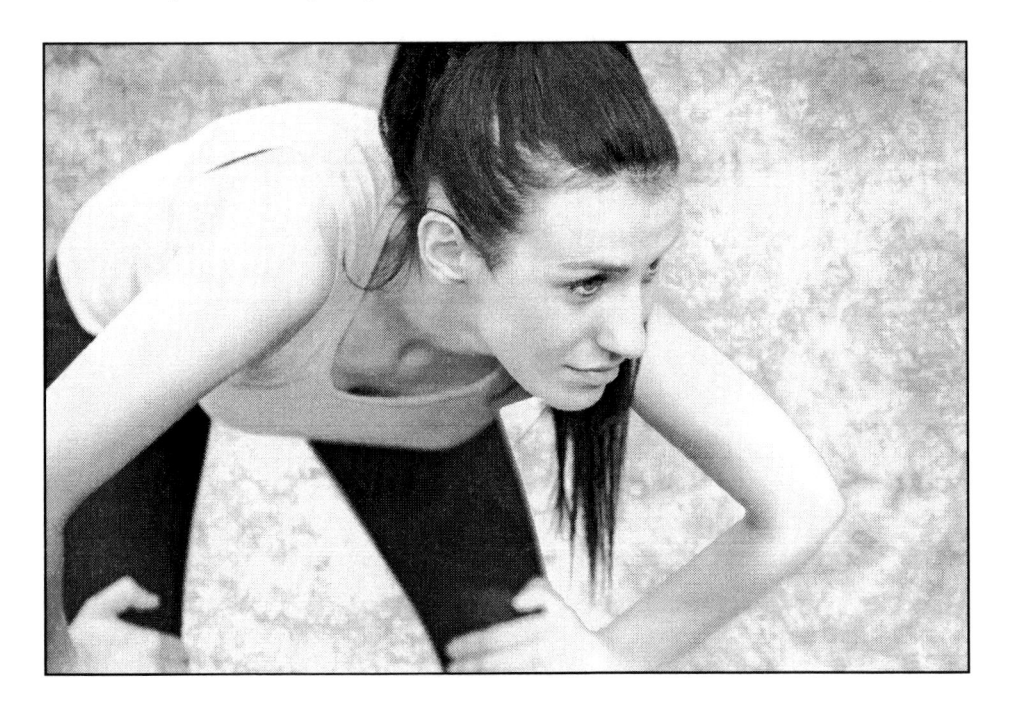

You just spent nine months growing a human being and then labored for hours to bring your child into the world. You may feel worn out, have pain, and feel extremely fatigued. Although common and expected, this type of pain can be managed and minimized with proper treatment. If you feel any of these symptoms:

1. Talk with your healthcare provider about the pain you're experiencing. It may or may not be normal soreness in the early postpartum period.

2. Find a women's health physical therapist that specializes in postpartum care.

3. Avoid heavy lifting and positions that exacerbate your pain. Use proper body mechanics and posture when handling your baby. Take a warm bath with Epsom salts if okayed by your healthcare provider. Baths may have to be avoided until you stop bleeding.

8. You may feel as if you're having the longest period ever, eight-weeks long to be exact.

In the first eight weeks after giving birth, you may still experience bleeding from the vagina. If this persists beyond eight weeks, or is an unusually heavy flow, take the following steps:

1. Talk with your healthcare provider to ensure the amount of bleeding you're experiencing is normal.

2. Find a women's health physical therapist that specializes in postpartum care.

3. Until you've stopped bleeding, avoid positions or exercises that elevate the hips above the heart level, including bridges and inversions.

9. You may feel as if something is falling out of your vagina.

Oftentimes, in the first eight to twelve weeks after giving birth you may feel heaviness in your pelvis, a feeling of pressure, or as if something is coming out of the vagina. Involution, or the process of the uterus returning to its original size, shape and position, can take up to eight weeks. In the meantime:

1. Don't panic! How you feel during the first eight to twelve weeks after giving birth is not how you will feel for the rest of your life. Talk with your healthcare provider to see if you may have weakness, prolapse, or instability leading to these sensations.

2. Find a women's health physical therapist that specializes in postpartum care so that you can learn the proper self-care tools and exercises to alleviate your symptoms.

3. Avoid any heavy lifting, pushing, or pulling which increases abdominal pressure. Use the pelvic brace with transitions, and you can Kegel as long as it is pain free.

10. Your baby may need to be extracted using a vacuum, resulting in your baby having a cone-shaped head.

Depending on the position of the baby, how long you've been pushing, and the health of you and your baby, your healthcare provider may use a vacuum to accelerate the birth of the baby. The pressure of the vacuum can oftentimes cause your baby to have a cone-shaped head, and may lead to additional pelvic floor muscle weakness for you. The cone shape is nothing to worry about. The head resumes its shape so don't panic; it's only a temporary thing. Consider taking children born with vacuum or forceps to a cranial-sacral therapist or a chiropractor that specializes in children. If you end up using a vacuum and find yourself with additional PFM weakness:

1. Talk with your healthcare provider about your options.

2. Find a women's health physical therapist that specializes in postpartum care to address any pelvic floor muscle weakness that could result from use of the vacuum.

3. Avoid any heavy lifting, pushing, or pulling which increases pelvic pressure. Use the pelvic brace with transitions, and you can Kegel as long as it is pain free.

11. If you're planning on breastfeeding, your nipples could bleed.

Breastfeeding is challenging and takes practice. If the baby latches onto the breast incorrectly, your nipples may crack and bleed. You can also get clogged milk ducts that cause discomfort, pain, and can lead to a serious infection called mastitis if not managed properly. If this happens: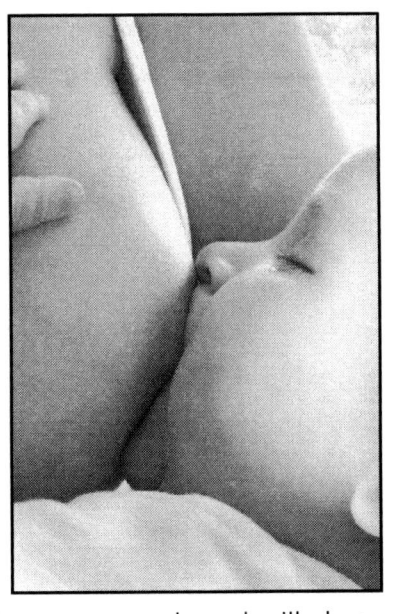

1. Talk with your healthcare provider about your options.

2. Find a lactation consultant as soon as you notice any unusual discomfort during breastfeeding—the sooner the better!

3. Find a women's health physical therapist to manage clogged milk ducts with modalities such as ultrasound, cold laser therapy, and manual massage techniques.

12. You will likely require stitches in the perineum following vaginal birth.

In an ideal world, all vaginal deliveries would involve a perineum that gracefully stretches, but does not tear, during delivery. Unfortunately, we find that most women at our healing center do require stitches, or sutures, following vaginal birth. Although stitches may cause pain or discomfort in the first few weeks following birth, they generally allow the vaginal tissue to heal in the best possible manner. Here are steps you can take to encourage full healing of the perineum:

1. Follow your physician's or midwife's instructions for postpartum perineal care, such as the use of a perineal bottle, cold compress and/or sitz baths.

2. At your postpartum check-up, ask if you may start to massage the scar tissue to increase the tissue extensibility. Find a women's health physical therapist who can teach you how to massage the vaginal scar tissue to achieve the optimal flexibility and strength.

3. You may think that the vaginal scar healed, until you experience pain with intercourse. Pain with intercourse may signal that the scar tissue needs more attention. It is never too late to see a women's health physical therapist to assess and treat vaginal scar tissue.

13. You may receive an episiotomy, even if it is not in your birth plan.

It is our experience that in general, episiotomies are more painful in recovery than natural tears. However, there may be situations during delivery when the physician is faced with difficult decisions on how to proceed based on the health of the mom and baby. If the baby needs to be delivered rapidly, your physician may choose to perform an episiotomy. With time and focused attention, you can heal your episiotomy scar. Here are steps you can take:

1. Follow your physician's or midwife's instructions for postpartum perineal care, such as the use of a perineal bottle, cold compress and/or sitz baths.

2. At your postpartum check-up, ask if you may start to massage the scar tissue to increase the tissue extensibility. Find a women's health physical therapist who can teach you how to massage the vaginal scar tissue to achieve the optimal flexibility and strength.

3. You may think that the episiotomy has healed, until you experience pain with intercourse. Pain with intercourse may signal that the scar tissue needs more attention. It is never too late to see a women's health physical therapist to assess and treat the episiotomy.

14. You will use a perineal squirt bottle instead of "wiping" after urination.

The tissues of the perineum will be very sensitive following vaginal birth, especially if you receive stitches from a tear or episiotomy. You will definitely not want to "wipe" this area with tissue after using the bathroom. The hospital staff will provide you with a squirt bottle that you will use to clean the perineum after urination and bowel movements. Do not fret. Most moms report that the perineal squirt bottle feels great on the perineum.

1. Follow the hospital staff's instructions for use of the perineal squirt bottle.

2. Make sure that you can take one of these bottles home for continued perineal care.

3. If you continue to have pain with urination or defecation at your postpartum check-up, discuss this situation with your healthcare provider. You would likely benefit from seeing a women's health physical therapist, who can help relieve pain from surrounding scar tissue or muscle spasm.

15. You may not be able to control your urine after delivery.

Tired muscles make it difficult to hold urine, while a catheter during delivery may temporarily disrupt the signal that you need to urinate. Many women are surprised and embarrassed that they cannot hold their urine at the hospital. This is common and will improve with time! You can take the following steps:

1. To reduce urinary incontinence, perform a pelvic brace (see Chapter 4, page 79) every time you move from sit-to-stand, cough, laugh, sneeze or lift your baby.

2. If performing a Kegel is not painful, you can begin to retrain your pelvic floor muscles. Refer to Chapter 9. Stop performing Kegels if they increase pain at the perineum or worsen your symptoms.

3. If you are experiencing incontinence at your six-week postpartum check-up, bring it to the attention of your physician or midwife and ask for a referral to physical therapy. All postpartum women should take part in a supervised pelvic floor and abdominal rehabilitation program so that they can regain their pelvic power.

16. You may have to sit on a donut cushion when your friends and family come to visit.

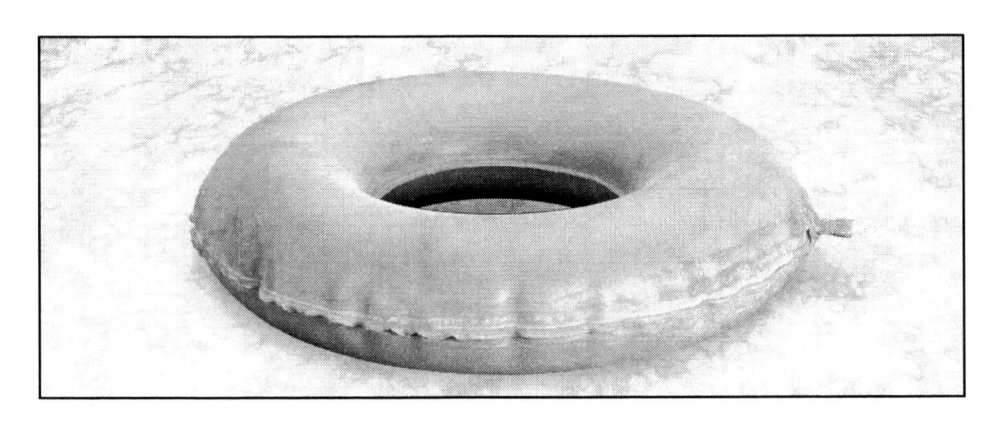

Most women do not picture themselves receiving guests while sitting on a special cushion after childbirth. However, the reality is that perineal tears, episiotomies and tailbone injuries can make sitting very painful after childbirth.

1. Speak with your healthcare provider to find the cause of your pain and to receive instructions for further treatment and self-care.

2. Send a trusted friend or family member to a pharmacy or surgical supply store to purchase a donut foam ring pillow. You can also order one online.

3. Seek out the care of a women's health physical therapist as soon as possible to begin your hands-on healing.

17. You may have difficulty controlling gas and bowel movements.

The same muscles that control urination also hold back gas and bowel movements when needed. These muscles are often weak following pregnancy and childbirth. Commonly a healing episiotomy or perineal tear prevents these muscles from performing at their best. If you experience a third or fourth degree tear, you are at high risk for experiencing the above symptoms. You can take the following steps:

1. When you feel the urge for a bowel movement, do not panic. Try to walk calmly to the nearest restroom. Becoming anxious often makes the stomach hurt worse and may decrease your ability to hold off a bowel movement.

2. If performing a Kegel is not painful, you can begin to retrain your pelvic floor muscles. Refer to Chapter 9. You can focus your Kegels at the anal sphincter by imagining that you are stopping the release of gas. If you are sitting, you can pretend you are lifting a pea off the chair with your anal sphincter. Stop performing Kegels if they increase pain at the perineum or worsen your symptoms.

3. If you are experiencing gas or fecal incontinence at your six-week postpartum check-up, bring it to the attention of your physician or midwife and ask for a referral to physical therapy. All postpartum women should take part in a supervised pelvic floor and abdominal rehabilitation program. You may also benefit from gentle massage of your healing perineal tear or episiotomy.

18. Your vaginal tear or episiotomy may require additional medical care due to granulation tissue.

Many women present to our clinic with perineal tissue that has become stuck in the healing process. The result is referred to as granulation tissue. This condition results in pain that is excruciatingly high for the healing perineum. The tissue appears bright red and may bleed. Steps you can take:

1. If you are experiencing constant pain at the perineum and have bright red, raw tissue, contact your healthcare provider immediately. Healthcare providers generally maintain that an examination is not necessary prior to six weeks postpartum, but you must be your own advocate and insist on being seen if you are experiencing excruciating pain. Your doctor can provide treatment for the granulation tissue.

2. You may require a donut cushion for sitting and feeding your baby as your perineum heals.

3. After receiving clearance from your healthcare provider, seek out the care of a pelvic floor physical therapist to ensure that the perineum and pelvic floor muscles regain their flexibility and strength.

19. You may develop an infection in your C-section scar and require additional medical care.

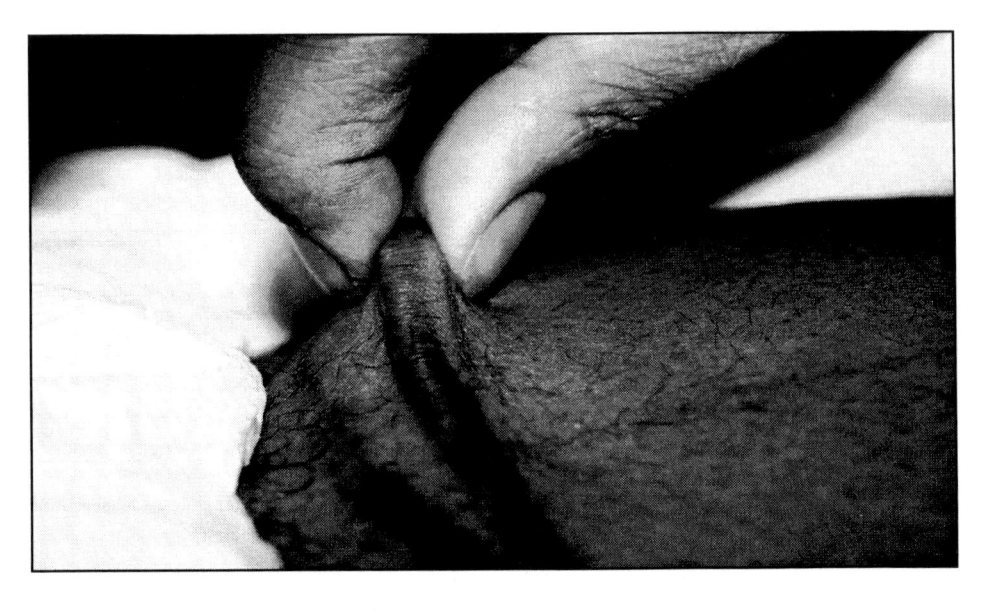

Many women acquire infections in the hospital that complicate and delay the healing of their Cesarean scar. If your scar becomes infected, you may need to stay in the hospital longer or receive care from a visiting nurse once you are home. Here are some steps you can take:

1. Report any signs of wound infection to your physician or hospital staff.

2. Use a pelvic brace, as described in Chapter 4, page 79 for all transitions and avoid jackknifing (p.59) to prevent excessive stress on the healing scar.

3. Once the infection has resolved, the sutures are removed and the Steri-strips have fallen off, you may begin to massage your own scar. (Numerous scar massage techniques are detailed in my other book, *Ending Female Pain*.) A pelvic floor physical therapist can also instruct you on effective scar massage techniques. Always receive physician clearance before beginning self-scar massage.

20. You may experience air escaping from the vagina during yoga class.

Weak vaginal muscles may cause some unpleasant noises and sensations with inverted yoga poses, such as plow and even downward facing dog. As shocking as this may sound, it is a very common postpartum complaint. Here are some steps you can take:

1. Do not return to yoga class or yoga practice until you are cleared by your physician/midwife and have stopped bleeding. It is dangerous to perform any poses in which the hips are higher than the head before the uterus completely returns to its prepregnancy position.

2. If Kegels do not cause pain, begin a pelvic floor strengthening program. Refer to Chapter 9. A supervised program with a pelvic floor physical therapist will provide you with the most targeted results.

21. Baby blues can be caused by the foods you are eating. You feel what you eat.

Inflammation could be the cause of your baby blues and other mood disorders. Inflammation appears to be a primary determinant of depressive symptoms such as flat mood, mood swings, slowed thinking, avoidance behavior, anxiety and altered perceptions. Wheat and gluten are powerful drivers of inflammation. Dairy products can also drive inflammation in the system. For postpartum women, wheat, gluten and dairy can lead to increased levels of inflammation and can be the underlying cause of their depression.

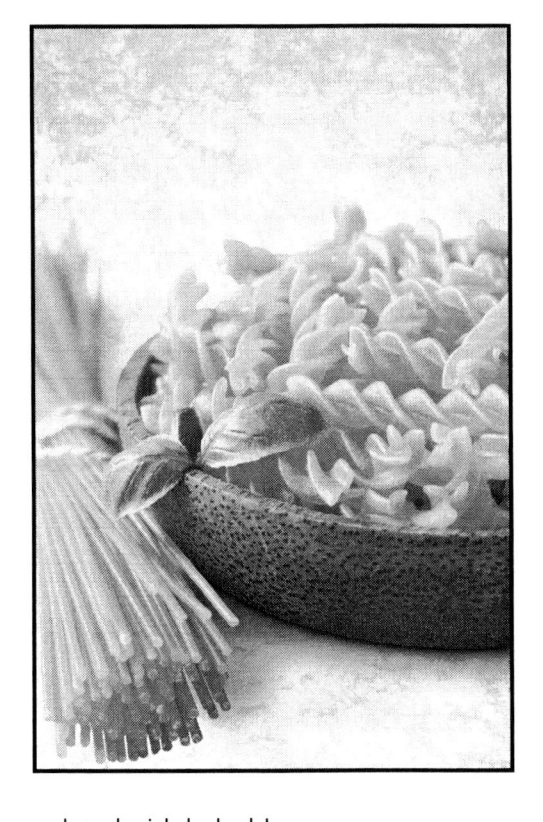

Postpartum women are more vulnerable to autoimmune disorders and inflammation due to the high demands of pregnancy and the quick hormonal shifts that happen after the baby is born. Cytokines, and other inflammatory by-products, are released in the blood when there is inflammation in the body. These inflammatory messengers are found in high numbers in the blood of postpartum women and have been directly correlated with baby blues.

Not every woman gets depressed. Why? Because you need the proper circumstances. Autoimmune conditions and disorders and high levels of inflammation in the body require three platforms:

- there needs to be a genetic susceptibility (it's in your genes);

- there have to be environmental triggers (we are swimming in a pool of toxins—pesticides, pollutions, GMO foods, processed foods);

- there has to be intestinal permeability (gut-brain connection disruption).

To combat the baby blues, food and lifestyle changes are very necessary. If you want to regain mental clarity and feel like your old self again, start with what you eat and then add some exercise and meditation into the mix. Below I have listed the top three recommendations that could help you regain your mental health in a holistic non-pharmacological way.

1. See your MD immediately if you are suffering from depression, anxiety or psychosis. Seek the right help from someone who knows how to treat baby blues.

2. Eliminate inflammatory agents and eat only real foods. No processed foods allowed. Dr. Kelly Brogan, holistic psychiatrist, recommends a diet free of wheat and gluten for at least one to three months or longer until you stabilize. Additionally, Dr. Brogan is a firm believer in helping the body reach homeostasis by including supplements and vitamins into the diet. Dietary supplements and vitamins and eating the right whole foods work to not only strengthen the body from the inside out, but also to provide a platform by which health can be achieved without the intervention of pharmacological agents. For more information on the food-inflammation-depression connection please visit *www.kellyBroganMD.com*.

3. Breastfeeding decreases the likelihood of postpartum depression. Breastfeeding is hard work and requires support. Get lactation help right away and have weekly lactation consultations if possible until breastfeeding has been established.

22. Your bottom will hurt (hemorrhoids).

Hemorrhoids are a real pain in the butt and you might get hemorrhoids that are so large you could mistake them for another unborn child. After my labor, I was shocked to learn that a lot of my pain was driven by hemorrhoids. I did everything to get rid of them and it took weeks before my bottom felt well again. Be aware that they can hurt pretty badly. For some women their anus will never be the same again.

THINGS YOU CAN DO ARE:

1. Continue your sitz baths and use your perineal bottle.

2. Try natural over-the-counter remedies or see an herbalist. See your physical therapist for low-level laser light therapy. Low-level laser works wonders for hemorrhoids and it's a natural solution. We use this modality at my healing center all the time with great results.

3. If necessary contact your doctor and get a medical prescription for steroidal cream to eliminate them.

23. Blood pooling can happen (hematoma).

Hematoma is a collection of localized blood outside the blood vessel that can occur in the vulva, vaginal/paravaginal area, and/or retroperitoneum. Women who develop hematomas usually complain about pain with sitting or an inability to void.

1. Don't despair, stay calm and see your OB/GYN or MD immediately if you discover that you have developed one.

2. Seek help from a physical therapist once you have healed to get the pelvic floor muscles back to optimal functioning.

24. Your baby may need help getting out.

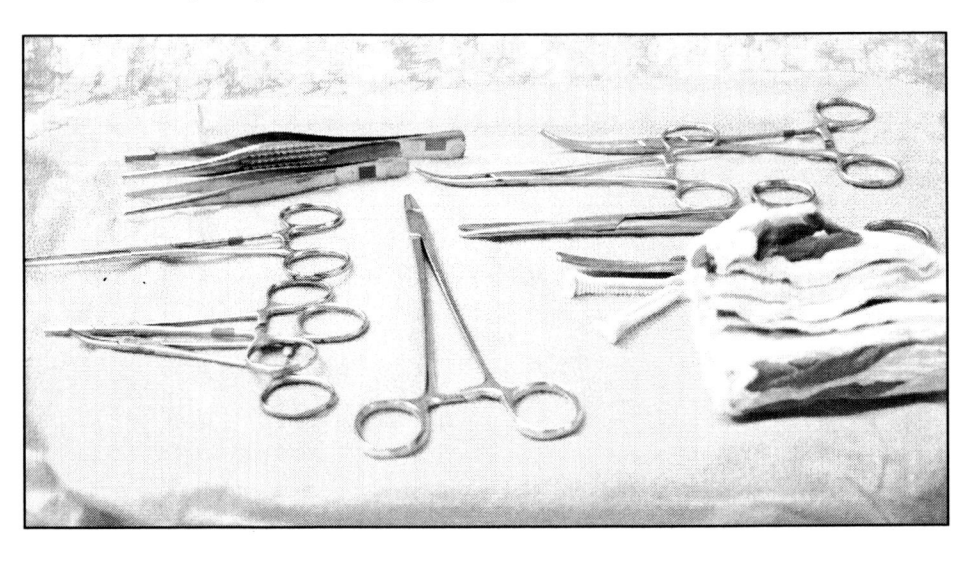

Assisted or operative vaginal delivery sometimes is necessary to get the baby out. Forceps delivery can result in tears to the perineum or vagina. Baby could have temporary bruising or cuts.

1. Make sure to discuss these types of delivery with your doctor or midwife and find out what experience they have in doing these types of deliveries. Before you consent, ask why assisted vaginal delivery is necessary and what instrument will be used.

2. Seek help from a physical therapist once you have healed (usually six weeks) to get the pelvic floor muscles back to optimal functioning. Scar tissue can also result; seek a physical therapist who can help you heal by performing scar massage.

3. Rest as much as possible so you can heal faster and don't lift anything heavier than the baby. Stay positive and know that you will heal but it could take a while.

25. When your water breaks, the experience may not be like what you see in the movies.

Many times your doctor may break your water at the hospital with a small instrument. I know that when I had my baby I was almost completely dilated and my water would not break. I imagined delivering my baby in a bubble of water! But after several hours of my doctor asking me to allow him to break it, I finally gave in. As soon as my doctor broke my water, the baby came. Here are some things you should know:

1. If your water breaks at home avoid the bathtub and stick with the shower for pain relief. Call your doctor or midwife immediately.

2. There is no sex if your water is broken so if you are imagining an orgasmic birth remember that sexual intercourse is a no-no.

3. You could be walking around for hours if not days with "broken waters." The baby has its own divine timing and it will come when it is good and ready to do so. So chill out and don't panic.

Now that we have learned about things that can happen in childbirth, let's go into the next section of the book. Here you will learn how to train your abdominals safely and correctly. We will also teach you a full body exercise program that will keep your body strong and powerful and prepare it for childbirth and the marathon of pushing the baby out. To help ease stresses related to pregnancy we introduce you to mind/body medicine and aromatherapy. Enjoy this part of *Ending Pain in Pregnancy* and learn how to create balance in three key areas: the body, mind and soul.

PART FOUR:

EXERCISES AND TOOLS FOR THE ABDOMINALS, BODY, MIND AND SPIRIT

"To keep the body in good health is a duty...otherwise we shall not be able to keep our mind strong and clear."

— Buddha

Chapter 12

THE NEW CORE FOR THE RESTORATION OF PREGNANCY POWER

Pregnant women are often concerned about what their abdominals will look like after birthing their child, but our abdominal muscles serve a far greater purpose than looking tight and awesome. This area is part of what I call the Pregnancy Pelvic Power relay station. Our abdominal muscles create stability in our hips, PFMs and lumbar spine. They also provide support for our internal organs, house the first two chakras and prevent energy leaks. If your abdominals are in a weakened state or are compromised by having a diastasis recti separation, you are at greater risk for pregnancy-related pelvic dysfunction and pain. These problems include an increase in urinary leaking, urgency and frequency of urination, hip pain, pelvic floor muscle weakness or spasms and pelvic/low back pain.

I cannot overstress the importance of intelligent core training during pregnancy. Many women love to work their abdominals, but are doing it all wrong. Performing the same old crunches during pregnancy will not improve your pregnancy pelvic power. In fact, traditional abdominal exercises can actually contribute to your pregnancy pelvic pain and symptoms. The exercises in this chapter do not require that you put your hands behind your head and lift your shoulders off of the floor. Instead you will be working on the deepest abdominal muscle, the transversus abdominis (TrA), while simultaneously engaging your PFMs. This co-contraction is called a pelvic brace and is the foundation of all the other exercises in this program. It creates power from within the body and can result in lifelong changes. Proper co-contraction of TrA and a low-level Kegel contraction can result in improved sexual power, better bladder and bowel control, and less pelvic, hip and low back pain. At the bare minimum, you should close up the diastasis and work on training your transverse abdominal muscles as this will help keep you strong during pregnancy.

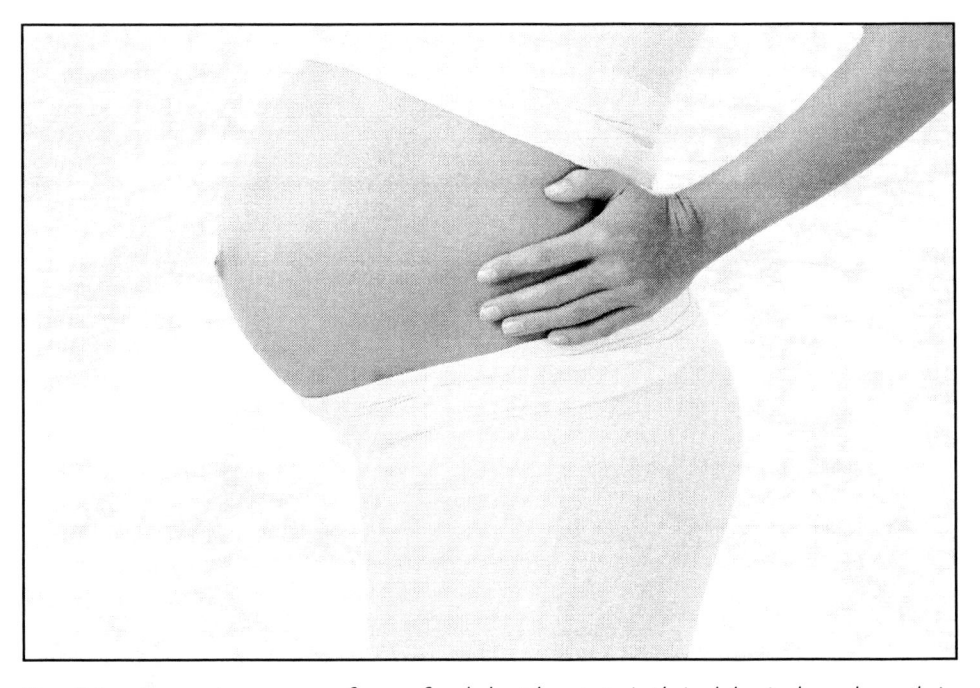

Description: Pregnant women are often confused about how to train their abdominal muscles as their pregnancy progresses.

Now is the time to reclaim your body and to work within your fitness and symptom levels. First, I will describe what a diastasis recti separation is and how to test for one. Then I will prescribe two corrective exercises to close up the separation and get you back on the road to reclaiming your pregnancy pelvic power. The New Core for Pregnancy Power Program includes six levels of exercises, which can be found in Table 12.2. As most abdominal exercises will require the alignment of neutral spine, practice this first and make sure you have it mastered before starting any of the other exercises.

The New Core for Pregnancy Power uses a physio ball. Table 12.4 provides guidance on how to purchase one. In pregnancy balance becomes challenged, so be careful not to fall off when using the ball. To maintain proper balance on the ball sit in good posture and keep the feet hip-width apart or wider. This creates a safe base of support. You can also place the ball on a ball stand or against the wall to give yourself better support.

Table 12.3 details the most common mistakes made while training the abdominal muscles using the New Core for Pregnancy Pelvic Power. Familiarize yourself with these common mistakes so that you don't repeat them as you progress in your core program. Once you have the proper foundation and your diastasis recti separation is closed up, you can begin the New Core training for stronger abdominal muscles and lifelong female pelvic power. Now let's get started.

Specific Considerations for Abdominal Diastasis Recti Separation during Pregnancy

Diastasis recti abdominis (DRA) is a separation of the rectus abdominis muscle at the linea alba. The outermost abdominal muscles, called the rectus abdominis, form two halves, called right and left recti muscles. These two halves are covered by fibrous connective tissue from other muscles and join at the central seam called the linea alba. Like a zipper, these abdominal muscles can separate due to incorrect biomechanics, pregnancy or with sudden weight gain. DRA can also result from performing abdominal exercises incorrectly or by suddenly sitting up straight in bed from a horizontal lying down position, called "jackknifing."

DRA has profound effects on the function of the pelvic floor muscles and bladder and bowel function. The PFMs and the abdominals have a synergistic relationship. When DRA is present, it decreases the ability of the PFMs to contract effectively, contributing to pelvic pain, urinary, stress and fecal incontinence and sexual dysfunction. DRA leaves the abdominals in a weakened state. When this separation is present in women with pelvic, hip and/or low back pain, the PFMs cannot function optimally which makes the contract/relax exercises more difficult than they need to be. Make sure to test for DRA as defined in the next section. I would recommend not beginning the core series until your DRA measures two-fingers wide or less. Ideally I like the DRA to measure one-finger width as I find too much dysfunction with the PFMs when the separation is bigger.

The function and insertion of the other abdominal muscles, called the transversus abdominis and internal/external obliques, are hindered when you have a DRA. This altered state of the abdominals can lead to the formation of trigger points in the abdominal wall. These abdominal trigger points can cause urinary urgency and pelvic pain. Many times these abdominal trigger points can lead to pain above the pubic bone and can cause the sensation of a bladder infection without actually having one. Always see a doctor if you have lower abdominal pain as this can be a sign of a serious problem.

Before beginning the New Core for Pregnancy Power Program, you must first determine if you have a DRA by performing the test described below. If you find a DRA, perform the corrective exercises to close the gap before progressing to the more advanced core program. There are two exercises that you can perform to correct your DRA, one seated and one lying down on your back. If you have very weak abdominal muscles, start with the seated exercise and then incorporate the lying down corrective exercise in one week. Many pregnant women are uncomfortable performing exercises on their back after the first trimester; the seated position for DRA correction exercises is also advisable in these cases. During pregnancy the goal is to make sure the DRA does not get bigger. After the baby comes test yourself and start to close the gap of your abdominals as soon as you can. It takes time to close up a DRA separation. Be consistent with the correction exercises and keep in mind the "Tips to Avoid Making the DRA Worse" that are discussed below.

Diagram Description: Notice diastasis recti separation at the linea alba and the wide gap between the rectus muscles. Source: Winston Johnson

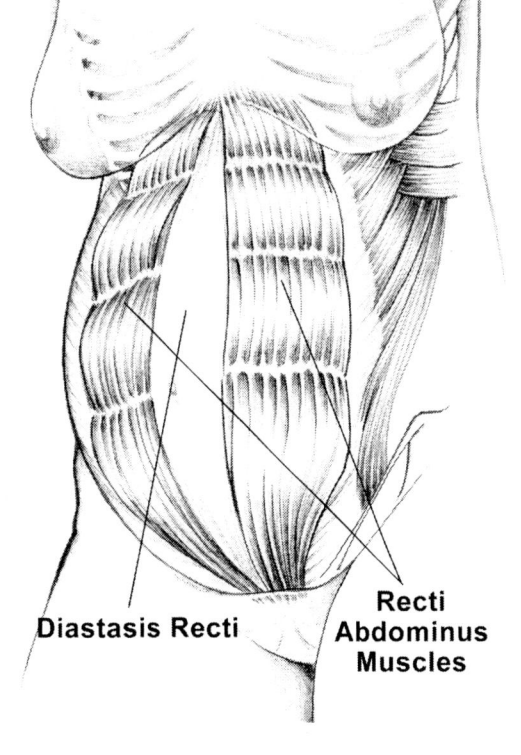

Diastasis Recti

Recti Abdominus Muscles

Table 12.1: DRA Tracking
Use this chart to keep track of your progress as you work to close your DRA.

DATE	2 INCHES ABOVE	AT UMBILICUS	2 INCHES BELOW

How to Test for DRA Separation

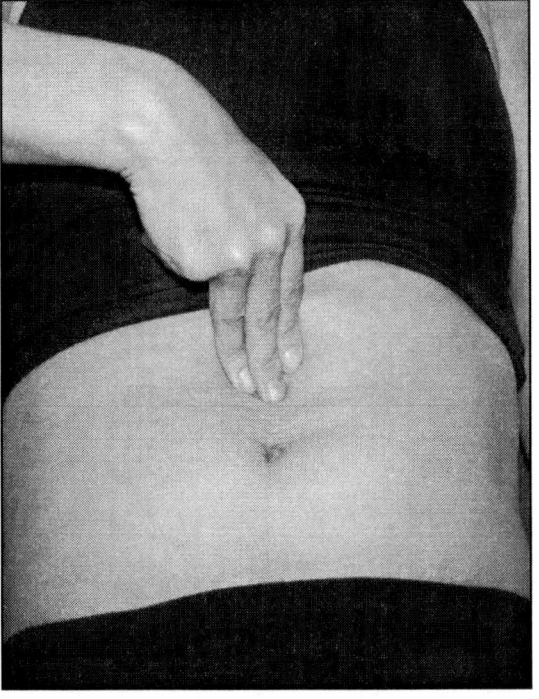

1. Lie on your back with your knees bent.

2. Exhale and slightly lift your upper back off the floor with your arms reaching forward. Check how many fingers you are able to insert horizontally two inches above the umbilicus, at the umbilicus, and two inches below the umbilicus. Make sure not to contract your TrA when testing DRA.

3. DRA of one- to two-fingers separation is considered normal. A three-finger separation requires correction. Corrective exercises are used to close up any separation of the abdominals. The closer the DRA is the less symptomatic you will be. If you still have symptoms at two-finger width, then you need to correct it further. DRA correction in my protocol is driven by symptoms; for some women, the separation must be closed up to one-finger width to find relief.

Tips to Avoid Making the DRA Worse

1. Avoid jackknifing out of bed. Instead, logroll out of bed by engaging your abdominals, turning completely to the side and then use your arms to push yourself to a seated position. A pelvic brace is ideal to do before changing positions.

2. Avoid sudden weight gains.

3. Avoid coughing or sneezing without first engaging your abdominals and PFMs.

4. Avoid traditional abdominal exercises such as abdominal crunches, which can make the DRA larger.

5. Avoid exercises at the gym or daily activities that make your belly pop out, also called the diastasis recti bulge.

6. Avoiding leaning forward such as bending from the hips to pick something up from the floor.

7. Avoid bending forward to pick up young children or to lift them out of their cribs.

Finding Neutral Spine (NS)

Before we start with the corrective exercise for DRA, you must understand how to maintain and achieve neutral spine. Neutral spine is the natural position of the spine when all the parts of the spine—cervical, thoracic and lumbar—are in excellent alignment. This position is the most favorable to be in when performing the Pregnancy Pelvic Power Core program because in this position your abdominal and PFMs can optimally contract and relax as needed while executing the core program. You must be able to find this neutral spine in all positions including lying down, seated and standing. In pregnancy NS is difficult to maintain because of the big pregnancy belly but it is not impossible. Focused awareness about your posture and making corrections so your spine is at neutral will be of great benefit to you.

Neutral Spine (NS)

WHAT TO DO:

1. Lie on your back with your knees bent and your feet flat on the floor. Make sure your lower extremity is in alignment. Imagine there is one continuous line from your hips to your knees to your feet. To accomplish this make sure your feet are parallel and not out to the side.

2. Keep your arms at your side and keep the body relaxed.

3. Exhale and use your abdominal muscles to press your lower back into the floor performing a posterior pelvic tilt (PPT). Inhale, release the PPT and return to NS.

4. Exhale and pull your lower spine up and away from the floor creating an anterior pelvic tilt (ANT). Inhale, relax and release the ANT.

5. Most women have their spines either in an anterior pelvic tilt or a posterior pelvic tilt because of muscle imbalances and weakness. Neutral spine is a place in between these two extreme positions. Practice this exercise and get a sense of what it means to be in neutral spine for you before moving forward.

Corrective DRA Exercises: Seated Splinted Holds

WHAT TO DO:

1. Sit in cross-legged position with correct posture, shoulders over hips or sit in a chair.

2. Crisscross your hands over your belly, or use a scarf or Dyna-Band to bring the abdominals together.

3. Inhale through your nose into your belly. Exhale through your mouth to initiate the belly button reaching toward the spine, engaging the abdominals while keeping a NS. Hold this position.

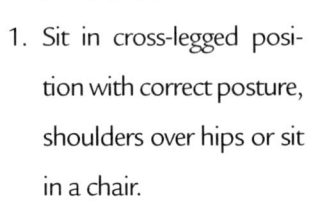

4. Simultaneously, pull the sides of your abdominals together with your arms to approximate the recti muscles. You should also do a gentle PFM contraction while doing this exercise to avoid bearing down into the PFMs.

5. Breathe naturally and hold for five seconds. Return to start position.

6. Perform twenty times, two to three times a day.

Corrective DRA Exercises: Lying Down Splinted Head Raises

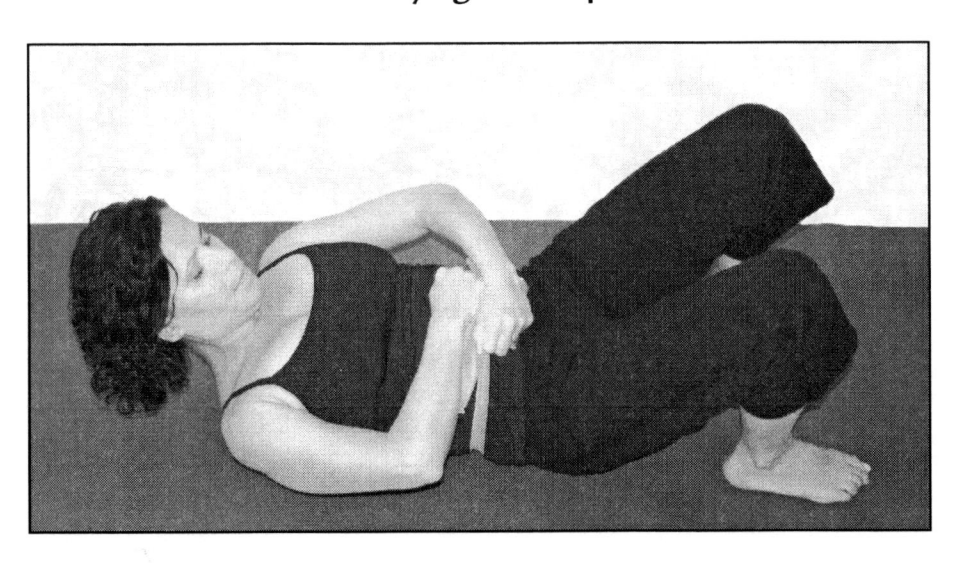

WHAT TO DO:

1. Lie on your back with your knees bent on the floor.

2. Bring your belly button to your spine while maintaining a NS.

3. Crisscross your hands over your belly, or use a scarf or Dyna-Band to bring the abdominals together.

4. Exhale very slowly, contract your abdominals and raise your head toward your chest just before the diastasis bulge begins. To begin, keep the shoulders in contact with the floor. To maximize the approximation of the recti muscles you can use a large scarf or wrap to bring the muscles together. You should also do a gentle PFM contraction while doing this exercise.

5. Breathe naturally and hold for five seconds. Return to start position. As you get stronger, you will be able to lift your shoulders off the floor.

6. Perform twenty times, two to three times a day.

Once you have become aware of your diastasis and have begun to take corrective measures, you will be ready to move ahead into the other exercises highlighted in the New Core for Pregnancy Pelvic Power Program.

Your Diastasis Recti Is Corrected: What Now?

Once you have corrected your diastasis recti and it is within a one to two-finger separation, you are ready to embark on the more difficult exercises of the New Core for Pregnancy Pelvic Power. All of the exercises in this amazing program involve a transverse belly hold. You must master this foundational exercise first, before progressing through the rest of the New Core for Pregnancy Power Program.

How to Progress through the Abdominal Program

There are several exercises to the New Core for Pregnancy Pelvic Power Program. Do not move to a more difficult exercise before you master the previous level. When you can perform twenty reps, two to three times in great form you have mastered an exercise and can move to the next level. You can be working at two levels at the same time on different exercises as long as you have mastered the previous level.

The New Core for Pregnancy Pelvic Power

Table 12.2: Trade Secrets: The New Core for Pregnancy Pelvic Power

Level 1: Corrective DRA Exercises, Seated or Lying Down
Level 2: Transverse Belly Holds: Foundational exercise for all other exercises
Level 3: Seated Leg Press or Lying on Back Leg Press
Level 4: Ball Marching or Lying on Back Marching
Level 5: Ball Arms
Level 6: Box Planks or Knee or Toe Planks (depends on your strength; these are advanced exercises)

Table 12.3: Common Mistakes: What to Avoid in Your Pregnancy Pelvic Power Training Program

1. Avoid holding your breath while performing your abdominal exercises. If you hold the breath, you will leak urine and not activate the core muscles correctly.

2. Do not advance to a more difficult abdominal exercise without first mastering the previous level.

3. Never leak urine. If you leak with your abdominal exercises, then the exercise is too difficult for you. You should return to the previous level and master that exercise without leaking.

4. Do not exacerbate your pelvic, hip or low back pain. There is a thin line between intelligent working out and creating more tension in the abdominal and PFMs. If you experience an increase in pain, you should return to the previous level and master those exercises without pain.

5. Avoid sticking your butt into the air when performing exercises such as plank. If you find that you are doing so, then you are using too much of your arm and leg power.

6. Do not flare out your ribs when doing the core program. Instead keep them pulled in toward your spine. If your ribs pop out, then you are not activating the core properly.

7. Avoid sagging the lower back when performing your plank exercises.

8. Do not over-contract your abdominal core muscles. Over-contraction activates the obliques instead of the deeper transversus abdominis muscle. You are over-contracting if you feel a bearing-down sensation in the pelvis or if your lower abdominals "pop out" with contraction. You may also feel increased pelvic pressure if you over-activate the abdominal core muscles.

9. Do not forget to co-contract the PFMs with the transverse holds while performing the New Core exercises. True core strength requires activation of both muscle groups through the entire set of exercises. This co-contraction is at about 30 percent of effort, not 100 percent. Remember: PFM is a low-level contraction.

10. Avoid rounding or arching the lower back while performing the core exercises. Keep your spine in neutral.

How to Purchase a Physio Ball

You will need to purchase a physio ball for the pregnancy abdominal strengthening series. The balls usually come in four different sizes depending on the height of the user. Use Table 12.4 as a reference when you purchase your physio ball. In addition to doing the abdominal exercises with the ball, it can also be used for stretching and as a support in labor and delivery. Many birth coaches recommend that you have one for the birth as well, so you will get plenty of use out of it. The ball is a great tool that will help support you if you find that a stretch or exercise is too difficult; it challenges your stabilizing and balancing muscles in unique ways. Be careful not to fall off the ball when you use it.

Table 12.4: Physio Ball Height Guidelines

HEIGHT OF USER IN FEET & INCHES	SIZE OF BALL IN CENTIMETERS
4' 7" – 5' 0"	45 cm ball
5' 1" – 5' 6"	55 cm ball
5' 7" – 6' 1"	65 cm ball
6' 2" – 6' 8"	75 cm ball

Proper Seated Ball Posture

Seated Ball Posture

WHAT TO DO:

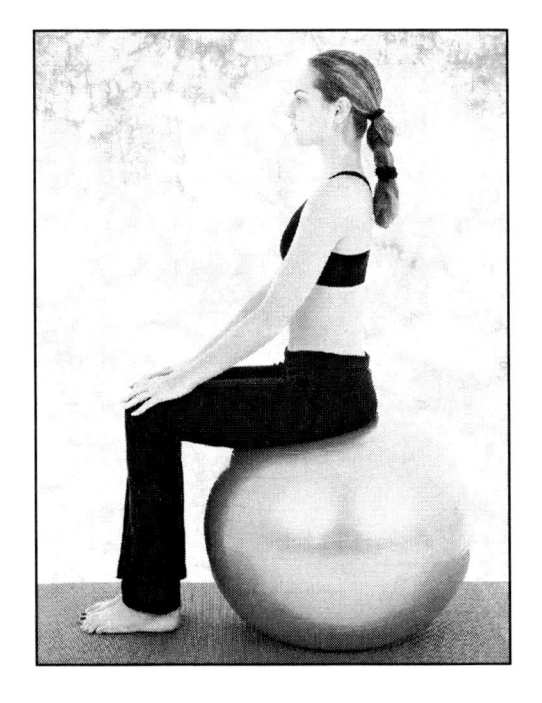

1. Sit tall on the ball with your weight evenly distributed on your sit bones, ears aligned with the shoulders, and abdominal muscles pulled in.

2. Your knees and hips should form a right angle with your feet flat on the floor. It's acceptable for your hips to be slightly higher than your knees, but not the other way around because it will put stress on your lower back and leg muscles.

3. Pull your shoulder blades back toward each other; imagine you are putting your shoulder blades into your back pockets, in and down.

4. Once comfortably in this posture, practice five to ten minutes of diaphragmatic breathing together with reverse Kegels or contract/relax Kegels, depending on where you are in your Kegel program as defined in Chapter 9.

5. This is called "good ball posture" and is the basis of many of the exercises in this series.

WHAT TO WATCH OUT FOR:

1. Incorrect ball size will put increased pressure and strain on muscles. Use Table 12.4 on page 300 to determine which ball is the proper size for your height.

2. Avoid rounding the shoulders or lower back and sticking your chin out, as these will cause pain or strain to your body and could lead to injury.

BENEFITS:

1. Provides good sensory input for the reverse and contract/relax Kegel exercises, as your PFMs are in direct contact with the surface of the ball.

2. Reinforces good sitting posture which will help decrease pain associated with poor sitting and/or slouching at work or home.

Transverse Belly Holds

Learning to activate your TrA during pregnancy will keep your core strong, minimize muscle weakness, and help you avoid excessive downward pressure through the pelvis. Once you learn how to tune into the TrA muscle, it is particularly important to use this skill during functional and transitional movements as a pelvic brace (see Chapter 4).

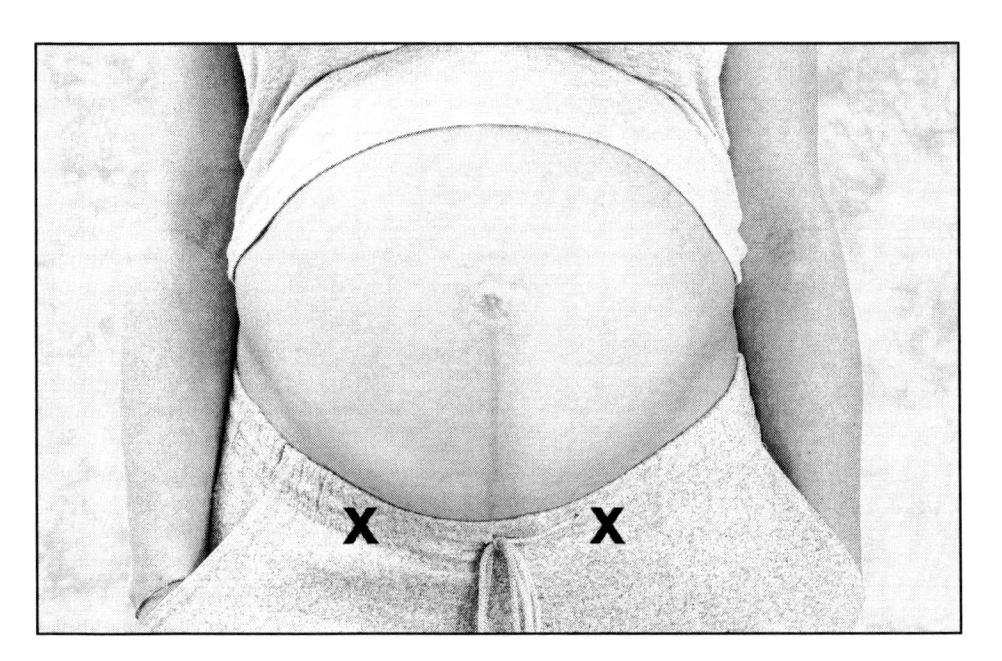

Diagram Description: X marks the location where you can feel and locate the transverse abdominal muscles

WHAT TO DO:

1. This exercise may be done sitting on a ball or chair, supine or standing. Keep a neutral spine as you take a full belly breath. As you exhale draw your belly closer and more firmly toward the spine. As you pull in your abdominals try to imagine that you are trying to squeeze into an old pair of jeans that don't fit. Make sure to keep a NS.

2. Additional cues that work well to activate and train the transverse muscle are:

    a. Imagine that you are doing a Kegel that moves all the way up to the lower part of your abdominals.

    b. Imagine that there is a guy wire from the right anterior hip bone to the left and imagine the guy wire becoming slack as you bring the two hip bones together.

    c. Practice activating your transversus abdominis facing sideways in front of a mirror. As your baby grows and the belly gets bigger, you will actually see the baby lift up and in toward your body. Check in with your oblique muscles by watching the area of the belly directly below the rib cage. If you feel or see tension develop here, you are most likely overactivating the superficial muscles and need to exert less effort.

3. Once you establish the above movement, hold for five seconds and repeat ten times. Do one to three sets per day. Use the different cues to help you. Although this exercise looks easy it is extremely difficult to train and isolate the transverse muscle.

WHAT TO WATCH OUT FOR:

1. Holding the breath, which can increase leaking or pain. Also watch out for supine hypotension when lying on your back during pregnancy.

2. Over-contracting the abdominals, which engages the more superficial abdominals, such as the rectus abdominis and external obliques.

3. Increased abdominal pain or trigger points in the abdominals and/or an increase in your symptoms. Check with your MD or midwife right away if you experience any unusual symptoms. Never ignore pain.

Seated Ball Leg Press

WHAT TO DO:

1. Seated in good ball posture with feet flat on the floor as explained above, engage your transversus abdominis and your PFMs. Keep this engagement at 30 percent of effort.

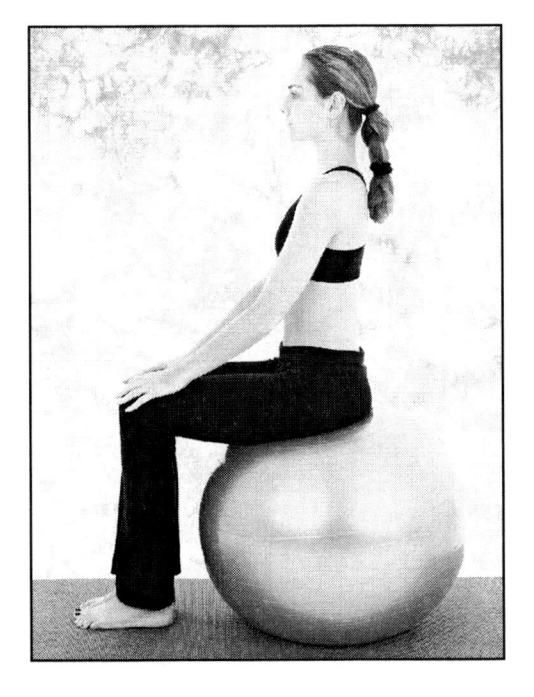

2. Bring your outstretched hands to your thighs. Inhale and exhale gently. Push your hands into your thighs making sure your legs don't move. Continue this pressing into your thighs for five seconds and then rest. Repeat ten times or as tolerated. This is an isometric abdominal exercise and it works wonders for your body. You can also do this exercise in a regular chair.

WHAT TO WATCH OUT FOR:

1. Moving the legs and pressing too hard. This exercise is a sustained hold with no movement.

2. Holding the breath. Breathe naturally as you hold the resistance against your thighs.

3. Allow the rectus abdominis to "pop out" during the exercise. If your belly bulges, then you have likely lost your transverse belly hold and the NS.

Lying Down Leg Press *(not recommended after first trimester for those women who suffer from supine hypotension)*

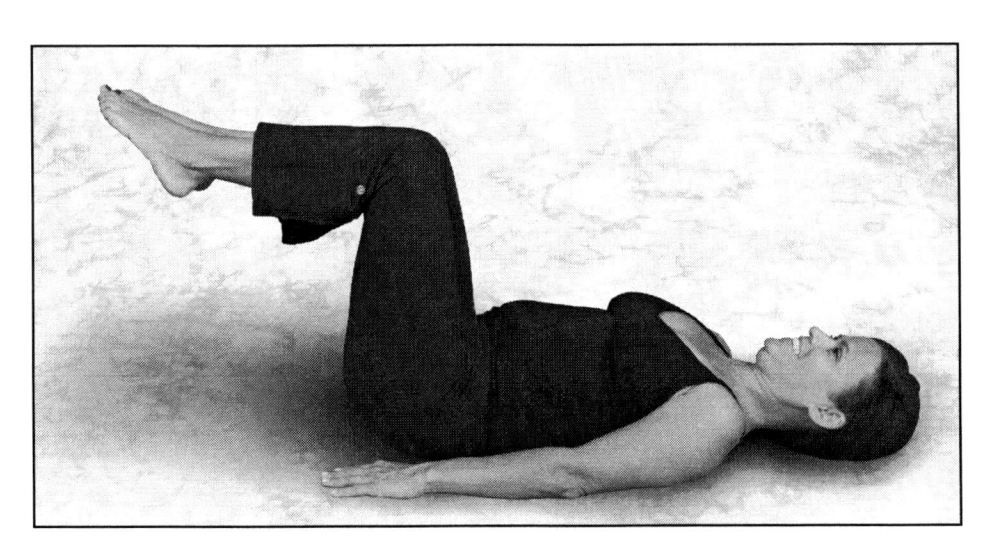

WHAT TO DO:

1. Lie flat on the floor with your lower back in NS and rest your arms on the side. Engage your transversus abdominis and your PFMs. Keep this engagement at 30 percent of effort.

2. Hug your knees into your chest; then release your knees slightly away from you until they form a 90 degree angle.

3. Bring your outstretched hands to your thighs and gently push your hands into your thighs making sure your legs don't move. Continue this pressing into your thighs for five seconds and then rest. Repeat ten times or as tolerated.

4. You may also try this in a seated position with your feet flat on the floor which is easier than doing it lying down.

WHAT TO WATCH OUT FOR:

1. Moving the legs and pressing too hard. This exercise is a sustained hold with no movement.

2. Holding the breath. Breathe naturally as you hold the resistance against your thighs.

3. Allowing the rectus abdominis to "pop out" during the exercise. If your belly bulges or your back comes off the floor, then you have likely lost your transverse belly hold and the NS.

Ball Marching

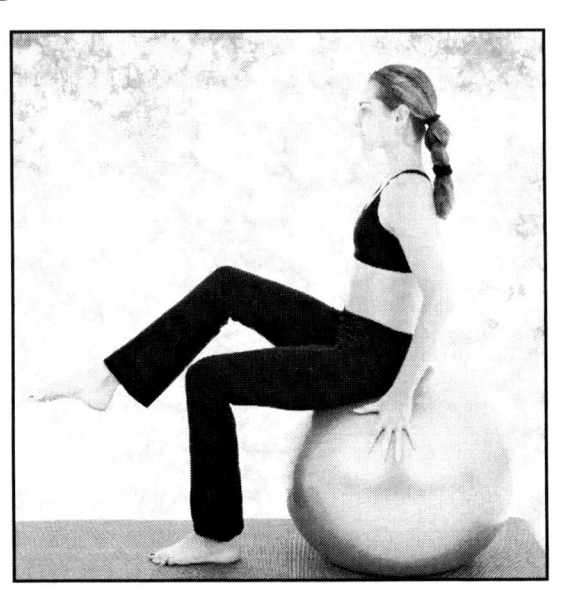

WHAT TO DO:

1. Sit on a physio ball in good balance posture or lie flat on the floor with a NS and rest your arms on the side. Engage your transversus abdominis and your PFMs. Keep this engagement at 30 percent of effort.

2. Slowly raise the right leg one to three inches from floor. Keep trunk rigid. Hold three seconds. Lower the right leg and then slowly raise the left leg one to three inches from floor. Keep trunk rigid. Hold for three seconds.

3. Repeat ten times on each leg.

WHAT TO WATCH OUT FOR:

1. Holding the breath, which can increase leaking or pelvic/low back pain. Also watch out for supine hypotension when lying on your back during pregnancy.

2. Over-contracting, which engages the more superficial abdominals, such as the rectus abdominis and external obliques.

3. Moving the pelvis and trunk and lifting the legs too high off the floor.

Ball Arms

WHAT TO DO:

1. Sit on a physio ball in good balance posture or lie flat on the floor with a NS and rest your arms on the side. Engage your transversus abdominis and your PFMs. Keep this engagement at 30 percent of effort.

2. While maintaining good posture and keeping your NS, raise your arms directly over your head and hold for five seconds. Slowly lower your arms. Rest for ten seconds and repeat ten times.

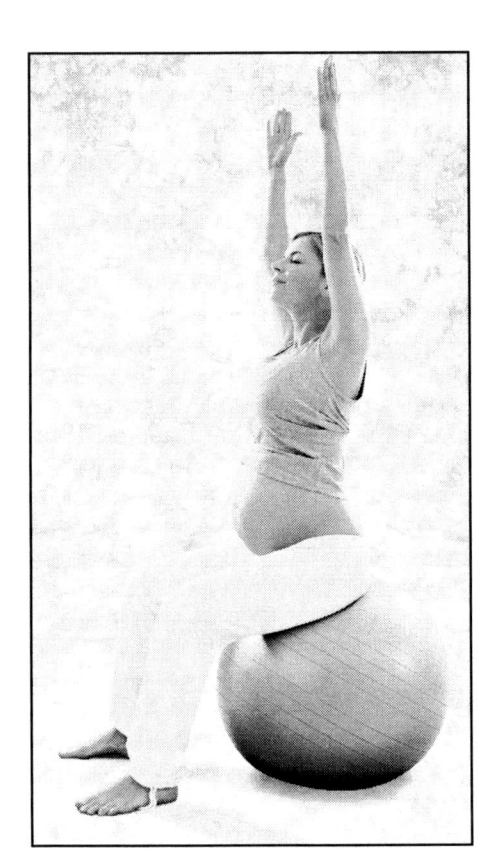

WHAT TO WATCH OUT FOR:

1. Holding the breath, which can increase leaking or pelvic/low back pain.

2. Over-contracting, which engages the more superficial abdominals, such as the rectus abdominis and external obliques.

3. Overarching the back and losing your neutral spine position.

4. Not maintaining the proper ball posture.

Pregnancy Box Planks

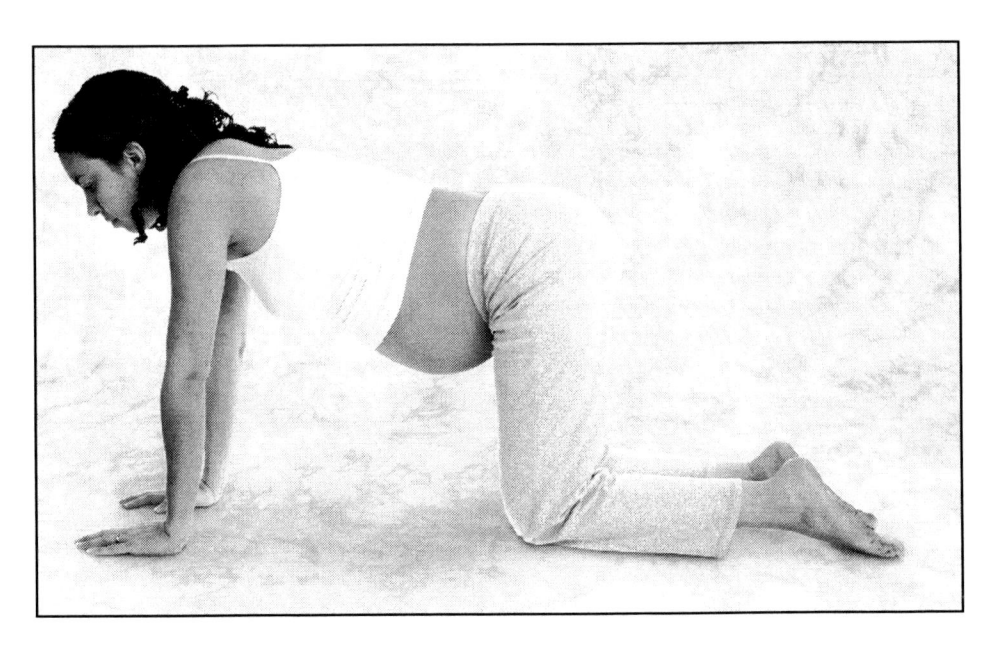

WHAT TO DO:

1. Get into an all-fours position on the floor. Engage your TrA and perform a low-level Kegel. Your elbows should be directly beneath your shoulders and your hips over your knees in a box form. Your body should form a straight line from your head to your hips.

2. Now turn the toes under and lift your knees from one to three inches off the floor and breathe naturally. Hold for up to ten to thirty seconds depending on your strength.

WHAT TO WATCH OUT FOR:

1. Keep your spine straight. Do not stick your butt into the air.

2. Avoid arching your low back, as this can cause a strain or injury to the lower back. Keep your spine in neutral.

3. Don't hold your breath.

Advanced Planks

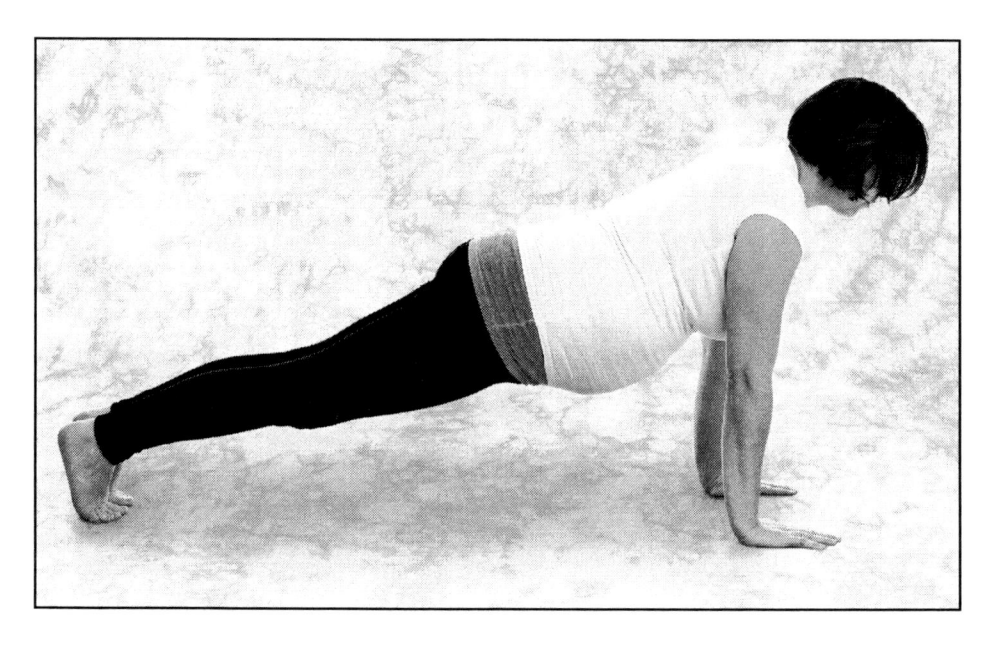

WHAT TO DO:

1. Get into pushup position on the floor. Your elbows should be directly beneath your shoulders, and your body should form a straight line from your head to your feet.

2. Hold the plank position for ten seconds or as tolerated. The goal here would be sixty-second holds. Repeat five to ten times. If this exercise is too difficult make it easier by placing your knees on the floor. Remember to lift the feet off the floor for this easier version. (Note: This version of the exercise is not shown in the photograph.)

WHAT TO WATCH OUT FOR:

1. Keep your spine straight and do not stick your butt into the air. Avoid holding your breath.

2. Avoid arching your low back, as this can cause a strain or injury to the lower back. Keep your spine in neutral.

Now that we have covered the abdominal training let's start the next phase: keeping your body strong during your pregnancy using our specific intelligent and targeted training (SITT) exercises. Read the next chapter for details on this amazing new way of working out and see your body transform into a strong and powerful one.

CHAPTER THIRTEEN

"Yoga practice can make us more and more sensitive to the subtler and subtler sensations in the body. Paying attention to and staying with finer and finer sensations within the body is one of the surest ways to steady the wandering mind."

—Ravi Ravindra

Chapter 13

AT-HOME EXERCISES THAT WORK IN EVERY TRIMESTER

Keeping your body strong during pregnancy does not have to be a complicated venture involving different exercise equipment, personal trainers or fancy classes. You can achieve a lot by doing what I call Specific Intelligent and Targeted Training (SITT). The SITT program serves four purposes: 1) to keep you out of pain; 2) to build your strength without bodily injury; 3) to improve lumbar, hip and pelvic stability; and 4) to prepare you for the marathon of labor. You will use a resistive Dyna-Band, your own body weight or a physio ball to do all the exercises where you choose—in the privacy of your home, in the park or at your job. The SITT workout programs listed here can be done throughout your entire pregnancy and target the muscles most affected by pregnancy. The SITT exercises, which incorporate an upper body, lower body and yoga flow stretching program, are safe and require little modification. (If an exercise does require modification I have indicated that under the heading "trimester modification" in the charts that follow.) The exercises chosen for the SITT program work on multiple muscles at the same time—that's good news because you don't have to spend hours working out. All three SITT exercise programs can be completed in less than twenty minutes. Remember to warm up before performing any of the SITT exercise programs: you can walk, bike or dance for ten to twenty minutes before getting started. When my patients graduate and are pain free I frequently give them this program to maintain the gains they achieved in physical therapy. The SITT exercises can be easily continued into the early postpartum period putting you on the road to reclaiming your body. (Modifications for the early post-partum period are also indicated in the charts listed below.)

Do the SITT program workouts and you will be better able to maintain a strong mind and body and be better prepared for labor and delivery. Table 13.1 is a sample workout breakdown. You can follow this sample or do all three SITT programs Mondays, Wednesdays and Fridays. Rest the area that you have just worked out for at least twenty-four hours. If you have a lot of soreness you may have to rest the area for longer than twenty-four hours. Listen to your body. Look at the photos and read the instructions carefully to insure that you are executing the exercises correctly.

Table 13.1: Exercise Program Sample Schedule

SITT PROGRAM	SAMPLE WORKOUT SCHEDULE
Upper Body Program	Monday, Wednesday, Friday
Lower Body Program	Tuesday, Thursday, Saturday
Yoga Flow Program	Daily if possible but listen to your body
Abdominals	Daily if possible but listen to your body (see Chapter 12 for more details)

Table 13.2: SITT Upper Body Exercises

SITT UPPER BODY EXERCISES	REPS AND SETS	TARGETED MUSCLE AND FUNCTION	TRIMESTER MODIFICATION
Brother, Can You Spare a Dime?	Beginner: ten reps/one to two sets Advanced: fifteen to twenty reps/two to three sets	Targets rhomboids and lower traps, helps improve posture and prepare the body for the demands of breast-feeding.	You can sit to do this exercise instead of standing. Okay for early postpartum.
Charm Walks	Beginner: Walk thirty seconds to one minute/one to two sets Advanced: Walk two to three minutes/two to three sets	Targets the whole body. Improves posture and re-trains the gait so there's no waddling and pain associated with walking	No modifications needed. Okay for early postpartum.
Chin Tucks	Beginner: five-second holds/ten reps/one to two sets Advanced: five-second holds/ten reps/two to three sets	Targets the neck muscles. Helps to keep the neck long and in good alignment. Helps to improve posture and reduce neck and upper back pain.	No modifications needed. Okay for early postpartum. If exercise increases neck and upper back pain stop and see your MD.
Lat Pull-Downs	Beginner: ten reps/one to two sets Advanced: ten reps/two to three sets	Targets the lats and the thoracolumbar fascia. Helps to stabilize the sacroiliac joint, low back and hips. Also helps to keep your waist narrow.	No modifications needed. Okay for early postpartum.
Rows	Beginner: Hold three to five seconds; ten reps/one to two sets Advanced: Hold three to five seconds/ten reps/two to three sets	Targets rhomboids and lower traps. Great exercise to help correct postural dysfunction. Promotes great posture. Helps to prevent neck and upper back pain.	You can do this exercise standing instead of sitting. Okay for early postpartum.

Brother, Can You Spare a Dime?

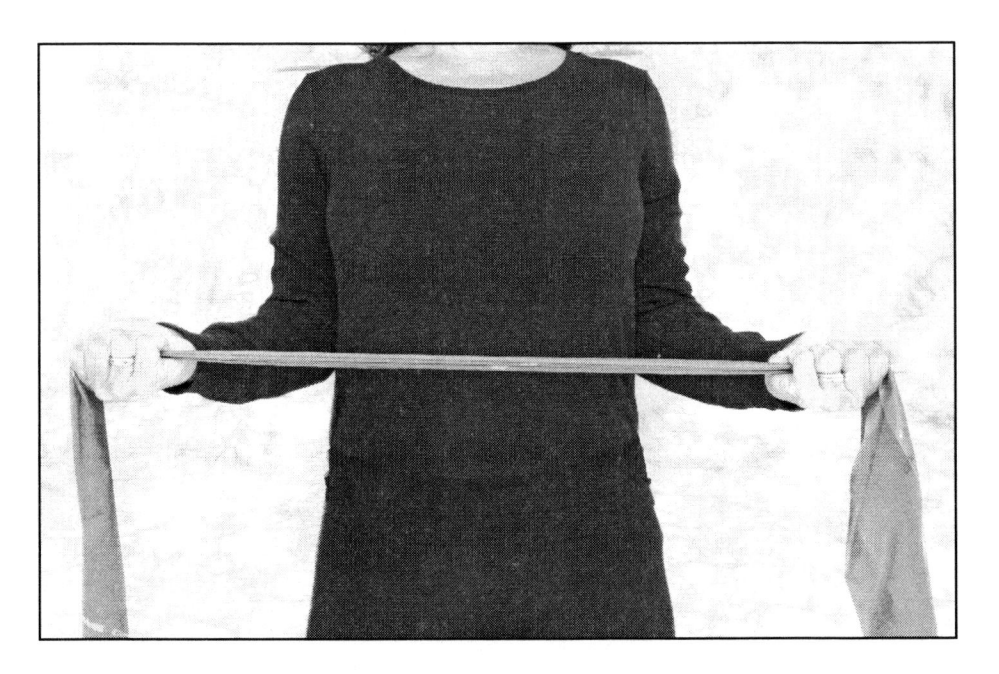

WHAT TO DO:

1. Stand in excellent posture remembering to keep the knees soft.

2. Wrap the Dyna-Band around your hands as in photo with palms up and elbows at your side aligned with your wrist.

3. Exhale. Pull the Dyna-Band outward while simultaneously squeezing your shoulder blades together and downward toward your back pockets. This is called scapular retraction (shoulder blade squeezing) and scapular depression (shoulder blades going downward).

4. Hold for three to five seconds and relax the shoulders. Rest three to five seconds.

5. Repeat ten times for one to three sets.

WHAT TO WATCH OUT FOR:

1. Not stabilizing the pelvis with a pelvic brace.

2. Too much tension on the band and overdoing it.

3. Not utilizing the whole scapular motion. Shoulder blades must come inward and downward as you pull the Dyna-Band outward.

4. Poor posture. Keep yourself in great posture while you do this exercise.

BENEFITS:

1. Helps correct postural dysfunctions that are common during pregnancy.

2. Helps alleviate neck and shoulder pain.

3. Promotes confidence and self-assurance on an energetic level because the body is in a more optimal position.

Charm Walks

Photo Description: This is good walking posture. Notice the alignment. If we drew a line from the ears to the shoulder and then to the hips the line would be straight. See Chapter 4 for more information on posture.

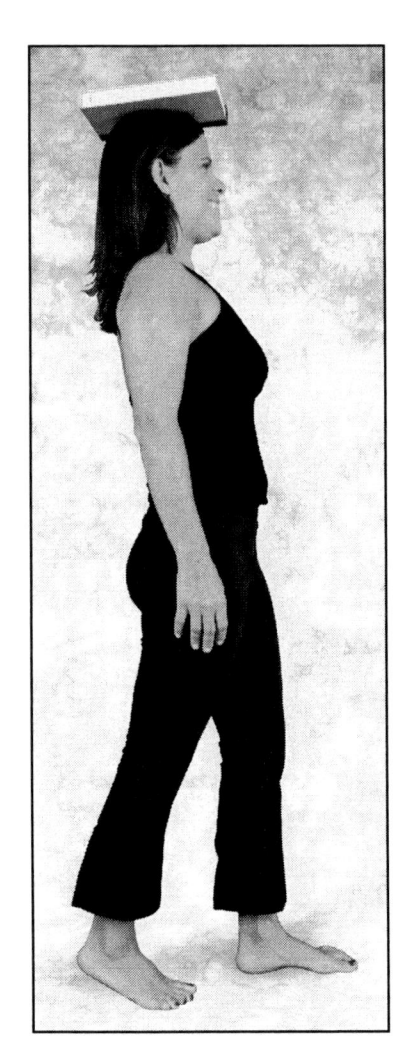

WHAT TO DO:

1. Place a small book on the top of your head. Keep your body in good posture as you walk with the book on your head.

2. Start with a small book and then progress to a larger book when you are able to walk for three minutes without the smaller book falling off your head.

WHAT TO WATCH OUT FOR:

Waddling gait or any other gait dysfunction will lead to the book falling off your head. Pay attention to where the book falls. It can be a clue as to the area of the body where you are having your gait problems

BENEFITS:

1. Promotes a better gait pattern thereby reducing pelvic pain and aches and soreness due to faulty gait mechanics.

2. Promotes awareness of your gait so that you can then start to correct yourself as you walk.

Chin Tucks

WHAT TO DO:

1. Stand or sit in great posture.

2. Gently place two fingers on your chin and pull your chin gently away from your fingers in a chin tuck motion.

3. Hold for three to five seconds and repeat ten times. Do one to three times a day or as tolerated.

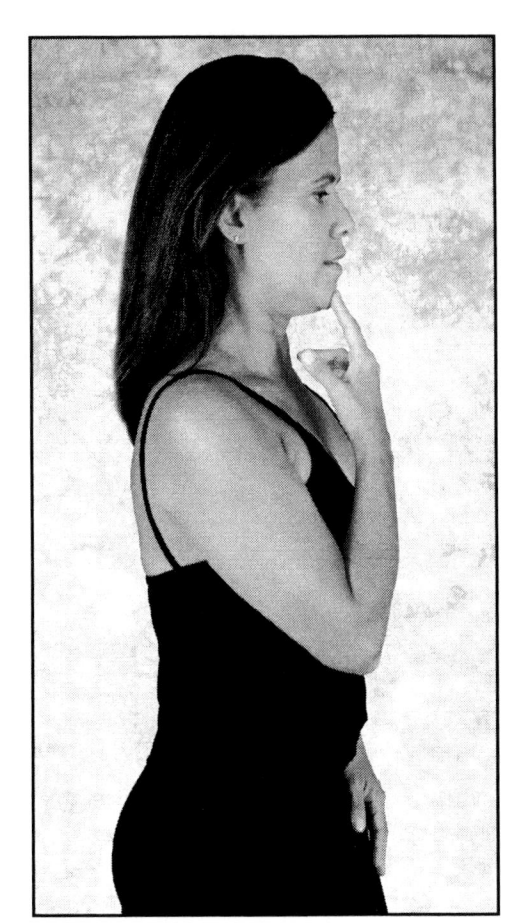

WHAT TO WATCH OUT FOR:

1. Pulling the chin down and back instead of purely back. The tucking of the chin is a backward pull-in motion in a straight line.

2. Pulling the chin in too aggressively. This motion is gentle and should be pain free. This should not increase your neck or shoulder pain but reduce it. If your pain increases you are doing your chin tucks too aggressively and you have to back off a little.

BENEFIT:

Promotes amazing posture and helps decrease neck and upper back pain.

Standing Lat Pull-Down

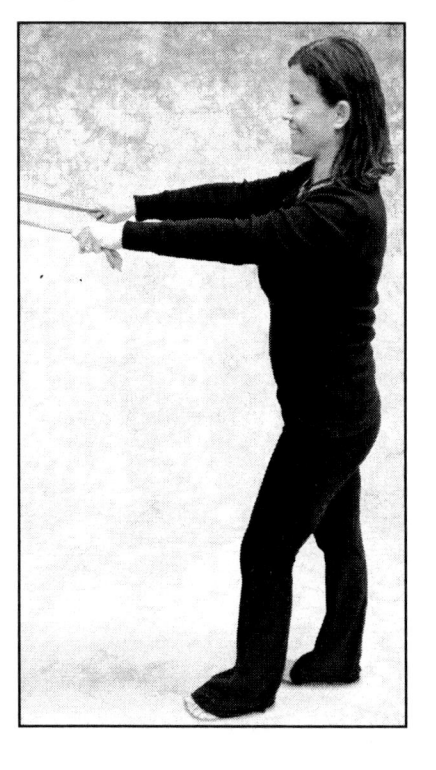 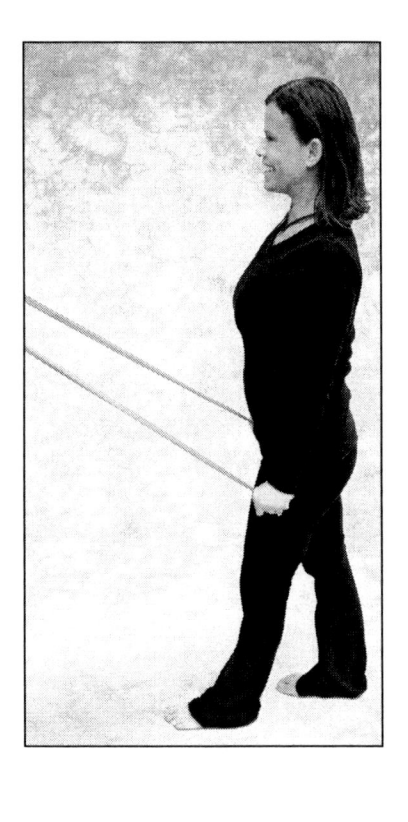

WHAT TO DO:

1. This exercise can be performed standing or sitting. Attach a Dyna-Band high on a doorway so that you have two ends of the band to grasp.

2. Your arms should be slightly in front of your body, elbows straight, and hands grasping the Dyna-Bands.

3. Contract your transverse abdominis muscle first (see Transverse Belly Holds in Chapter 12).

4. Keeping your arms straight, pull your arms down and back just until they are at the side of your waist.

5. Hold three to five seconds and envision you are keeping your shoulder blades down and back as if you were going to put them in your back pockets. Repeat ten times; do one to three sets per day.

WHAT TO WATCH OUT FOR:

1. Holding the breath, which can increase abdominal pressure and cause leaking, pain, and pressure.

2. Keeping your shoulders rounded or hunched in front which places the cervical spine and upper back in a compromised position. Your chest should be up and shoulders back in excellent posture.

BENEFITS:

1. Tenses and strengthens the latissimus dorsi muscle and its fascial extension, the thoracodorsal fascia, which provides support and stability to the sacroiliac joint, lumbar spine, and hips.

2. Can be used to facilitate proper posture and body awareness.

3. Assists in balancing and increasing strength in the posterior aspect of the body. As the baby grows and shifts the center of mass anteriorly, strengthening the posterior column muscles is extremely important to keep your back stable and supported.

BENEFITS:

1. Helps to stabilize the sacroiliac joint thereby reducing pain and promoting lumbar hip and pelvic stability.

2. Helps to improve posture and reduce low back pain.

Rows

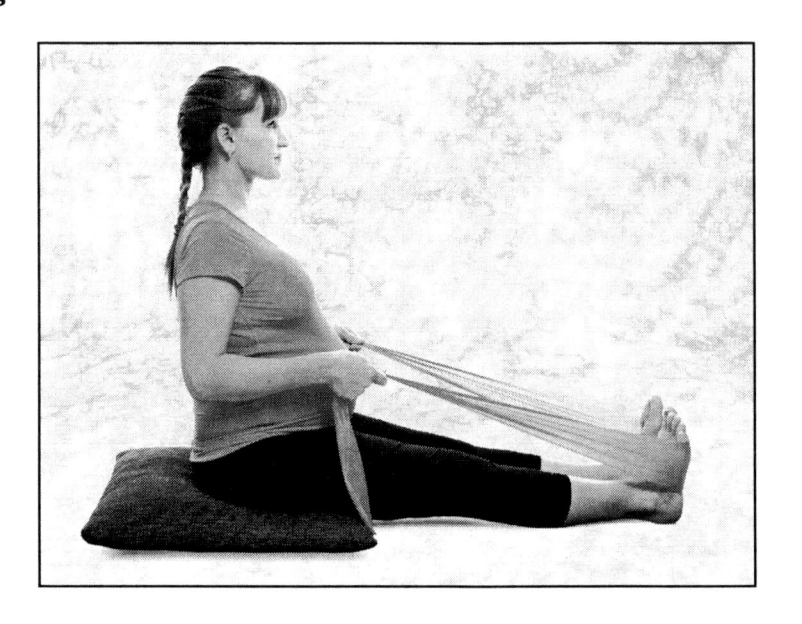

WHAT TO DO:

1. Sit in good posture with your knees slightly bent, legs outstretched in front of you, and wrap the Dyna-Band around both feet.

2. Wrap both ends of the Dyna-Band around your hands with palms facing inward toward each other and elbows at right angles.

3. Do a pelvic brace and gently pull the arms back while simultaneously bringing your shoulder blades together. Hold for three to five seconds and release to start position. Repeat.

WHAT TO WATCH OUT FOR:

1. Slumped posture.

2. Pain in the lower back. If this occurs do this exercise sitting in a chair and attach the Dyna-Band around a sturdy immovable object.

BENEFITS:

1. Strengthens the mid-back muscles and promotes great posture.
2. Helps to alleviate neck and upper back pain.
3. Promotes excellent posture.

Table 13.3: SITT Lower Body Exercises

SITT UPPER BODY EXERCISES	REPS AND SETS	TARGETED MUSCLE AND FUNCTION	TRIMESTER MODIFICATION
Ball Squats	Beginner: ten reps/one to two sets Advanced: fifteen to twenty reps/two to three sets	Strengthens the legs and prepares the body for all labor positions. Will also keep your legs toned and in shape.	To make this exercise easier hold on to a sturdy immovable object and use it to help you lift your body up and down. Okay for early postpartum.
Clams	Beginner: ten reps/one to two sets Advanced: fifteen to twenty reps/two to three sets	Strengthens and stabilizes the hip, pelvic girdle and lumbar spine and muscles.	No trimester modification necessary. Okay for early postpartum.
Seated Abduction	Beginner: Hold three to five seconds; ten reps/one to two sets Advanced: Hold three to five seconds; fifteen to twenty reps/two to three sets	Strengthens the outer thigh muscles and helps to stabilize the sacroiliac joint, low back and hips.	No modifications needed. You can always use a lighter band. Okay for early postpartum.
Seated Adduction	Beginner: Hold three to five seconds; ten reps/one to two sets Advanced: Hold three to five seconds; fifteen to twenty reps/two to three sets	Strengthens the inner thigh muscles and helps to stabilize the sacroiliac joint, low back and hips and pubic symphysis.	No modifications needed. You can always use a lighter band. Okay for early postpartum.
Bridging	Beginner: Hold three to five seconds; ten reps/one to two sets Advanced: Hold three to five seconds; fifteen to twenty reps/two to three sets	Strengthens your lower back and gluteal muscles. The abdominal muscles co-contract with the lower back muscles in this exercise. Helps to prevent backache.	If you experience any signs of supine hypotension, stop this exercise immediately. Caution should be used after first trimester. Avoid in postpartum until bleeding has stopped.
Alternating Arm and Leg	Beginner: ten reps/one to two sets Advanced: fifteen to twenty reps/two to three sets	Strengthens back and gluteal muscles. Stabilizes the hip, pelvic girdle and lumbar spine. Prevents backache.	Start with alternating arms. Then if you can execute properly do the leg part of the exercise. Avoid in postpartum until bleeding has stopped.

Ball Squats

WHAT TO DO:

1. While standing with feet hip-width apart, knees slightly bent and in good postural alignment, place one hand on each hip bone.

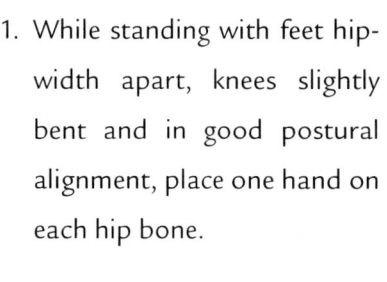

2. Imagine you are about to sit in a chair and perform a mini-squat, while focusing on inhaling into your PFM and simultaneously visualizing your sit bones coming apart. Lower your body and hold for three to five seconds as you breathe naturally. Return to start position as you exhale.

3. Repeat ten times. This exercise is great because it works with gravity to get the PFMs to release and at the same time strengthens your legs for labor and delivery.

4. Perform one to three sets.

WHAT TO WATCH OUT FOR:

Watch out for your knees. Make sure that they stay in alignment with your ankles and don't let them move forward past your toes.

BENEFITS:

1. Strengthens the lower body muscles and prepares the lower extremity for the rigors of birth.

2. Shapes and tones your legs.

3. Strengthens your gluteal muscles.

Clams

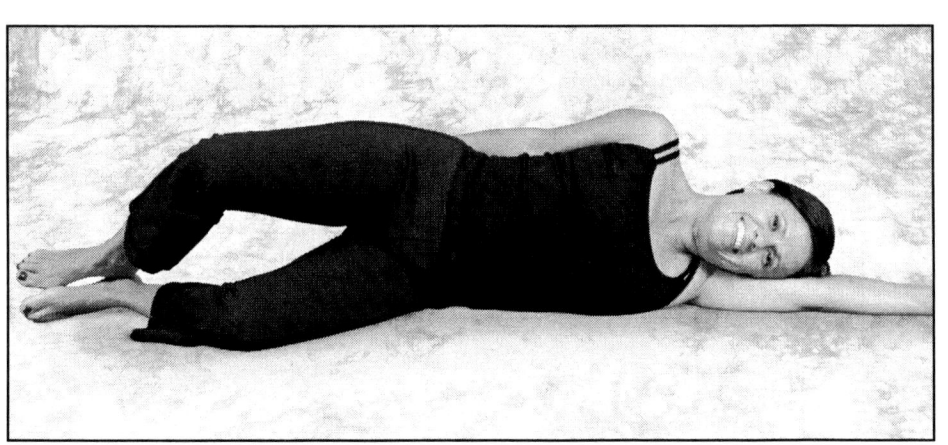

WHAT TO DO:

1. Lie on your right side and bring your knees together up to a 45 degree angle. Keep your feet together and without moving your top hip raise your top leg upward. Hold for three seconds and lower slowly. Rest for three seconds at the bottom.

2. Remember to maintain a TrA and low-level Kegel as you raise and lower your top leg.

3. Repeat ten times and switch sides. Perform one to three sets.

WHAT TO WATCH OUT FOR:

Be careful with excessive hip movements. The hips remain stable and should not move as you raise and lower your leg.

BENEFITS:

1. Improves hip, pelvic girdle and lumbar spine stability.

2. Keeps you walking straight and prevents the "waddle gait" that pregnant women are famous for.

3. Shapes and tones your outer thigh muscles

Seated Abduction

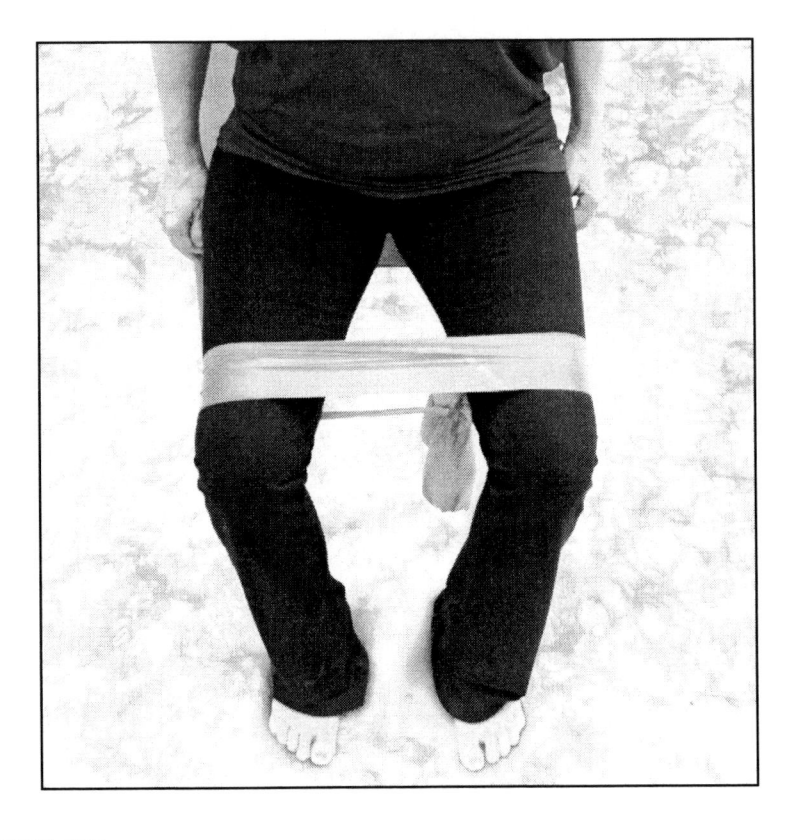

WHAT TO DO:

1. Wrap a Dyna-Band around the upper part of your thigh. Sit in good posture with your feet together. Remember to maintain a TrA and low-level Kegel for the active part of this exercise.

2. Exhale and pull your thighs out against the Dyna-Band (active part of the exercise) until you feel resistance against your inner thighs.

3. Hold for three to five seconds and then bring your thighs together and rest for three to five seconds. Repeat ten times; complete one to three sets or as tolerated.

WHAT TO WATCH OUT FOR:

1. Slouching and poor upper and seated body posture.

2. Using too much resistance with the band.

BENEFITS:

1. Promotes good gait pattern and helps to alleviate lumbar, pelvic and hip pain.

2. Helps to stabilize the lumbar hip and pelvic girdle regions.

3. Helps keep the legs in good shape and tones the outer thigh muscles.

Seated Adduction

WHAT TO DO:

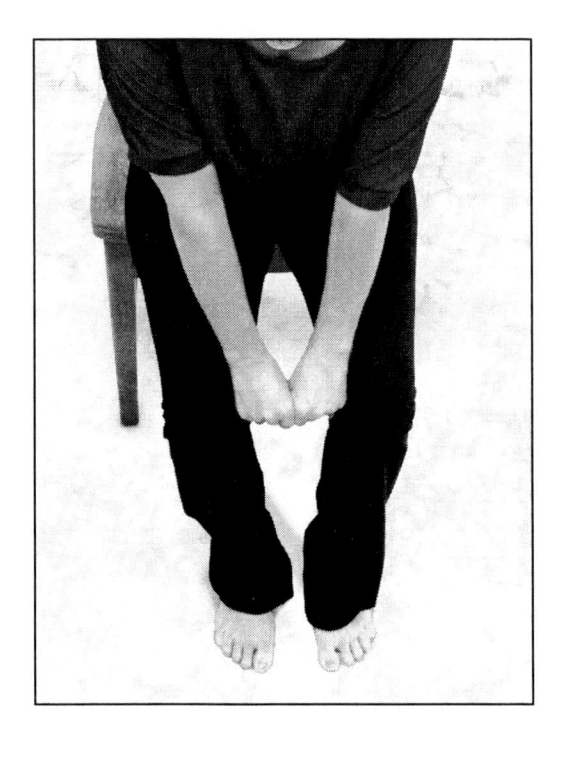

1. Sit in good posture with your feet together. Remember to maintain a TrA and low-level Kegel for the active part of this exercise. Place a yoga block, pillow or hands between your knees.

2. Exhale and bring your thighs together and press your thighs into the yoga block (active part of the exercise) or your hands.

3. Hold for three to five seconds and then bring your thighs apart and rest for three to five seconds. Repeat ten times; complete one to three sets or as tolerated.

WHAT TO WATCH OUT FOR:

1. Pressing too hard into the block and increasing your groin or pubic bone pain. This is a gentle yet firm squeeze.

2. Slouching and poor upper body posture.

BENEFITS:

1. Helps stabilize the pubic bone and sacroiliac joint

2. Shapes the inner thighs.

3. Promotes good gait mechanics.

Bridging

Proceed with caution after the first trimester unless you can perform the exercise without experiencing signs and symptoms of supine hypotension.

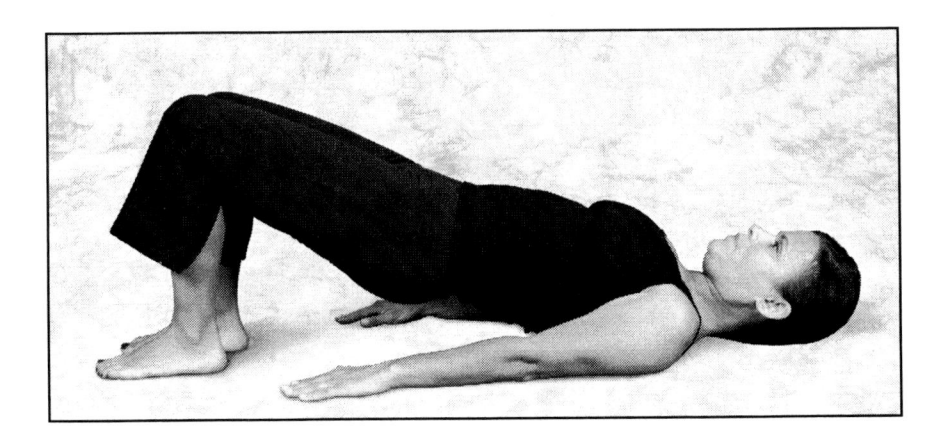

WHAT TO DO:

1. Lie on your back, with knees bent and feet hip-width apart and keep your arms close to your side.

2. Exhale and lift your pelvis off the floor until it is aligned with your knees. This forms the bridge position. Hold the bridge position for three to five seconds and then lower to start position. Rest for three to five seconds. Repeat ten times; do one to three sets of ten repetitions.

WHAT TO WATCH OUT FOR:

This exercise should be pain-free. If pain persists, check and correct your alignment (see Chapter 5), do fewer repetitions, hold for fewer seconds at the top, or stop completely.

BENEFITS:

1. Strengthens the lower back, gluteal muscles and promotes hip extension.
2. Helps you to walk better and minimizes gait dysfunctions.
3. Strengthens the hamstring muscles.
4. Helps shape the gluteal muscles and back of thighs.
5. Stabilizes the hip, pelvic girdle, and lumbar spine.

Alternating Arm and Leg

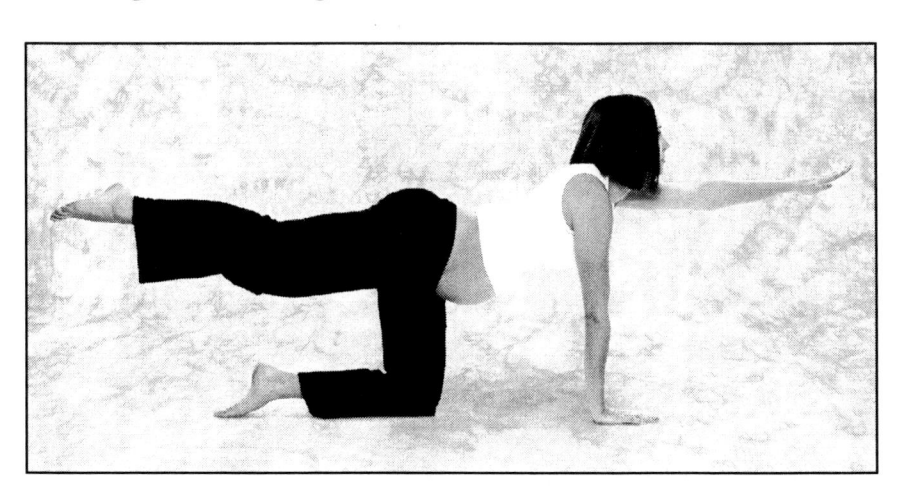

WHAT TO DO:

1. Get onto your hands and knees. Your arms and hands should be aligned with your shoulders. Your knees should be aligned with your hips (hip-width apart).

2. Perform a pelvic brace and extend your right arm outward. Hold this position. Extend your left leg straight back and lift it until it's in alignment with your hips.

3. Hold for five to ten seconds; return arm and leg to start position. Rest for five to ten seconds and switch sides. Lift the left arm and right leg until it is aligned with your hip. Hold five to ten seconds. Rest five to ten seconds and return to start position.

WHAT TO WATCH OUT FOR.

1. Unstable execution of the exercise. The hips should not waver but stay straight, stable and in alignment with each other.

2. Hyper extension of the elbows.

3. Dropping the head. Keep the head and neck aligned with the spine.

4. Sagging in the lower back. Keep your back straight.

SITT Yoga Flow: (Adapted from Renew PT Prenatal P.R.E.S.S. Yoga Series)

As a result of the changes that occur in pregnancy many muscles respond by becoming tight or inflexible. Painful areas can also become tight. Stretching and yoga promote relaxation, circulation and create supple muscles. In the exercises that follow, I advise that you go into a stretch and to feel the stretch, but avoid pain when stretching and never override a pain signal. These exercises can be performed as stand-alone stretches or you can flow them into your own yoga flow class. To do so first start with standing exercises then process to seated and then to prayer squat followed by child's pose and relaxation pose. Always warm up your muscles before doing the yoga flow stretches. You can walk for ten to twenty minutes or you can put on some good music and dance for ten to twenty minutes. The yoga exercises highlighted here are adapted from our prenatal P.R.E.S.S. Yoga Series, which empahasizes yoga for pelvic floor stabilty.

Table 13.4: SITT Yoga Flow

SITT UPPER BODY EXERCISES	REPS AND SETS	TARGETED MUSCLE AND FUNCTION	TRIMESTER MODIFICATION
Split Leg Pose: Hip Flexor Stretch	Beginner: Hold ten to thirty seconds Advanced: Hold thirty seconds to one minute	Stretches the hip flexors, helps to maintain proper posture and pelvic hip alignment, and prevents posterior pelvic pain.	Hold on to a sturdy or immovable object for balance support. Okay for early postpartum.
Standing Modified Sugarcane Pose	Beginner: Hold ten to thirty seconds Advanced: Hold thirty seconds to one minute	Stretches the front of the thighs and helps maintain proper posture and pelvic hip alignment. Prevents posterior pelvic pain.	Hold on to a sturdy or immovable object for balance support. Okay for early postpartum.
Seated Modified Heron Pose	Beginner: Hold ten to thirty seconds Advanced: Hold thirty seconds to one minute	Stretches the hamstring muscles, helps maintain proper posture and pelvic hip alignment and prevents posterior pelvic pain.	No trimester modification necessary. Okay for early postpartum.

Table 13.4 (cont.): SITT Yoga Flow

SITT UPPER BODY EXERCISES	REPS AND SETS	TARGETED MUSCLE AND FUNCTION	TRIMESTER MODIFICATION
Standing Modified Table Top	Beginner and Advanced: Hold ten to thirty seconds	Takes pressure off the back and stretches the hamstrings. Can relieve back pain.	No trimester modification necessary. Avoid in postpartum until bleeding has stopped.
Seated Side Bending Mountain Pose	Beginner: Hold ten to thirty seconds Advanced: Hold thirty seconds to one minute	Stretches intercostal rib muscles and quadratus lumborum. Prevents back and rib pain and promotes rib mobility.	No trimester modification necessary. Okay for early postpartum.
Seated Half Ankle to Knee	Beginner: Hold ten to thirty seconds Advanced: Hold thirty seconds to one minute	Stretches the gluteal muscles and helps prevent sciatic and low back pain.	No trimester modification necessary. Okay for early postpartum.
Seated Hero Heart Opener Pose	Beginner: Hold ten to thirty seconds Advanced: Hold thirty seconds to one minute	Stretches chest muscles and promotes good posture. Helps maintain posture with breastfeeding.	No trimester modification necessary. Okay for early postpartum.
Cat Cow Pose	Beginner and Advanced: Hold ten to thirty seconds	Stretches low back muscles and prevents backaches.	No trimester modification necessary. Avoid in postpartum until bleeding has stopped.
Prayer Pose	Beginner: Hold ten to thirty seconds Advanced: Hold thirty seconds to one minute	Targets PFMs, calves, glutes and helps prepare the body for labor.	Support yourself against a wall with a couple of pillows underneath your buttocks or hold on to an immovable sturdy object. Avoid in postpartum until bleeding has stopped.
Child's Pose	Beginner: Hold ten to thirty seconds Advanced: Hold thirty seconds to one minute	Stretches low back muscles, promotes relaxation and helps with reverse Kegel exercises.	No trimester modification necessary. Avoid in postpartum until bleeding has stopped.
Relaxation Pose	Five minutes at the end of your stretching session	Targets the mind and helps bring the body back into harmony and promotes relaxation.	In the later part of your pregnancy you may have to prop your upper back on pillows to avoid supine hypotension. Okay for early postpartum.

Split Leg Pose: Hip Flexor Stretch

WHAT TO DO:

1. Stand in great posture.

2. Take a small step forward with the right foot and bend the right knee slightly; the distance between the front and back leg does not have to be large or wide.

3. Make sure both feet are facing forward and the hips are squared to the front.

4. Gently tuck the pelvis under until a stretch is felt on the front of the left hip.

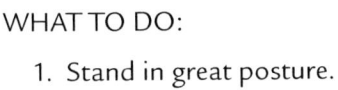

5. Hold ten to thirty seconds; then switch sides.

WHAT TO WATCH OUT FOR:

1. Slouching. Keep your chest lifted.

2. Having the legs too far apart

3. Balance issues. Use a wall for support.

Standing Modified Sugarcane Pose (Quad Stretch)

WHAT TO DO:

1. Stand and touch wall or stationary object for balance. Grasp your right ankle or foot with your right hand.

2. Pull ankle or foot gently toward buttocks. Don't worry about how close your foot is to your buttocks.

3. Hold ten to thirty seconds; then switch sides.

WHAT TO WATCH OUT FOR:

1. Slouching. Keep your chest lifted.

2. Pulling the foot too vigorously toward the buttocks.

3. Balance issues. Use a wall for support.

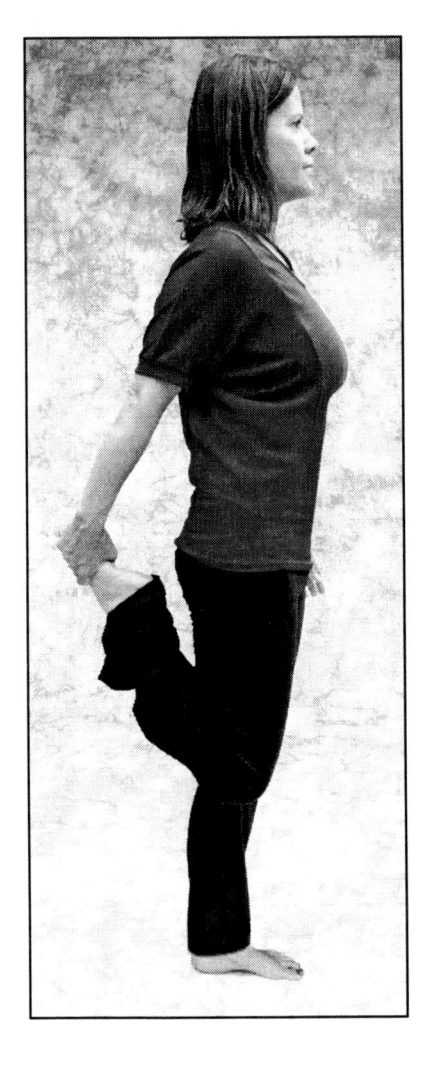

Modified Table Top Pose

Photo Description: This great pose gives your back a chance to breathe by "unweighing" it.

WHAT TO DO:

1. Stand close enough to the ball or wall so that you can reach the wall with your arms.

2. Bend with a straight back— do not round the back at all—and put your hands on the ball or wall. I prefer the wall for this exercise but many women want to use a ball. The ball has to be tall enough that you can reach for it while maintaining a straight back.

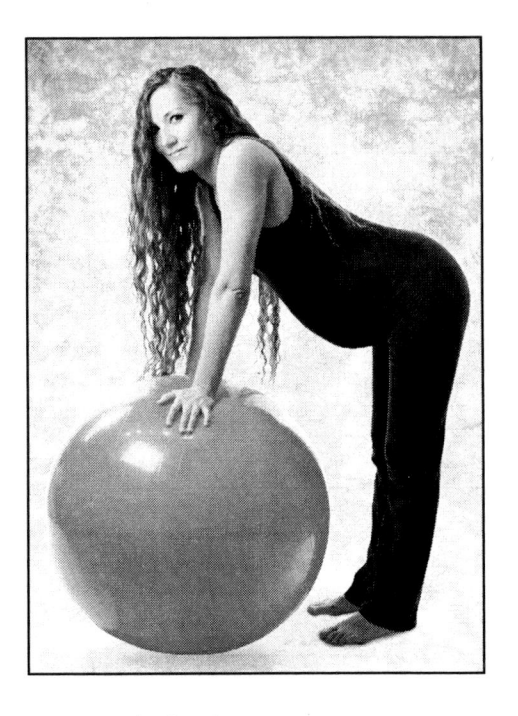

3. Hold the position ten to thirty seconds without collapsing and rounding the back.

4. To focus on stretching the hamstrings imagine that your sit bones are reaching for the ceiling.

WHAT TO WATCH OUT FOR:

1. Slouching in the lower back

2. Overarching the back. The back should be straight and the neck and back should be aligned.

3. Dropping the head. Keep the head and neck aligned with the back.

4. Locking the knees. Keep the knees slightly bent.

Seated Modified Heron Pose

WHAT TO DO:

1. Adopt a good seated posture at the edge of your seat.

2. Straighten out your right leg and point your toes toward your head until you feel a stretch behind the back of your leg and calf.

3. For deeper stretching, bend forward from the hips while keeping your back straight and shoulders square. Hold ten to thirty seconds.

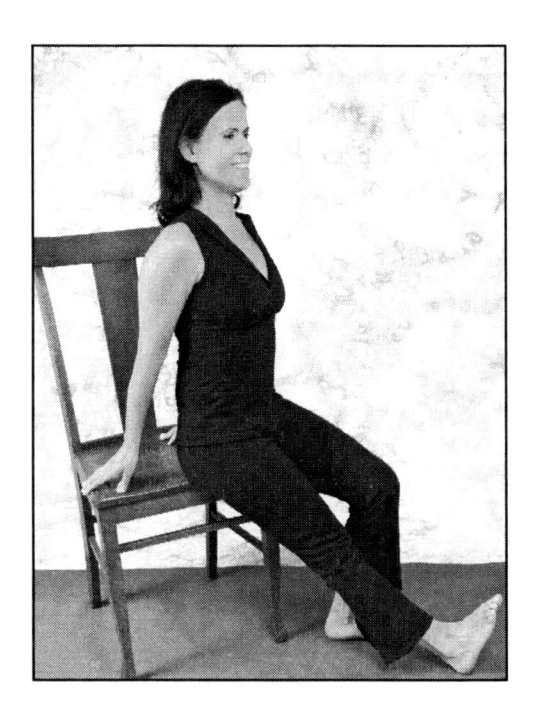

4. Switch legs and repeat.

WHAT TO WATCH OUT FOR:

1. Watch out for pain radiating into the toes. If this occurs, stretch less aggressively, keeping the foot in a more neutral position instead of pointing it up. Stop immediately if pain persists despite modification.

2. If you experience pain or discomfort in the lower back, make sure you remain upright instead of leaning forward. If pain continues in the lower-back muscles, stop.

3. Poor postural alignment while doing this stretch can put excessive strain on your upper and lower back muscles. Make sure you don't overarch your back as well.

BENEFITS:

1. This stretch improves hamstring and calf flexibility.

2. Helps to decrease lower back pain encouraging good posture and pelvic/
   hip alignment.

Seated Side Bending Mountain Pose

WHAT TO DO:

1. Start in a seated position at the front of your chair, using good posture as
   outlined earlier in the chapter.

2. Raise your right arm up toward the ceiling and place
   your left arm at your hips.

3. Bend your upper body to
   the left while reaching up
   and over with your right
   arm. Hold ten to thirty seconds.

4. Bring your body back to the
   center and repeat the pose
   on the other side.

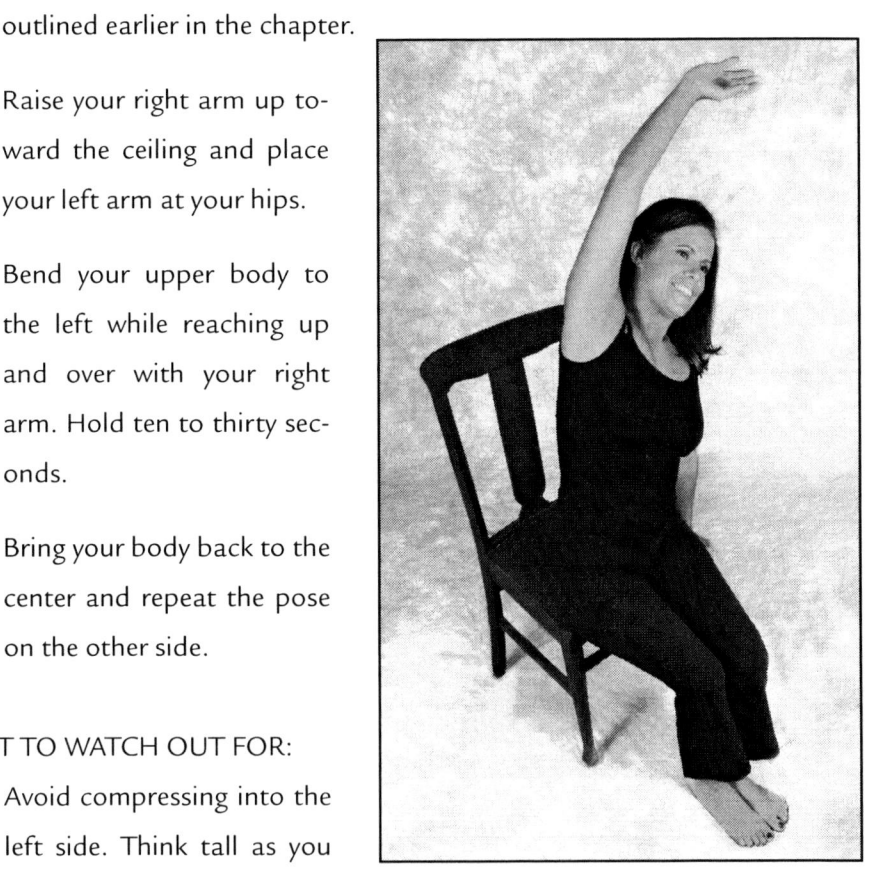

WHAT TO WATCH OUT FOR:

1. Avoid compressing into the
   left side. Think tall as you
   bend sideways.

2. Avoid overstretching and forcing the side-bend as this can cause pain to the intercostal or side muscles.

BENEFITS:

1. Helps increase the flexibility of your spine, arms, and rib cage.

2. Helps to realign pelvic bones and maintain lumbar spine and sacral alignment.

3. Enhances nerve function.

4. Facilitates rib expansion which will help get more oxygen into your lungs and promote better breathing.

Seated Half Ankle to Knee (AKA the Figure Four Stretch)

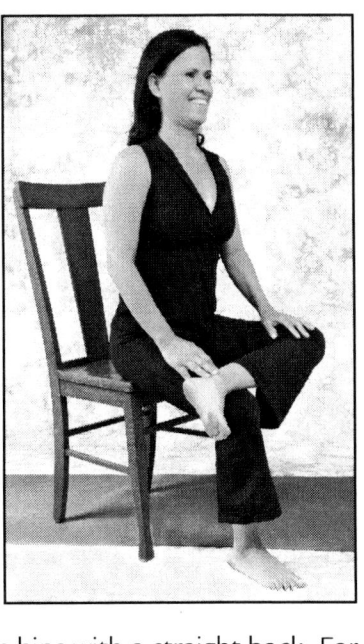

WHAT TO DO:

1. While seated in good posture at the edge of your seat, place the left ankle lightly on the thigh of the right leg making a figure four. Keep your hips square, your shoulders down and back as you sit straight.

2. If you are able, gently press your crossed leg down but not lower than your thigh.

3. For a deeper stretch, lean forward from the hips with a straight back. For an even deeper stretch rotate your upper body slightly toward your feet.

4. Hold ten to thirty seconds, then bring your body back to center and repeat the pose on the other side.

WHAT TO WATCH OUT FOR:

1. Don't torque the ankle bone. Remember to keep the ankle bone slightly off the resting thigh to avoid stressing it.

2. Avoid slouching in this posture to prevent stress on the lumbar spinal nerves and to make this stretch more effective.

3. If your pain increases and/or radiates into your thigh or lower leg/foot, or persists for thirty minutes or longer, discontinue this stretch and consult your healthcare professional.

BENEFITS:

1. Helps prevent sciatica.

2. Helps to stretch the piriformis muscle and maintain pelvic alignment.

3. Helps increase the mobility and function of the major nerve roots of the lumbar and sacral spine which innervate the pelvic floor muscles and internal pelvic organs.

4. Improves blood flow to the hip and pelvic muscles.

Seated Hero Heart Opener Pose

WHAT TO DO:

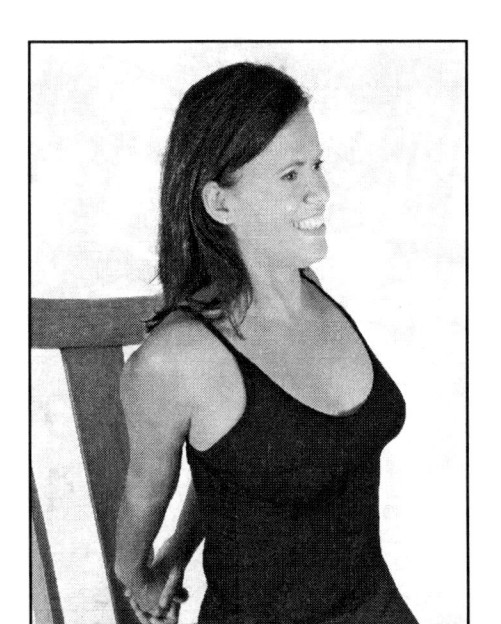

1. Sit with good posture on the edge of your seat.

2. Clasp your hands behind your back, interlocking your fingers.

3. Roll your shoulders down and back, stretching your chest upward.

4. Raise your arms slightly upward, tucking your chin under.

5. Hold for ten to thirty seconds.

WHAT TO WATCH OUT FOR:

1. Don't stick out your chin as this puts pressure on your neck.

2. Don't slouch in this pose. Sit up straight.

BENEFITS:

1. Improves posture.

2. Decreases upper and lower back pain.

3. Psychologically opens you up and puts you in a position of confidence.

Cat Cow Pose

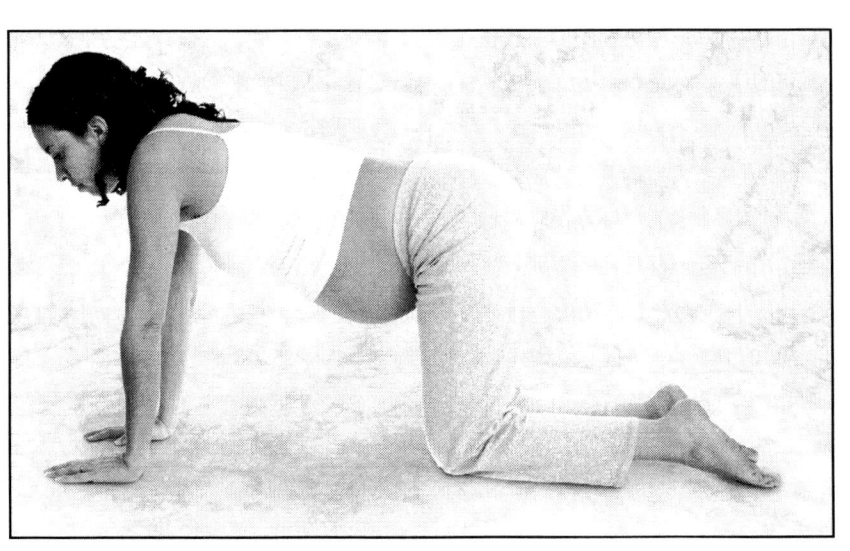

WHAT TO DO

1. Get onto your hands and knees. Your arms and hands should be aligned with your shoulders. Your knees should be aligned with your hips and about hip-width apart.

2. Make sure your head and neck are aligned with your spine.

3. Start with a flat and straight back.

3. Inhale; round your back forming a C-shape curve while simultaneously tucking your head and chin. Hold for ten to twenty seconds.

4. Exhale; arch your back, lift your head and tilt your pelvis upward toward the ceiling. Hold for ten to twenty seconds. Slowly return to your original flat back position.

WHAT TO WATCH OUT FOR:

Pain in the low back and gluteal area, increase in sciatica and abdominal pain are all signs to stop this stretch. Most likely you will feel these types of pain when you round your back.

Prayer Squat Pose

WHAT TO DO:

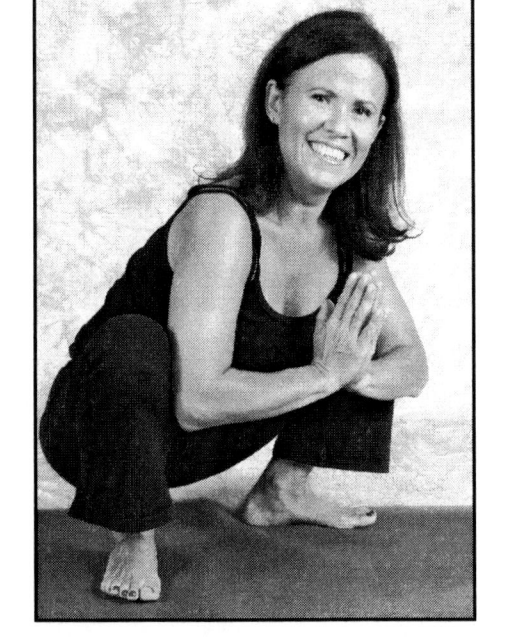

1. Adopt a squatting position as in the photo.

2. Place your arm across your chest in prayer position or hold onto a sturdy immovable object

3. Breathe diaphragmatically

4. Focus on releasing your pelvic floor muscles.

WHAT TO WATCH OUT FOR:

This can be a very stressful position for women who lack flexibility in the hips and calves. To make the Prayer Pose easier, put some pillows under your feet. You can also do the Prayer Pose against the wall for back support. It might also be helpful to place a pillow underneath the buttocks to take pressure off the body and to make the Prayer Pose easier to handle. If you sufer from pudendal nerve neuralgia avoid this pose.

BENEFITS:

1. Opens up the hips, leg and calf muscles.

2. Stretches the calf, back and hip muscles.

3. Relaxes the PFMs as they are relaxed in this pose.

4. Can help to relieve back and hip pain.

Child's Pose

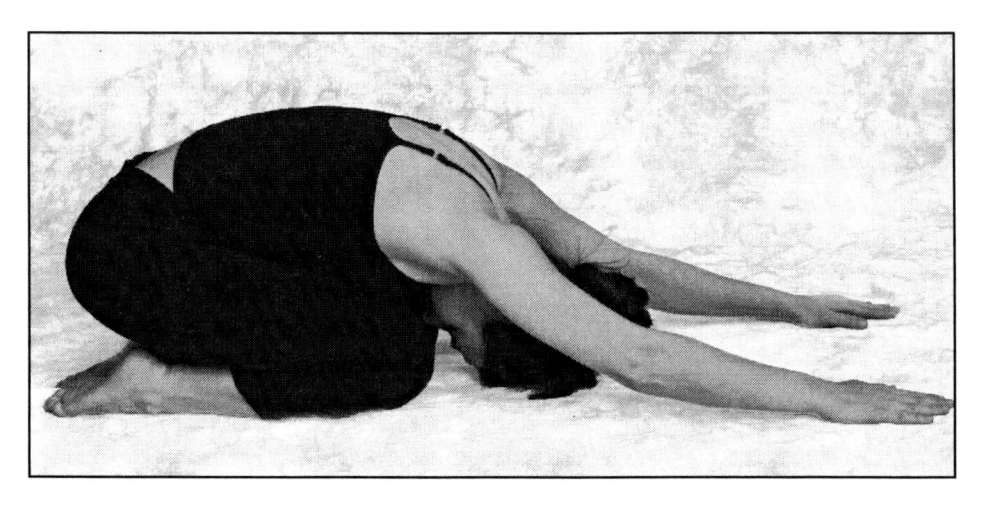

WHAT TO DO:

Get on your hands and knees and then bring your body into child's pose as in the above photo.

WHAT TO WATCH OUT FOR:

1. Pain in the abdominal and/or low back area is a signal to stop and get out of this pose. Make sure you widen your legs to accomodate the baby.

2. Pain in the ankles can occur. Place a pillow under your feet if needed to relieve your ankle and/or foot pain.

BENEFITS:

1. Stretches the low back and helps to relieve back pain.

2. Great pose for practicing reverse Kegels.

3. Promotes relaxation and a sense of peace.

Relaxation Pose

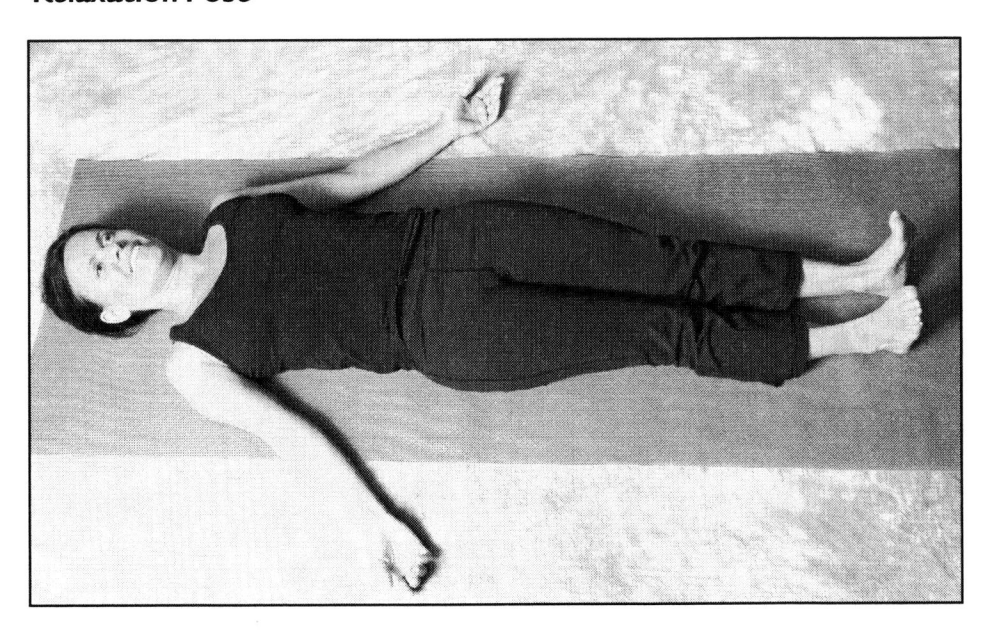

WHAT TO DO:

Lie on your back with your legs straight and your arms at your side.

WHAT TO WATCH OUT FOR:

1. Supine hypotension symptoms. To resolve this, turn to the left side and wait for symptoms to go away. Make sure to prop your upper back and neck with a couple of pillows so that you are in an inclined seated position.

2. Low back or sacral pain. To resolve this, place a pillow under your knees.

BENEFITS:

1. Promotes relaxation.

2. Calms the mind and restores the body.

Now that you have done the hard work and know how to train your body safely and effectively, it is time to take care of the mind and the spirit. In the next chapter you will learn how to relax and use imagery to create the birth and laboring experience you want. You will be introduced to tools that promote relaxation and are helpful in times of stress. The information provided in Chapter 14 will be invaluable even in the period beyond your pregnancy; it can be implemented in the postpartum recovery period when caring for a new baby can be very stressful. Mind/body medicine will not only help you now but will also help you to cultivate mindful parenting.

CHAPTER FOURTEEN

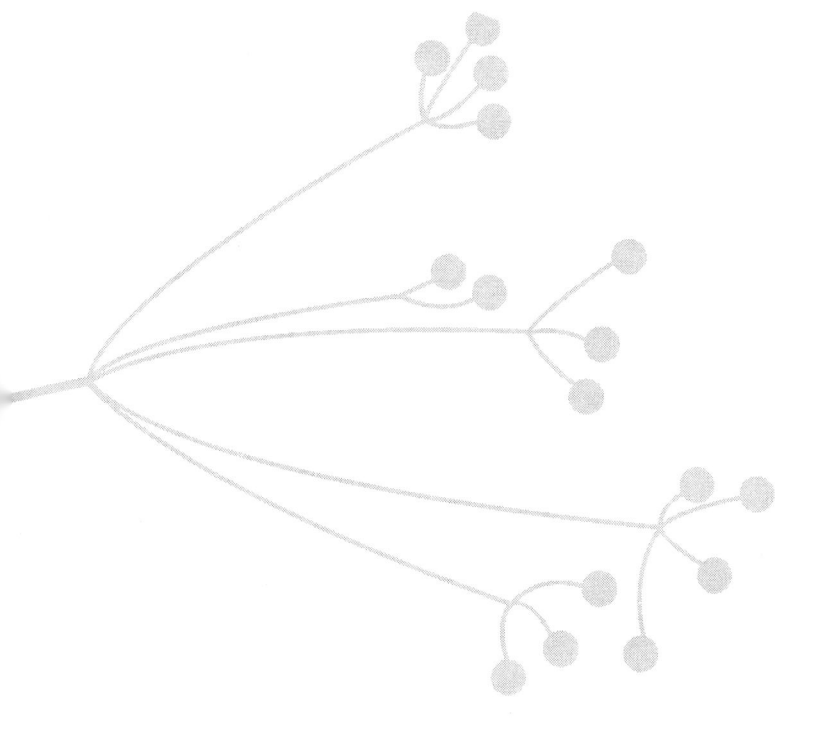

"The course of our lives is determined by how we react—what we decide and what to do—at the darkest times. The nature of that response determines a person's true worth and greatness."

—Daisaku Ikeda

Chapter 14

MIND/BODY MEDICINE

Chronic pregnancy pain can have devastating effects on a pregnant woman's life. Working with patients I have observed that if you don't address the mental component of your pain, your condition will wreak havoc on your mind, soul and body. Although chronic stress does not cause pregnancy pain, it can worsen your pain and symptoms, making you more sensitive and thus causing more flare-ups. I also find it very difficult to treat patients successfully when they are chronically negative and in a state of stress. Many times I have to get them to relax during their treatment sessions before we can even begin any treatments. When I incorporate mind/body relaxation techniques into a pregnant woman's self-care and home exercise programs, they always do better in the long-term. What I have also noticed is that women who do the best with my treatments are those who are able to defeat negativity by incorporating stress reduction mind/body techniques as part of their healing program.

The Physiology of Stress

Your body undergoes many physiological changes when you become stressed out. The first thing that happens is that your endocrine system reacts by releasing many different types of stress hormones into your bloodstream including adrenaline and cortisol. These hormones awaken you mentally and physically and prepare your body for an emergency response. The body goes through physical changes as well, including increased heart rate, tightening of the muscles, increased sharpness and keenness of the five senses, elevation of blood pressure, increase in perspiration, and shunting of blood from the small muscles to the large muscles of the arms and legs. In addition, your physical strength increases, your reaction time gets faster, and your focus is sharper. These bodily changes prepare you to either fight or flee from a dangerous situation. When real danger is present, stress is a good thing and can motivate you to perform better in life. But when stress is an everyday occurrence it can be detrimental to your health and relationships, eventually clouding your thinking and leading to feelings of being overwhelmed. If you're stressed over a busy schedule, an argument with a friend, a traffic jam, or a mountain of bills, your body reacts just as strongly as if you were facing a life-or-death situation. If you have a lot of responsibilities and worries, your emergency stress response may be "on" most of the time. The more your body's stress system is activated, the easier it is to fall into a pain response or flare-up and the harder it is to shut it off.

Long-term stress can even rewire the brain, leaving you more vulnerable to anxiety and depression. Researchers at the Northwestern University Institute of Neuroscience found that people suffering with chronic back pain, for example, not only demonstrate abnormal brain chemistry, particularly in the emotional center of the brain, but also experience actual brain shrinkage (*The Journal of Neuroscience*, November, 2004).

For pain sufferers it is extremely important to manage stress and keep it in check. I have included several techniques and exercises that I use as part of my Ending Pain in Pregnancy Program, helping my patients manage their stress and overcome catastrophic thinking. These stress reduction techniques, meditations, affirmations, and visualizations are easy to do and require no special equipment and can be done anywhere and anytime.

Table 14.1: Stress Reduction Techniques
Frequency: Daily

NAME OF TECHNIQUE
1. Relaxation Breathing
2. Cardiovascular Stress Reduction
3. Progressive Relaxation with Jacobson's Techniques
4. Positive Thinking vs. Negative Self-Talk
5. Mantras and Meditation
6. Journaling
7. Affirmations
8. Keep It Simple – Stop Taking on Too Much
9. Join a Self-Help Group
10. Gratitude Training – Rock and Walk
11. The Present Moment – Staying in the Power of Now
12. Creative Visualizations
13. Positive Birth Visualization: Visualizing the Birth That You Want
14. Talking to Your Unborn Baby

Relaxation Breathing

Focusing on your breathing can have tremendous benefits for your overall stress level. It also helps you to quiet your mind and centers your attention on the present moment. Most people don't take the time to focus on their breathing during the course of the day, but this powerful yet simple exercise can help you release tension, stress, and anxiety. Pregnant women in particular will be challenged with breathing because the baby is taking up a lot of space making lung expansion more difficult. Many of the pregnant women that I treat breathe incorrectly and are upper-chest breathers. Pregnant women need to focus on expanding the entire rib cage including the front, sides and back of the rib cage. This will allow for a bigger breath and will keep the rib cage flexible. Many women experience rib pain because the rib cage is not expanding optimally, they have poor posture or the ribs are out of alignment.

This breath exercise focuses on the length of the inhalation and exhalation. Exhaling for longer than inhaling has a positive effect on the nervous system and promotes deep relaxation.

WHAT TO DO:

1. Sit cross-legged, stand or lie down in a relaxed comfortable position.

2. Slowly inhale through your nose, expanding the rib cage in all directions while counting to five in your head.

3. Exhale from your mouth, counting to ten in your head. The exhale counting depends on your comfort. Some women may find that exhaling for ten seconds is too long and causes anxiety or shortness of breath. Breathing this way enhances relaxation and it's a natural way to breathe.

TIPS:

1. As you breathe, let your lower abdomen expand outward, keeping your upper shoulders quiet and without excessive moment. Avoid raising your shoulders as you inhale and exhale. Breathing this way also helps fill your lungs more fully with fresh air and helps to release old stagnant air.

2. Repeat several times a day for five to ten minutes. This exercise is great to do at work, during stressful situations, and while meditating. It also complements all the exercises in this book.

3. To release more tension, purse your lips and exhale so the air comes out like a whisper. This kind of breathing is done in many yoga classes.

4. Focus on releasing your stress with your exhale; imagine you are attaching your stress to your breath as it leaves your body.

Cardiovascular Stress Reduction

Cardiovascular exercise for at least thirty minutes a day is a great stress-buster, and it also helps to release natural endorphins that help relieve pain. The one exercise that anyone can do is walking, which is why I always recommend a walking program to release stress. Practice the relaxation breath described above as you walk. It will do wonders for your mood and "bust" that stress right out of your body. Also follow the exercise guidelines in Chapter 3 so you are safe in your walking program. Listen to your body and avoid pain in your walking program.

WHAT TO DO:

1. Walk during your lunch hour instead of having lunch at your desk.

2. Take an evening walk after dinner instead of sitting in front of your computer or TV.

3. Join a gym and walk on the treadmill in bad weather. You can also do a walking program in a mall when it's cold outside.

4. Combine your walking with your gratitude meditation, which I will describe later in this chapter. This is a really positive way to build a permanent change to your overall thought patterns.

5. As an alternative to walking, try stationary biking and then see how you feel.

Progressive Relaxation with Jacobson's Techniques

Progressive muscle relaxation was developed by Dr. Edmund Jacobson more than fifty years ago. Dr. Jacobson discovered through his work with his patients that a muscle could be relaxed by first voluntarily tensing it for a few seconds. This voluntary contraction and subsequent muscle relaxation of various body areas produces a deep state of relaxation. Dr. Jacobson found that this technique of progressive relaxation was capable of relieving a variety of conditions, from high blood pressure to ulcerative colitis, to overall pain.

General Guidelines

This relaxation technique requires that you alternately tense and relax your muscles. Try to practice this relaxation at the same time each day for fifteen to thirty minutes. Find a comfortable position such as supported incline sitting or side-lying. Start with the relaxation breathing technique described above for five to ten minutes. The best way to start is to work with groups of muscles in the following sequence, but you can also develop a system that works for you.

Basic Jacobson Contract/Relax Sequence

WHAT TO DO:

1. Contract the right arm for ten seconds and then relax your right arm for ten to fifteen seconds. Do the same for the left arm.

2. Contract both shoulders for ten seconds and then relax your shoulders for ten to fifteen seconds.

3. Contract your neck muscles for ten seconds and then relax your neck muscles for ten to fifteen seconds.

4. Contract your lips and eyes by closing them tightly for ten seconds and then relax your lips and eyes for ten to fifteen seconds.

5. Contract your whole right leg including toes and ankle tightly for ten seconds and then relax your whole right leg for ten to fifteen seconds. Do the same for the left leg.

6. This is a basic sequence, but you can separate out the body parts and tense and relax as many body parts as you want. The more body parts you individually contract and relax the longer this relaxation will take.

Positive Thinking vs. Negative Self-Talk

Oftentimes, my patients can be their own worst enemies. Self-sabotaging thoughts in the form of negative self-talk prevent them from doing the things they need to do to get better. Sometimes the self-sabotaging thoughts are even subconscious, and my patients don't even realize what they are doing habitually until I point it out to them.

I am a firm believer that the body will follow the mind. What you think is what you are. The way we talk to ourselves can make a situation sunny and bright or can make the same situation dark, cloudy and gloomy. Pay attention to the story that your thoughts are creating about your life. Acknowledge your thoughts, but don't always take them as gospel. You can change your entire life by first changing your negative self-talk into more positive, focused and optimistic thought patterns.

Start by examining your thoughts and knowing that many of the statements you are thinking are from habitual patterns or from past conditioning. This is the acknowledgement phase. Then ask yourself: "How can I change this thinking so it does not feed my negativity and old ways of being?" The ego can be difficult to overcome and the shadows in our lives can perpetuate our faulty patterns leading us to a place of inaction and acceptance of thoughts that are not true. Some of our thoughts keep us in the dark. The search for the light and for conscious living is not easy but it can be done. You can fight back. You can change your life by changing your thoughts.

Mantras and Meditation

I give my patients mantras to get them through the day. A mantra is a repeated word, syllable, phrase, or sound that can help you relax during times of stress or as a precursor to your stretching, strengthening or dilator work. Saying a mantra during meditation or at various times throughout the day will help quiet your mind and bring inner peace to you. The most basic mantra is *OM*. This mantra can be repeated

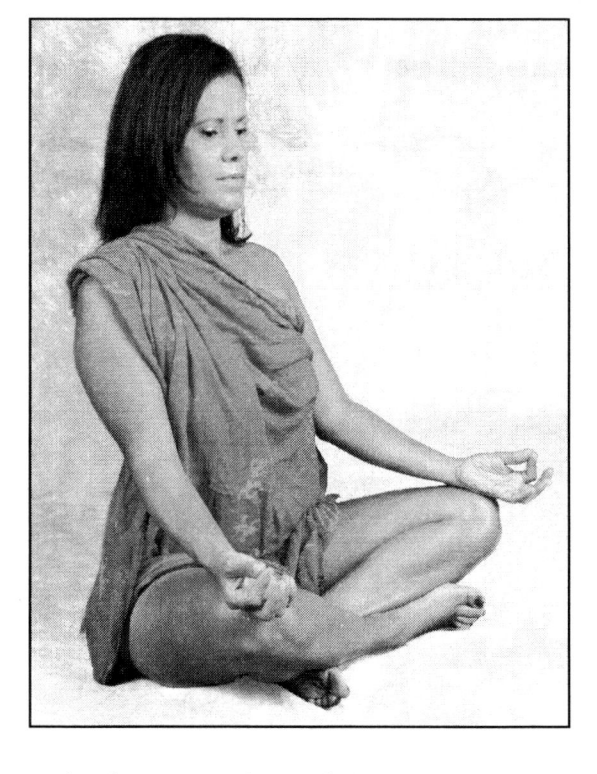

slowly for three to five minutes and it brings a calming feeling to your entire body. Allow the syllable or syllables of your mantra to resonate slowly inside your head and body like a bell, using it to clear out the "thought clutter" that often prevents us from staying in the present moment. The main objective is to quiet down negative thoughts to make room for positive thoughts to sprout into your consciousness. Remember: you must believe in your mantra, and then your body will follow. I like to have my patients meditate for three to five minutes while quietly repeating their mantra. This meditation technique with mantras has been shown to lower cholesterol, reduce stress, pain, and blood pressure, and improve heart function. You can choose your own mantra; *OM* is just an example.

WHAT TO DO:

1. Sit or lie down on your side, usually with your eyes closed.

2. Focus on deep diaphragmatic breathing for five to ten breaths as you slow down your mind. Many of my patients report holding their breath or breathing shallowly when they experience pain, which limits oxygen to the tissues and results in more pain. You must do the opposite during your meditation.

3. Begin repeating your mantra with conviction, allowing it to permeate into your being.

4. After three to five minutes of diaphragmatic breathing, repeat the mantra *OM* or try a different one.

MANTRA EXAMPLES

My baby and I are safe

I-Am-Pain-Free

I-Am-Healed

I-Am-Fearless

Journaling

I often tell my patients to keep a journal of their journeys up to the present moment. I tell them to write down the stories of their pain as they perceive it. Sometimes the pain is a result of a traumatic incident from childhood or emotional experience. I had a patient tell me she had pain since she fell off a horse as a youngster. Other patients don't tell me, but I get a sense that their pain is the result of sexual abuse. Oftentimes they don't completely remember what happened, but they feel that their body's response has been one of "closing down" in an effort to protect itself.

Whatever the story of your pain may be, I encourage you to write it down and track feelings as you journey forward with the Ending Pain in Pregnancy Program. Once my patients have written down their feelings, I often suggest they perform a ceremony where they burn or shred their story and release the past from their body and mind. I first did this after a painful, late-stage miscarriage. My husband and I were filled with pain and anguish, and thought we could not move forward. We ended up journeying to the mountains in Spain where we burned the printouts of the sonograms of our baby, releasing the past from our psyches. It was hard to do but it ended up being a wonderful experience that brought us tremendous feelings of peace and acceptance, and cleared out the past. Once you let go of the mental burden of your own pain story, you can free your consciousness to spring forward to positive thoughts and allow the healing energy of the universe to flow once again through your body and mind. Burn your story and free yourself. It will be like a new beginning for you.

Affirmations

It is always remarkable to me how powerful your words can be in shaping your actions and your life. I am a firm believer that your body will follow what you say you are. So if you are a person who suffers from chronic pain, you might not realize that what you say could be perpetuating your suffering as much as your thoughts. As you go through your day, try to see yourself from the outside and actually listen to the words you use to describe yourself and your various situations in your life, from your job, to your relationships, to your perception of your own existence. You might find that you are actually saying out loud that you won't get better, you are destined to be in pain, or that it is your fate to be afflicted.

By using affirmations to change your spoken words about your perceived life situations, you can create powerful forces of change that your body will eventually follow. I like to have my patients write down their affirmations and say them while looking themselves in the eye in the mirror. Repeat the affirmations every morning before brushing your teeth and every evening before going to bed, and you will find your words will change your life. Say them with conviction and the changes you desire will come more quickly. I always recommend my patients read Louise Hay's great book, *You Can Heal Your Life*, to get a more in-depth analysis of the power of affirmations. I have included here some great affirmations for women with pregnancy pain, but it is also great if you write some of your own as well. Remember to write your affirmations in the present tense with words like "I am" or "I have" so that your mind can tell your body that these are states of life that you already are in, not some distant place where you hope to be in the future.

Table 14.2: Affirmations for Pregnancy Pain

AFFIRMATION
1. I am healed.
2. I am having a great and active pregnant life.
3. I have healed from my back pain.
4. I am in a loving and satisfying relationship.

Keep It Simple: Stop Taking on Too Much

Are you taking on too much work or find yourself overscheduled? Are you not sure how to say no to other people's demands on your time? If the answer is yes, then you can put yourself in a state of chronic stress and you habitually will tend to take on more than you can handle. Do you find you are constantly putting yourself last on your own list? If this is the case, you might be subconsciously sabotaging your healing and causing yourself undue stress, tension and pressure.

If you keep telling yourself you just don't have time to do your Ending Pain in Pregnancy Program healing techniques, then you have to break the cycle of taking on too much. If necessary, schedule time for yourself during the day and in the mornings and evenings. Even fifteen minutes during the day to do a quick meditation, breathing, mantra, and workplace stretching program will work wonders for your body, mind, and soul. You will also find that once you begin to carve out time for yourself, it becomes easier to keep on doing it because your body and your mind will gravitate to the positive way it makes you feel.

Tips for Keeping It Simple and Not Taking on Too Much

1. Say no to family and friends if what they are asking of you puts you under stress.

2. Make sure that your work schedule does not interfere with your healing work.

3. Space out your social calendar so that you have *ME* time.

4. Do something that brings you joy and happiness everyday, even if it is as simple as looking at flowers for five minutes.

5. Surround yourself with positive energy and avoid being around negative people.

Join a Self-Help Group

I find that the women who do the best in my practice have someone to talk to about their emotional pain. Many of my patients tell me they feel better and are less stressed after being surrounded by women who have the same problems they do.

TIPS:

1. Join a self-help group and keep with it for several months.

2. Get a life-coach.

3. See a psychotherapist for your emotional pain.

4. If there are no groups near you, then start one yourself or join an Internet blog.

5. Ask your physical therapist if she could help you arrange a self-help group with other patients.

Gratitude Training - Rock and Walk

When I first saw *The Secret* by Rhonda Byrnes, I was captivated by the part in the DVD that mentions having an "Attitude of Gratitude." Another great source for gratitude training is Deepak Chopra, who talks about gratitude and how it needs to be the foundation of your overall outlook. I constantly find that my patients come to me so focused on their pain and how it pervades their whole life that it is the only thing on their minds. I always tell them—although they often look at me like I am crazy at first—that they need to think about all of the things they are grateful for instead. I tell them that, in order to get on the road to healing, they have to first focus on things that are positive in their lives instead of focusing only on the pain and what they don't have.

Gratitude Rocks

When my patients come to me on their first visit, I give them a gratitude rock. This rock serves to remind them of the beauty, love and joy that they currently have in their lives.

WHAT TO DO:

1. Find a rock small enough that you can carry with you everyday. I carry mine in my pocket or purse. I collect rocks from the ocean or streams because they are smooth and have all of the rough and symbolically "painful edges" smoothed off by the power of water. I let my patients pick a rock that catches their eye.

2. When you are having a hard day and a pain flare-up, touch your rock and repeat to yourself: "I am grateful today for _____." Think about your statement and feel it. Feel the joy, happiness and elation around your statement. Send these feelings to all your cells, all body parts and muscles.

3. Put the rock next to your bed, and when you wake up, roll up and sit on the edge of your bed. Take your rock in your hand and think about something you are grateful for. Set the tone for your day as one of gratitude, one in which your pain and negativity, if it comes, will only be a fleeting part of your day.

4. Remember that the universe will not give more than you can bear, so stay grateful for things as simple as having enough air to breathe, and you will have a powerful transformational effect on your existence.

Gratitude Walks

As part of your cardiovascular training, incorporate gratitude into your walking program. Be conscious of how your thoughts are taking up space in your mind while you are walking Make sure to take notice of the beauty around you: birds, flowers, kids playing, the sunlight shining through the trees, or any other visuals or sounds that should make you feel grateful. Instead of thinking about how much you hate your boss or how much pain you are in, think about how grateful you are to be working at all, and how grateful you are to be on the road to healing, even if you are currently only making the smallest of steps forward in your program. The momentum will build and you will be amazed at the results.

The Present Moment — Staying in the Power of Now

Misery, stress and unhappiness are usually caused by thinking about events that are in the future or in the past. I find that when my patients stay present "in the now" they have less stress and anxiety. A personal favorite is Eckhart Tolle, a great author and lecturer who has written many books including a wonderful one called *The Power of Now*. I recommend this book to my patients, and they tell me they now understand how the constant flurry of activity that occurs in their minds affects their health and overall outlook. It is not difficult to be in the present, but you must make an effort to be in the now.

Tolle talks at length about how the mind creates "the story of me," and how your ego tries to interpret events and actions in your life within this context. So if your mind has created "a story of me" that is one of perpetual pain, then your mind and ego will seek out events and people and interpretations of what has happened to you to keep going with this story. Once you let go of the past and the future, which are only creations of the mind, you can embrace the present moment, which you will find is actually quite manageable and one in which you can make conscious decisions to move forward down the path to your ultimate healing.

TIPS:

1. When thinking about future or past events, bring your mind to the present moment and focus your energy on your current breath. You can acknowledge your thoughts and thank your brain for trying to interpret every perception in the context of "the story of me," but let your mind know that you are going to focus on the present moment right now and enjoy it without interpretation.

2. Get a copy of Eckhart Tolle's book, *The Power of Now*, and read it at least two times.

Creative Visualizations

As discussed earlier, you are what you think and say you are, so be careful because the universe will lovingly give you what you think and declare you are. Why not start by thinking and visualizing yourself well, free from excess mental chatter, happy, and pain-free? Creative visualization is a great tool to use to reduce stress related to your painful condition. It's quite easy to do and can consist of almost any visualization. Below are two examples I have found that work great for my patients.

The Mirrored Hallway

Several times a day, whenever you are able, take a moment for a mental break and try the mirrored hallway visualization exercise. Repeat the exercise at least once per day for two to four weeks and track your progress. You should begin to see just how powerful your mind can be in keeping you in a state of pain if you let it, even subconsciously keeping you from declaring that you are better each day.

WHAT TO DO:

1. This exercise can be done sitting or lying down. I like to do this on the subway on my way home.

2. Close your eyes and focus on your breathing for five breaths. Focus on slowing down your breathing. Release the thoughts of the day up until that point, inhale through the nose and exhale through the mouth. Don't think about the future or the past.

3. Imagine the lights are being turned on and you find yourself in a short six to eight foot hallway with a door on one end. You are just entering the hallway so the door is at the other end of the hallway.

4. You then notice that there are floor to ceiling mirrors on both sides of the hallway. On the left, see yourself or your situation, allowing your reflection to be your state of pain, your misery, your negative outlook, anything in life, which you wish to overcome.

5. Then look to the right and allow your reflection to be the exact opposite from the left. See yourself in a pain-free state, happy, filled with positive thoughts, having overcome that which your mind says you cannot overcome. Focus and remember how good you will feel once you have overcome your pain.

6. Then turn back to the left mirror; notice that there is a large wooden staff in the corner of the hallway. Take the staff and smash the mirror on the left in one forceful blow, bringing your mind into that moment, telling your mind that you will not tolerate these reflections to exist any longer.

7. Focus back on the right, and then walk through the hall seeing your reflection, open the door and continue on your journey as a pain-free person.

Mental Suds Visualization

I like to use this visualization as a gauge to help me get a sense of how many thoughts are actually "on my mind." At first you will find how amazingly filled your mind is even when you think you are in the moment. I often use this visualization as I prepare to do a meditation and mantra to calm down my mind.

WHAT TO DO:

1. Sit comfortably, with your eyes closed, with your focus slightly upward toward your third eye. Your third eye is the area above your nose and in between your eyebrows.

2. Allow the thoughts in your head to flow freely into this area of focus. Don't worry whether the thoughts are good or bad; simply take notice of them as they cross your focus.

3. As each thought passes into your gaze, place it into a bubble and allow it to float in your perception. Don't let it float away, but keep it within your gaze.

4. Repeat this for each thought that is currently "on your mind." You may find in a short while that all of the bubbles you have created have made what I call "mental suds," where the bubbles are so close together that they look like suds in a bubble bath. If this is the case, don't worry; you have just created a mental picture of what is whizzing through your mind at the present moment.

5. Make an effort to pop bubbles in your field of view, releasing the thoughts contained in each bubble, which are not important to your present moment.

6. Try to pop all the bubbles that relate to your past or to things you have to do or that relate to relationships and how you need to talk to this person or that person, or how you are always going to be in pain, etc. Leave just a few bubbles in your field of view: maybe one bubble filled with a thought about your breath and how it can heal you, and maybe another bubble filled with a thought about something you are grateful for, and maybe one bubble with a thought about how great it is to be pain-free.

Positive Birth Visualization: Visualizing the Birth That You Want

Many women are understandably afraid about childbirth and spend too much time watching births on TV or listening to other people's birth stories. It's okay to learn about a friend's experience but I find that people always want to tell you the bad parts of their birth instead of what happened that was good.

WHAT TO DO:

1. Get into a comfortable position and start to breathe naturally and slowly.

2. Next comes imagination "play" at its best. Think about the birth that you want. See the birth, feel the contractions and see yourself holding the baby. Visualize as much of the birth as you can in as much detail as you can.

3. Practice this for five minutes a day. Always see the birth and outcome that you want. Focus on the positive outcomes only. Nothing else will do here.

Talk to Your Unborn Baby

Pregnant women are incredibly intuitive and have a high level of awareness. I find that communicating with baby before it is born is a nice meditation that allows for bonding to occur in the womb. Babies have ears and they can hear. Why not have a dialogue with the baby? Many times in our quiet moments we can receive messages or intuitive "hits." In much the same way, you can experience moments in which you feel intimately connected with your baby.

WHAT TO DO:

1. Start a dialogue with your baby; ask the baby questions and see what happens.

2. Listen quietly so you can receive your baby's messages. You'll be surprised what the baby will tell you.

In the next chapter, *Aromatherapy for Today's Pregnant Woman*, you will learn the ins and outs of using essential oils to enhance your pregnancy and labor experience.

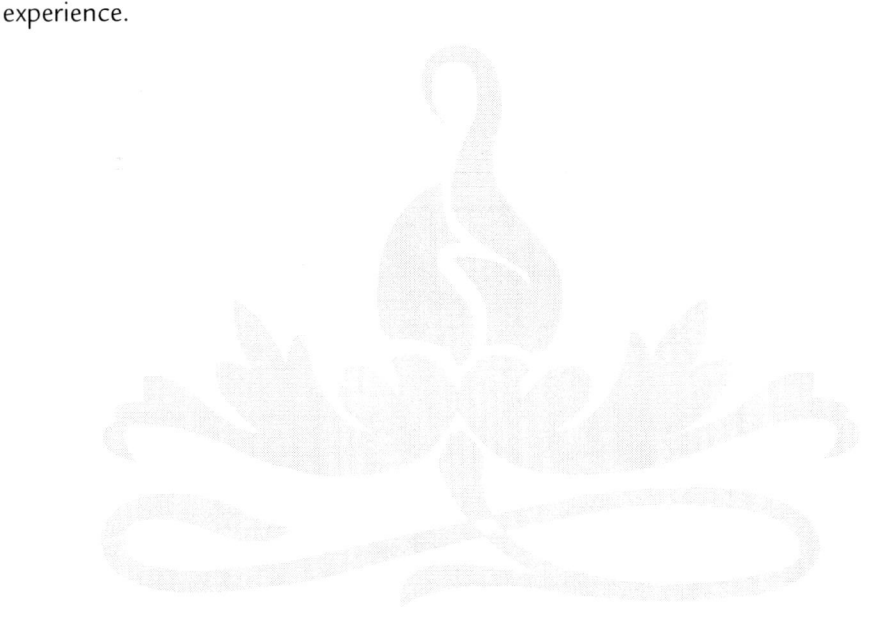

CHAPTER FIFTEEN

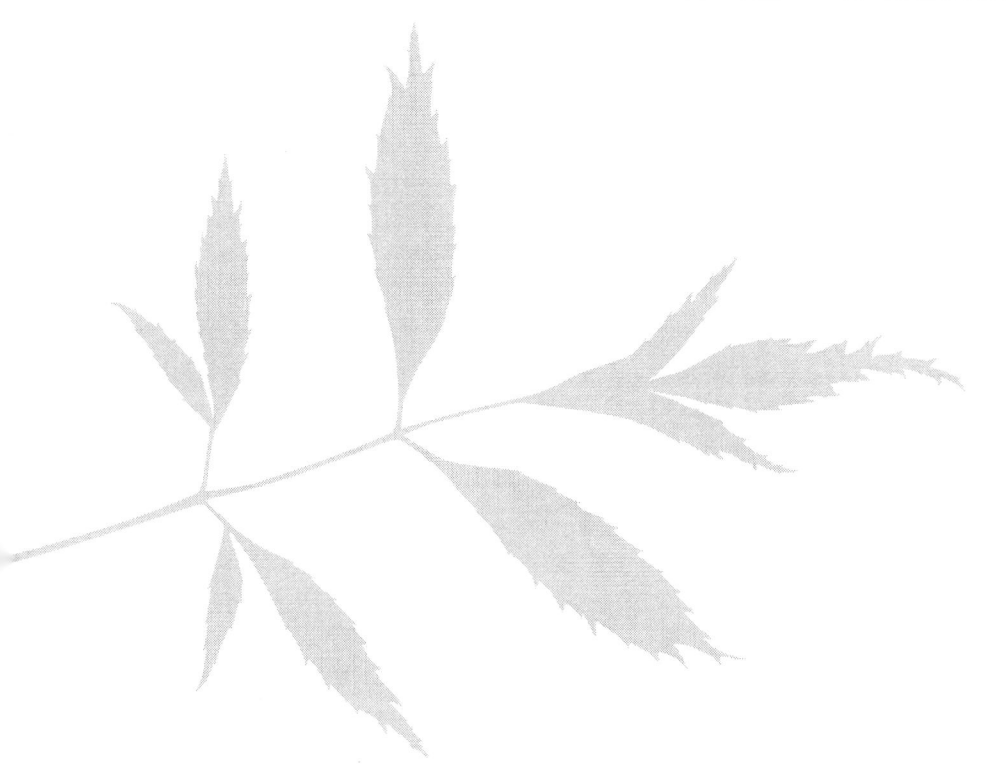

*"Mother love is the fuel that enables a
normal human being to do the impossible."*

– C. Garrety

Chapter 15

AROMATHERAPY FOR TODAY'S PREGNANT WOMAN

Aromatherapy is gaining popularity and many women find it helpful to use essential oils, which are both safe and non-toxic, during the childbearing year. Aromatherapy is not a new age fad; in many countries clinicians have to study for years and take numerous exams to be certified in aromatherapy. Many of the pregnant women that we treat at Renew Physical Therapy already use oils as part of their pregnancy self-care program. But we find that they are often confused about which oils are safe and how to use them while pregnant. Aromatherapy works in three ways including inhalation, topical application and ingestion. Aromatherapy involves the sense of smell: through the scent of the oils tremendous healing can occur. Oils, of course, can be applied topically. Since the skin is the largest organ in the body and the oils can be absorbed through the skin, the healing effects of skin application can be profound.

There is a great deal of information on the market today, but it can be very difficult to make sense of it. Many individuals have their own spin on aromatherapy. With this chapter we want to give you the facts regarding the use of oils during pregnancy. We want to educate pregnant women so that they feel more comfortable using aromatherapy to combat the aches, pain and other symptoms that come along with growing a baby inside your body. First, we will introduce you to the concept of aromatherapy and provide you with the most up-to-date information.

Pregnant women experience an array of symptoms and essential oils offer a safe and alternative choice to over-the-counter drugs and prescribed medications. Today essential oils are available in pharmacies and can even be found in supermarkets. The problem is that all oils are not the same and during pregnancy women need to be very careful about what they put on their bodies since most things affect the baby. It is our recommendation that only high-quality therapeutic grade essential oil be used during pregnancy. Why? Because these oils are typically very pure and not mixed with additives and other compounds that may not be safe in pregnancy. What you put on your skin has a direct effect on your growing baby. Don't risk using lower quality oils. Instead, look for brands that can be trusted such as the Young Living brand. We've found their oil to be safe and therapeutic: in fact, we use it to make our Renew PT proprietary blends. At our practice we use lavender for spasms related to pubic bone pain and sciatica. For pregnancy blues and depression we use Renew PT Sunshine in a Bottle. Many of our patients rave about Renew PT Labor of Love. Used only during active labor, this oil helps to maintain the efficiency of contractions while promoting positivity and fearlessness

Essential oils can provide many positive effects for pregnant women. They can help deal with stress and anxiety by promoting relaxation and can be effective for relieving pregnancy-related symptoms such as morning sickness, heartburn, edema, constipation and allergies. Essential oils can boost a pregnant woman's immune system and help her fight colds, flu and infections. They are amazing for back pain and muscles spasms. Essential oils can also help to prevent stretch marks. Many pregnant women have trouble sleeping and oils can definitely help improve insomnia. Essential oils can fight fatigue: they can energize you so you can complete your task or get through a work day. In the next section we will cover essential oil application, safety and benefits.

How to Apply the Oil:

Careful application of essential oils is necessary and must be followed very strictly—especially during pregnancy. Read the criteria below and make sure to adhere to the recommendations. There are several ways that oils can be used: They can be inhaled, diffused, or applied to the skin (either directly or in the bath). Note that when using essential oils on the skin, they must be diluted with a carrier oil. See Table 15.3 for sample carrier oils.

Essential Oil Application Methods:

Inhalation Techniques:

- Five to six drops in a diffuser (in a cold air or ultrasonic diffuser).

- Inhale from the bottle.

- Place one drop in your hands, rub hands together, cup hands over nose and mouth and inhale.

Topical Technique (directly on the skin):

- Apply one to two drops to the desired area in ten milliliters (10ml =.68 tablespoons) of carrier oil.

- Dilute fifty/fifty (one drop of essential oil to one drop of carrier oil, such as coconut, almond, or olive oil) especially if the essential oil is being applied to a sensitive area or you have sensitive skin. Do not use more than ten drops oil whether alone or in combination.

Ingestion: Not advised during pregnancy.

Massage Techniques:

- Apply one to two drops to the desired area in ten milliliters (10ml =.68 tablespoons) of carrier oil.

- Massage areas with the oil.

Baths:

- Use two to three drops of essential oil in two to four tablespoons of bath salts. Always swish the water around to disperse the oil. Mix together and then add to bath —only after getting medical clearance from your care-giver.

Diffusion/Vaporization:

- Four to six drops of essential oil in a diffuser.

Foot Rubs:

- Feet transport oils very quickly into the body, so less is more when using the feet as a vehicle for oil transport.

- Apply one to two drops to the desired area in ten milliliters (10ml =.68 tablespoons) of carrier oil.

- Massage areas with the oil.

Table 15.1: Essential Oil Safety and Precaution Information

1. Keep oils away from eyes.
2. Keep oils out of the reach of children.
3. Consult your midwife or doctor before using essential oils. Work with a trained aromatherapist.
4. If you have had vaginal bleeding in the pregnancy consult your doctor and/or midwife before using any essential oil.
5. Avoid essential oils during high-risk pregnancies. Consult your MD and/or midwife.
6. If you have a history of miscarriage consult your doctor and/or midwife before using essential oils.
7. If you have heart problems consult your doctor before using essential oils.
8. Essential oils must always be diluted in a carrier oil before applying to your skin.
9. There are some exceptions such as lavender oils that can be used directly on the skin but sparingly and in small amounts. Consult a certified aromatherapist when using oils.
10. If you get an essential oil in a sensitive area (genitals or eyes) flush the area with a fatty carrier oil (almond, coconut, or olive). Avoid flushing with water as it will drive the essential oil further into the area and increase the pain.
11. If an oil feels hot on the skin dilute it with a carrier oil. This will help reduce the skin irritation and burning.
12. Avoid all topical use of oils during the first trimester. Instead, inhale or diffuse the oil but you MUST first get clearance from your doctor and/or midwife.
13. Always do a skin patch test before using an essential oil on a larger area of your body or using it for massage. Add two drops of essential oil to half tablespoon of carrier oil. Put on inner part of elbow. Wait twenty-four hours. If any redness, burning or itching occurs, this is not the oil for you and you should not use it.
14. During pregnancy NEVER ingest essential oils by mouth.
15. If you suffer from epilepsy, consult an aromatherapist. Do not use fennel, hyssop, sage, or rosemary. Seek help from a trained professional as you can trigger an epileptic attack.
16. Essential oils are flammable and should be kept away from direct contact with flames from candles, fire, matches, cigarettes, and gas cookers.
17. Peppermint oil is contraindicated with the use of cardiac stabilizing medications, including quinidine. Peppermint oil interferes with calcium channel blockers. Also avoid using peppermint oil with and Gastroesphageal Reflux Disease (GERD) and heartburn. Peppermint oil can also increase the activity of NSAIDS and naproxen. Do not use this oil if you have poor liver enzymes or suffer from liver disease.
CAUTION: Do not use peppermint oil around children younger than three years old because this oil has led to respiratory collapse in children.

Table 15.2: Pregnancy and Oil Use: Trimester Recommendations

Essential Oils in the first trimester – Avoid all oils during the first trimester unless okayed by your OB/GYN or midwife.
Second Trimester and onwards – Use primarily through inhalation and only use small amounts of essential oils topically. Increase the amounts of essential oils used; use more topically as the pregnancy progresses and they must be diluted.

Table 15.3: Carriers Oils for the Dilution of Essential Oils

1. Sweet Almond Oil
2. Avocado Oil
3. Coconut Oil
4. Grapeseed Oil
5. Jojoba Oil
6. Olive Oil
7. Calendula Oil
8. Wheat Germ Oil

Table 15.4: Oils That Can Be Safely Used during Pregnancy

ESSENTIAL OIL	PURPOSE AND BENEFITS	HOW TO APPLY AND IN WHAT TRIMESTER
Lemon (Citrus limon)	Helps to restore energy when fatigued. Helps with memory and helps aid in circulation. Avoid sunlight for twenty-four hours after applying lemon. Avoid using lemon under the nose.	Diffusion; Inhalation; and Massage. *Avoid in first trimester.*
Lavender (Lavandula angustifolia)	An anti-spasmodic that helps relieve pain and muscle spasms in muscles. Helps with insomnia and sleeplessness. Can be used for stretch marks. Helps reduce indigestion and heartburn. Great for headaches.	Diffusion; Inhalation; and/or Topical. *Avoid in first trimester.*
Roman Chamomile (Chamaemelum nobile)	Helps reduce indigestion and heartburn. Helps with insomnia and sleeplessness. Also works well on itchy skin.	Diffusion; Inhalation. *Avoid in first trimester.* Ask your midwife and/or doctor about using this oil in the first trimester for morning sickness. Some may permit and others may not allow it.
Peppermint (Mentha piperita)	Helps reduce nausea and morning sickness. Helps reduce indigestion and heartburn. Great for headaches. Peppermint is a great anti-viral. Do NOT use it around children less than three years old.	Inhalation. *Avoid in first trimester.* Ask your midwife and/or doctor about using this oil in the first trimester for morning sickness. Some may permit and others may not allow it.
Ginger (Zingiber officinale)	Helps reduce nausea and morning sickness.	Inhalation. Ask your midwife and/or doctor about using this oil in the first trimester for morning sickness. Some may permit and others may not allow it.
Spearmint (Mentha spicata)	Helps reduce nausea and morning sickness.	Inhalation. Ask your midwife and/or doctor about using this oil in the first trimester for morning sickness. Some may permit and others may not allow it.

Table 15.4 (cont.): Oils That Can Be Safely Used during Pregnancy

ESSENTIAL OIL	PURPOSE AND BENEFITS	HOW TO APPLY AND IN WHAT TRIMESTER
Myrrh (*Commiphora myrrha*)	Helps with stretch marks and can be used for perineal massage. Fifty/fifty dilution with carrier oil and no more than two to five drops for perineal massage.	Topical. *Avoid in first trimester.*
Ylang-Ylang (*Cananga odorata*)	Reduces nervous and emotional tension and promotes relaxation.	Inhalation; Massage. *Avoid in first trimester.*
Tangerine (*Citrus reticulate*)	Great for stretch marks and aiding sleep.	Inhalation. *Avoid in first trimester.*
Eucalyptus globulus (*Eucalyptus globulus*)	Great for colds and flu. A decongestant that helps you to breathe better.	Diffusion; Inhalation. *Avoid in first trimester.*
Frankincense (*Boswellia carteri*)	Can be used for stretch marks and for relaxation. Great to use toward the end of first stage of labor. Great for headaches.	Inhalation; Massage; and Topical. *Avoid in first trimester.*
Neroli (*Citrus sinensis*)	Reduces stress and promotes relaxation. Helps with aches and pains.	Diffusion; Inhalation, Massage; and Topical. *Avoid in first trimester.*

Table 15.4 (cont.): Oils That Can Be Safely Used during Pregnancy

ESSENTIAL OIL	PURPOSE AND BENEFITS	HOW TO APPLY AND IN WHAT TRIMESTER
Pettigrain	Calming and soothing.	Inhalation. *Avoid in first trimester.*
Geranium *(Pelargonium graveolens)*	Helps with aches and pains and elevates the mood.	Topical or Inhalation *Avoid in first trimester.*
Sandalwood	Anti-depressant.	Diffusion; Inhalation; Massage; and Topical. *Avoid in first trimester.*
Orange *(Citrus sinensis)*	Combats fatigue and improves mental awareness and clarity. Photosensitive oil. You must wait twenty-four hours after using it before exposing skin to sun. Avoid applying it to skin that is exposed to sun.	Diffusion; Inhalation, Massage; and Topical. *Avoid in first trimester.*
Renew PT *Sunshine in a bottle*	Used to combat the blues and depression during pregnancy. Photosensitive oil. You must wait twenty-four hours after using it before exposing skin to sun. Avoid applying it to skin that is exposed to sun.	Diffusion; Inhalation, Massage and Topical. *Avoid in first trimester.*
Renew PT *Labor of Love*	Helps with labor by promoting effective and strong contractions while promoting positivity and fearlessness.	Used during Active Labor only. Not to be used in pregnancy.

Table 15.5: Essential Oils to Avoid during Pregnancy

1. Juniperus sabina *(Savin)*
2. Spanish Sage *(Juniperus pfitzeriana)*
3. Parsley seed *(apiol)*
4. Basil *(Ocimum basilicum)*
5. Clay Sage *(Salvia sclarea)*
6. Jasmine *(Jasminum offcinale)*
7. Rosemary *(Rosmarinus officinalis CT cineol)*
8. Lemongrass *(Cymbopogon flexuosus)*
9. Thyme *(Thymus vulgaris)*
10. Cassia *(Cinnamomum cassia)*
11. Fennel *(Foeniculum vulgare)*

Table 15.6: Essential Oils Only to Be Used in Active Labor—Never in Pregnancy

Many women find the usage of essential oils for labor and delivery very helpful and purposeful. I frequently hear: "The oils helped me stay calm and relaxed while I was in labor." Listed below are the two most effective oils for labor and delivery.

ESSENTIAL OIL	PURPOSE AND BENEFITS	HOW TO APPLY AND IN WHAT STAGE OF LABOR
Clary sage *(Salvia sclarea)*	Helps maintain the rhythm of contractions and labor.	To be used in active labor only once contractions and labor have been established.
Jasmine *(Jasminum offcinale)*	Helps maintain the rhythm of contractions and labor. Promotes positivity.	To be used in active labor only once contractions and labor have been established.

Essential oils can help women overcome the common ailments they experience in pregnancy. They are real medicines and should be used with caution and under the supervision of a clinical aromatherapist and with the clearance of your caregiver. Although I use oils with my pregnant patients I am very conservative and follow the guidelines I have put forth in this chapter. Don't be afraid to use the oils, but please learn what you can before using them. This chapter is a brief introduction to aromatherapy. It is not intended to diagnose or treat you, but to inform you of the possibilities that are out there.

Conclusion

You've done it! You've gone all the way through my book. If this is your first read, go back and begin to absorb the nuances as you experiment with crafting your program from your new sets of tools. Armed with information and determination, embark on your journey to relieving your pregnancy pain and don't look back.

Be sure to check out the resource page. It has information on where to get important products that you will need to complete the Ending Pain in Pregnancy Program. Remember to keep on track by exploring my website, *www.RenewPT. com*. I am always adding new material to my great site and invite you to get involved in spreading the word to others who have suffered for too long.

Use the tools, information, exercises, and recommendations in *Ending Pain in Pregnancy* and become the heroine of your own story. May your healing journey be long lasting.

Isa Herrera, MSPT, CSCS

APPENDICES, GLOSSARY, BIBLIOGRAPHY & INDEX

"You may not always have a comfortable life and you will not always be able to solve all the world's problems at once but don't underestimate the importance you can have because history has shown us that courage can be contagious and hope can take on a life of its own."

– Michelle Obama

Appendix I

SEX DURING PREGNANCY: TRADE SECRETS FOR SUCCESS

Pregnancy has its challenges when it comes to love making. Some women are turned on and have increased libido and the best orgasms of their lives. There is so much blood flow to the vaginal area that it makes sense that women who have never had an orgasm report that they are having them during pregnancy. Other women cannot even think about sex and have little or no desire. This paradigm is reflected in men also. Some men are turned on by the pregnancy and the voluptuousness of the pregnant body and want to engage in sexual intercourse and others are not interested.

In addition to the physical changes there are fears that are associated with sex and pregnancy. These fears and thoughts relating to the baby's getting hurt or triggering premature labor need to be examined and discussed as a couple and with your OB/GYN or midwife. There are times when sex should be avoided and they are listed in the table below.

Many women want to feel close to their partners and have sexual desires that they want to fulfill. Many pregnant women also feel sexier and want to have more sex but are unsure about how to accommodate the physical changes with a sexual romp. The first trimester is a challenge for sexual relations because most women are nauseous, fatigued and just not feeling like their normal selves. During the second trimester most pregnant women start to feel better, and this is when the libido returns and their desire for sex often increases. My patients have told me that during this period of time they became multiorgasmic. The third trimester can be a big challenge for those who want to have sex because the belly is getting bigger making certain positions uncomfortable. Despite all its challenges, sex during pregnancy can be very gratifying and can enhance the bond between the soon-to-be parents. With some experimenting and with the suggestions listed below, both you and your partner will be able to find a position that works during any trimester of your pregnancy.

Precautions and Contraindications for Sex during Pregnancy

1. Placenta Previa
2. Twin or multiple pregnancies
3. Premature labor or risk of premature labor
4. Bleeding during pregnancy
5. Uterine Irritability
6. Your MD has stated you should avoid sex. Please be in communication with your doctor or midwife and ask them if there are any reasons that you should abstain from sexual intercourse during pregnancy.

Recommended Positions for Sex during Pregnancy

Side-Lying Spoon:

Lie on your most comfortable side with your partner side-lying behind you. This position allows your partner to keep most of his weight off your pregnant belly. You can also add clitoral stimulation as a way to heighten your sexual response. Your partner can also control the depth of penetration in this position.

Crisscross:

Place one to three pillows under your head to increase comfort and decrease weight of uterus, your organs and blood vessels. Your partner is side-lying next to you as you drape your legs over his upper thighs. Keeping your legs together also helps ease back pain.

Woman on Top:

This position adds no weight on your abdomen and you can control the depth of penetration. To lessen penetration, place a pillow on partner's thighs. You can also try facing toward your partner's feet to see if this is more comfortable.

All Fours:

This is a great position since there is no weight on your uterus. This position allows for deep penetration of the penis. Communicate with your partner at all times. Let him know if you are uncomfortable with the depth of his penis and modify the depth so that you are comfortable.

Reverse Cow Girl:

Have your partner sit on a place that's safe and where there is no risk of falling. Sit on your partner's lap facing forward (you can also face away) as you gently guide his penis into your vagina. This position allows for deep penetration of the penis.

Outercourse:

Some women are unable to engage in sexual relations during their pregnancy. There are other ways to enhance intimacy and at the same time feel sexually gratified. Focusing on OUTERCOURSE gets you intimacy, orgasms and emotional connection without the penile penetration. Outercourse can include masturbation, oral sex, kissing, cuddling, slow dancing and massaging each other, lap dancing rubbing your parts on each other. The possibilities are endless.

When it comes to sex during pregnancy the rules are set by you, your partner and your comfort levels. There is no right way to do it during pregnancy and avoiding it altogether might not be work for most couples. The most important thing is to keep an open mind and to enjoy every moment and to be at peace with any decision you choose to make.

APPENDIX 2

RESOURCES

Renew Physical Therapy Website: *www.RenewPT.com*. Free information, blank PDFs of EFP book charts for your pain mapping, pain journaling, DRA testing, Q-Tip test, voiding diary, custom oil blends for pelvic pain, blogs, research, and other important tools. Also published case study on scar therapy at Renew PT, *http://tinyurl.com/kfllqrw.*

American College of Obstetricians and Gynecologists. Resource Guide *www.acog.org.*

American Physical Therapy Association. 1-800-999-APTA. Physical Therapy for the pelvic floor- Select Women's Health. *www.APTA.org.*

The Business of Being Born. Great information for all women planning to have a baby. *www.thebusinessofbeingborn.com.*

Dilator Sets. Available on this site. *www.vaginismus.com.*

Doulas of North America. It is our philosophy that all women should have a doula for prenatal and postpartum care. *www.dona.org/*

Endometriosis Association. *www.endometriosisassn.org.*

Health Organization for Pudendal Education. *www.PudendalHope.info*

Herbal and Flower Products. For herbal and flower remedies *www.mountainrose-herbs.com.*

Holly Herman & Kathe Wallace. Best teachers in pelvic floor rehab. Call to get a recommendation for a pelvic floor rehab specialist. Telephone - 646-355-8777. *http://hermanwallace.com.*

Interstitial Cystitis Network. *www.IC-network.org.*

Interstitial Cystitis Association. *www.IChelp.org.*

International Cesarean Awareness Network. *www.ICAN-online.org.*

International Society for the Study of Vulvovaginal Disease. *www.issvd.org.*

IPPS: The International Pelvic Pain Society. *www.PelvicPain.org.*

Kelly Brogan, MD. Holistic psychiatrist with tons of great information on post-partum depression and a great blog. *www.kellybroganMD.com.*

Midwives Alliance of North America. *www.mana.org.*

My Best Birth. Ricki Lake and Abby Epstein's great resource for women. *www.mybestbirth.com.*

National Fibromyalgia Association. *www.fmaware.org.*

NVA: National Vulvodynia Association. *www.NVA.org.*

Penny Simpkin. The original pioneer physical therapist for childbirth education and labor support. *www.PennySimpkin.com*

Pudendal Neuralgia Association, Inc. *www.pudendalassociation.org/*

Vulvodynia Online Resource. *www.vulvodynia.com.*

Young Living Essential Oils:

www.youngliving.com/en_US/. For medical/therapeutic grade essential oils, shop at Young Living. This is the brand I trust the most. Please use my subscriber number ID #1422496 to get a wholesale membership. There is a small membership enrollment fee to buy oils at wholesale that ranges from $40 to $275.

GLOSSARY

Abduction (Hip): Movement of hips away from midline.

Alcock's Canal: A structure within the pelvis through which the pudendal nerve, internal pudendal artery and internal pudendal veins travel. This structure is like a canal formed by the obturator internus fascia.

Anemia: A condition in which there is an abnormally low number of red blood cells in the bloodstream, leading to low iron levels.

Annulus Fibrosus: The outer ring of the intervertebral disc made of tough connective tissue. Supports and encases the jelly-like nucleus pulposus.

Anterior Innominate: A pelvic malalignment in which one innominate is rotated anteriorly, or forward, relative to the opposite side.

Anterior Superior Iliac Spine (ASIS): A bony projection on the front of the ilium that serves as an important anatomical landmark.

Biofeedback: Biofeedback training is a nonmedical treatment that helps people improve their health by taking conscious control of their muscles using real-time body signals. Physical therapists use biofeedback to help retrain the pelvic floor muscles.

BMI: Body Mass Index. A formula for determining obesity. An adult with a BMI of 25 to 29.9 is considered overweight, while a BMI of 30 or greater indicates obesity.

Body Mechanics: The way an individual moves his or her body when carrying and lifting objects.

Breech Position: The breech position describes a fetus that is feet-down or buttocks-down prior to birth. A baby in the breech position is often delivered via Cesarean section.

Carpal Tunnel Syndrome (CTS): Inflammation or irritation of the median nerve as it travels through the wrist within the carpal tunnel. Common symptoms of CTS include pain, numbness, tingling, and/or weakness in the thumb, index, and middle fingers.

Centralization: Related to low back pain; a process in which distal pain in the lower extremities moves up toward the low back in a more localized area. A sign of improving condition.

Cervical Cerclage: A surgical procedure in which a stitch is placed in the cervix to prevent premature labor in the presence of a weak or incompetent cervix.

Cervix: The lower end of the uterus that extends into the vagina. The cervix dilates, or expands, during a vaginal birth.

Cesarean Section: Incisions are made through the abdominal muscles and uterus to deliver the baby.

Chakra: Chakras are force centers that pulsate subtle energy. Seven major chakras are believed to exist within the body.

Chronic Pelvic Pain: A pelvic pain condition that persists for longer than three months. It is poorly understood and many times requires a multidisciplinary approach for successful treatment.

Coccyx: This bone is found above the anus and in between the gluteal muscles.

Coccyxdynia or Coccygodynia: Pain in the area of the tailbone and its associated structures.

Connective Tissue Rolling (Skin Rolling): A type of massage that is superficial in nature and can be performed on any part of the body, including but not limited to, the abdomen, thighs, buttocks and lower back.

Daily Voiding Log: A diary that helps you keep track of bowel and bladder habits. This tool allows you to quantify urge, leaking, and eating and drinking habits.

Diastasis Recti Abdominis: Separation of rectus abdominis muscles away from the midline that occurs during pregnancy and/or with improper exercise technique and poor body mechanics.

Electrodes: Sensors/pads that can be placed on the body to transmit electrical stimulation with a TENS unit.

Episiotomy: An episiotomy is a surgical incision made at the perineum to enlarge the vagina. This incision can be midline or medial-lateral. It is a common cause of sexual pain and can cause scar tissue in the perineum.

Fascia: A complex web-like system of soft connective tissue that surrounds your organs, muscles, nerves, blood vessels, and other visceral structures and holds your body together. Fascia helps maintain structural integrity, provides support and protection, and acts as a shock absorber.

Fetal Growth Restriction: A condition in which the fetal weight is found to be in the fifth percentile or lower for gestational age.

Gestational Diabetes: A form of glucose intolerance that occurs during pregnancy.

Gluteus Medius: This is a gluteal muscle that is under the gluteus maximus and can be found to the outside of the butt cheek near the top of the hip bone. This muscle can refer pain to perineum, labia, hip, posterior thigh and sit bone. It can also refer sciatica-like symptoms.

Greater Trochanter of the Femur: This is not a muscle but a very important area that tends to have trigger points and can be a big source of pelvic and hip pain. Many of the posterior hip muscles insert into this bone and it is necessary to reduce or eliminate pain in this area.

Hamstrings: The muscles of the back of the thigh that bend the knee and extend the hip.

Herniated Disc: Extrusion or protrusion of the jelly-like material between bones of the spine; can occur in different degrees and compress surrounding nerves. The inner nucleus pulposus bulge through the tough annulus fibrosus outer ring.

Hip Flexor Muscles: The muscles of the front of the hip that bring the thigh to the trunk.

Homeostasis: A state of balance in the internal environment of the body.

Hypermobility: A condition of excessive flexibility of the joints, allowing them to be bent or moved beyond their normal range of motion.

Hypertension: A condition of abnormally elevated blood pressure.

Hyperthyroidism: A condition of excessive production of thyroid hormones.

Iliac Crest: Prominent bones located at the level of the navel, felt with hands at the waist. The most superior aspect of the innominate bones.

Iliac Crest Line: This is not a muscle but an area where many muscles live. It is the top of hip crest.

Incompetent Cervix: When the cervix dilates before a baby is ready to be born.

Incontinence: Any involuntary leakage or loss of urine.

Innominates: The two bones that form the sides of the pelvis. The innominates are made up of three fused segments: the ilium, ischium and pubis.

Intervertebral Disc: Donut-like structure found between each vertebra of the spine in the cervical, thoracic, and lumbar regions. It functions as a shock absorber and cushions the spine during activities of daily living. Comprised of a hard outer ring (annulus fibrosus) and jelly-filled inner substance (nucleus pulposus).

Intra-Abdominal Pressure: Pressure within the abdominal cavity.

Intrauterine Constraint: A restriction that prevents normal fetal movement. Intrauterine constraint may be affected by pelvic alignment and may lead to breech positioning.

Intrauterine Growth Restriction: A condition in which the growing fetus is found to be at or below the tenth weight percentile for his or her age (in weeks).

Isometric Contraction: A type of muscle contraction in which the muscle contracts but does not shorten or change length.

Jackknifing: The act of sitting up straight out of bed; similar to doing a sit-up or crunch.

"Just in Case" (JIC) Urination: This occurs when one urinates out of habit instead of waiting for a proper bladder signal or urinating when the bladder is full. JIC urination is dysfunctional and needs to be eliminated to properly retrain the bladder back to health.

Kegel: An exercise named after Dr. Arnold Kegel that consists of contracting and relaxing the pelvic floor muscles.

L1-L5: L1 through L5 represent the five lumbar spinal vertebrae. The lumbar vertebrae are found between the thoracic and sacral vertebrae in the spinal column. Many times, women with pelvic pain will have some kind of associated dysfunction with L5 and the lumbar spine.

Labia Majora: The outer labia, or outer lips, of the vulva.

Levator Ani Muscles: The muscles that make up the pelvic floor.

Levator Ani Syndrome: Consists of pain, pressure, discomfort or deep dull ache in the vagina and rectum, including the sacrum and coccyx. Levator ani syndrome can also cause burning or radiating pain into the thighs and buttocks. Pain with sitting and defecation are common complaints. Many times the pelvic floor muscles are in spasms and have multiple trigger points in them.

Ligaments: Ligaments are structures that hold bones together and prevent excessive movement of the joint.

Lithotomy: Common position for childbirth and gynecologic/pelvic exam; lying flat on back, with feet above or level with hips.

Lumbar Lordosis: The natural curvature of the lower spine in a slightly arched posture. Lumbar lordosis can become excessive during pregnancy, also known as the "sway back" posture.

Lumbar Shift: A compensation seen with low back pain in which the upper body shifts away from the lower body in order to take pressure off of a painful segment in the low back.

Lumbar Spine: The segment of the human spine above the pelvis and below the ribs that is involved in low back pain. There are five vertebrae, or bones, in the lumbar spine.

Lymphedema: Fluid retention and swelling caused by a buildup of lymph fluid due to a blockage in the lymphatic system.

Muscle energy technique (MET): MET is an osteopathic technique that involves gentle muscle contraction performed against gentle resistance in a specific direction.

Myofascial Release: This is a connective tissue hands-on therapy for the treatment of muscle pain and immobility.

Neutral Spine (NS): Neutral spine is the natural position of the spine when all the parts of the spine—cervical, thoracic and lumbar—are in excellent alignment.

Nucleus Pulposus: Jelly-like center of the intervertebral disc, made mostly of water, which acts as the cushioning support of the spine.

Obturator Internus Muscle: The obturator internus muscle is found within the pelvis and within the hip-joint. This muscle helps to externally rotate the leg, extend the thigh and abduct the flexed thigh. It also helps to stabilize femoral head in the acetabulum. This muscle can cause sexual pain, hip pain and/or a deep ache in the pelvis. The obturator internus can refer pain to anywhere within the pelvic girdle. This muscle can be accessed through the vagina and rectum and can frequently have spasms and trigger points causing sexual and pelvic pain.

Osteopathic: Osteopathic techniques use the hands, rather than machinery, to diagnose, treat and prevent injury.

Pelvic Floor: A complex set of muscles, nerves and connective tissue that form the cradle or basket of your being.

Pelvic Floor Muscle Dysfunction: Abnormal or impaired function of the pelvic floor muscles.

Pelvic Floor Muscle Hypertonicity: Muscular hypertonicity is a disorder in which muscles continually receive a message to tighten and to contract. This causes excessive stiffness or tightness and interferes with their normal function.

Pelvic Floor Muscle Incoordination: A lack of normal and harmonious muscle action in the pelvic floor muscles.

Pelvic Floor Muscle Spasm: Involuntary contraction of a pelvic floor muscle.

Pelvic Floor Muscles: The pelvic floor muscles consist of three layers of muscle that support your pelvis, control urination and defecation and allow for optimal sexual function.

Pelvic Girdle: The pelvic girdle is the bony ring that makes up the human pelvis. The pelvic girdle consists of two innominates and one sacrum.

Pelvic Release: A lengthening release of the pelvic floor muscles that can be performed with either inhalation or exhalation.

Perineal Body: The central area between the rectum and the vagina in the perineum. It is also the area where most of the pelvic floor muscles are attached.

Perineal Tearing: Tears to the perineum (the area between the genitalia and anus) that can cause damage to the anal sphincter causing fecal incontinence, urgency, pain during intercourse or other problems.

Perineal Tears in Degrees: Tears are rated from 1st to 4th Degree. 1st Degree is tearing of the vaginal mucosa skin at or around the perineal body. 2nd Degree is tearing vaginal mucosa and submucosa through the pelvic floor muscles. 3rd Degree is tearing of the 1st and 2nd Degree tissues and the external sphincter. 4th Degree is all of the above levels of tearing plus the internal sphincter and the lining of the rectum.

Perineum: The diamond-shaped area between the legs that houses muscles and rectum, and in females, includes the vagina. This can also refer to both the superficial or deep structures in this region.

Peripheralization: Related to low back pain; a process by which pain in the low back spreads or radiates into the lower extremities. A sign of worsening condition.

Piriformis Syndrome: A disorder that occurs when the sciatic nerve is compressed, pinched or irritated by the piriformis muscle. This compression can cause pain, tingling and numbness in the buttocks and along the sciatic nerve path.

Placenta Abruption: A condition in which the placenta separates from the uterus before the baby is ready to be delivered. Placental abruption is a medical emergency. Any vaginal bleeding during pregnancy requires immediate medical attention.

Placenta Previa: A condition in which the placenta grows in the lowest part of the uterus, covering the opening to the cervix. Although common in the early stages of pregnancy, placenta previa later in the pregnancy may necessitate that a woman stop exercising and is often cause for a Cesarean section.

Posterior Innominate: A pelvic malalignment in which one innominate is rotated posteriorly, or backward, relative to the opposite side.

Posterior Superior Iliac Spine (PSIS): Bony prominence on each hip bone palpable where the "dimples" in the lower back can be found on many men and women.

Preeclampsia: A condition of hypertension occurring in pregnancy, typically accompanied by swelling and excessive amounts of protein in urine.

P.R.E.S.S. Prenatal Yoga Series: Renew PT Prenatal Yoga Program. P.R.E.S.S. stands for Pelvic Relaxation and Elongation of Structural Sytems, and focuses on rehabilitation of the pelvic floor while promoting flexibility, strength, and balance.

Preterm Labor: Labor that occurs before the thirty-seventh week of pregnancy.

Prolapse: An organ moves down into and protrudes through the vaginal canal or anal opening, resulting in the sensation of pressure or visible protrusion. The uterus, rectum, bladder or urethra can prolapse into the vagina and cause pelvic floor muscle weakness.

Psoas Muscle: This is deep muscle that cannot be seen from the outside of the body. It comes from lumbar spine and inserts into the top of the leg bone. This muscle can be a source of pelvic pain and many times has trigger points in it that refer pain to the hip, low back and vulvar-vaginal area.

Pubic Bone: This bone forms the anterior aspect of the pelvis and hip bones.

Pubic Symphysis: Cartilaginous joint located between two pubic bones, connects the two pelvis bones.

Pudendal Nerve: This nerve arises from the ventral rami of nerve roots S2 to S4 and from the pudendal nerve trunk. The pudendal nerve is a mix nerve with sensory, motor and autonomic fibers. It has three terminal branches that include dorsal nerve of the clitoris, perineal branch and inferior rectal branch. The pudendal nerve is the main nerve of the perineum and supplies the PFMs, vagina, urethra, skin of labia, external anal sphincter, urethral sphincter, anal canal, anal skin, clitoris and sensory to the lower vagina. Sometimes this nerve can be injured in childbirth.

Pudendal Nerve Neuralgia (PNN): A shooting, stabbing and knife-like pain that can occur anywhere in the distribution of the pudendal nerve. Some women experience this kind of condition after childbirth.

Quadratus Lumborum: This muscle can be found posterior in between the lower ribs and the top of the hip bone but lateral to the paraspinal muscles. Once you are in this area you have to press in toward the spine to find the trigger point. This muscle can be a big pelvic pain generator and must be addressed.

Rectus Abdominis: This is the six-pack abdominal muscle; it runs from below the breast bone to the pubic bone. There are two sides, one to the right of the belly button and one to the left that are connective via the linea alba. A separation of this muscle at the linea alba is called diastasis recti.

Relaxin: A hormone that facilitates birth by causing relaxation of the pelvic ligaments. Relaxin levels peak during the first trimester and again at delivery.

Reverse Kegel: This exercise is an elongation and relaxation exercise for the PFMs.

Round Ligament: Ligament that connects the uterus to the groin, often stretched in pregnancy and a common site of pain.

Round Ligament Pain: A sharp, stabbing pain that occurs due to a sudden tightening of a ligament that travels from the uterus to the labia majora.

Rupture of Membranes: Rupture of amniotic sac, commonly referred to as "water breaking" that occurs before the baby is delivered.

S2-S5: S2 through S5 are vertebrae of the sacral spine. The sacral spine is below the lumbar spine and is located at the base of the spine.

Sacral Torsion: A sacral torsion is a rotation of the sacrum that disrupts the normal mechanics of the SI joint.

Sacroiliac (SI) Joint: The joint formed in the back of the pelvis by the sacrum and innominates. This joint is often a source of pain during pregnancy due to misalignment, hypermobility and muscle weakness.

Sacrum: The sacrum is a triangular-shaped bone that forms the back of the pelvis; it is inserted like a wedge between the two hip bones. Its upper edge connects to the last lumbar vertebra, and its bottom connects with the coccyx (tailbone). The sacral nerves exit through small holes in the sacrum.

Scar: A scar is part of the natural healing process of wound repair in the skin and other tissues of the body.

Sciatic: Relating to the nerve roots that come from the spinal cord, forming a bundle of nerves that travel down the legs, passing beneath the muscles, where they can become compressed and cause pain.

Sciatica: Irritation to the sciatic nerve in the low back or buttock region causing pain, numbness, and/or tingling into the lower extremities.

Shotgun Correction: The shotgun correction is a pelvic MET that aligns the joint of the pubic symphysis.

Sit Bones: Also called ischial tuberosity, sit bones are the bones that we sit on. These bones have surrounding fascia that are intimately connected with the gluteal and hip muscles. Many times women suffering from pelvic pain experience pain at these bones. The gluteal muscles, adductor muscles, PFMs and PNN can refer pain to the sit bones. An exhaustive investigation is required to find out the exact cause of sit bone pain.

Skin Rolling: Also know as connective tissue rolling, this is a type of massage used for releasing and clearing barriers, and fascial restrictions and trigger points in muscles.

Stress Incontinence: Urinary leakage that occurs as a result of pressure on the bladder with changing positions, coughing, laughing, sneezing, lifting or exercise.

Supine Hypotension: A drop in blood pressure that can occur when a pregnant woman is lying on her back.

Symphysis Pubis Dysfunction: A painful condition that is caused by excessive movement in the pubic symphysis joint.

Tendinous Arch of the Levator Ani: A thickened portion of the obturator fascia where some of the levator ani muscles originate. This fascia can be painful to the touch. Let an experienced PT show you how to correctly release this fascia.

TENS (Transcutaneous Electrical Nerve Stimulation) Unit: A unit used to deliver electrical stimulation to the skin for pain relief.

Tension Release Breathing (TRB): A breathing technique—coined by author Isa Herrera—using mind/body connection to release pain and tension of a painful muscle. The individual inhales into the painful body part while thinking about collecting her pain as she inhales. Then the individual exhales and visualizes the pain leaving her body. This type of breathing should be performed for five breaths.

Thorax: Central region of the body which is partially encased by the rib cage and contains many vital organs such as the heart and lungs.

Transverse Abdominis: The innermost, deepest abdominal muscle that acts like a "corset" and provides significant stability to the trunk when activated appropriately.

Transversus Abdominis Muscle: This is the deepest abdominal muscle and it has an intimate relationship with the PFMs.

"Tucked Tush" Posture: Decreased lumbar lordosis, or flattened low back, caused by shortening of the gluteal muscles and shift in center of gravity during pregnancy.

Type 1 Diabetes: Common in children and younger individuals; a condition in which the body does not produce insulin, resulting in increased blood glucose levels.

Urge Incontinence: Urinary leakage that occurs following a sudden, intense urge to urinate.

Urgency or Frequency of Urination: Frequent urination (urinating at intervals less than three to four hours, or more than eight voids per day) or urgency of urination without an increase in the total urine held in the bladder. This condition may result from infections, a small bladder capacity, other structural abnormalities, from food irritants, or trigger points.

Uterosacral Ligaments: Ligaments that connect the uterus to the sacrum. When the sacrum is not in proper alignment, these ligaments may affect the position of the uterus.

Valsalva Maneuver: A forced exhalation where breath is held and air does not leave the body, resulting in increased pressure in the abdominal cavity.

Varicosity: Swollen, painful veins.

Vertebrae: The bones that form the spinal column.

Vertex Position: The vertex position describes a fetus that is head-down prior to birth.

Vulvodynia, Provoked: A type of vulvodynia that occurs with direct contact with the vulva.

Vulvodynia, Unprovoked: A type of vulvodynia that causes vulvar pain, burning, and discomfort without direct contact to the vulvar area.

Young Living Oils: An online company that sells therapeutic grade essentials oils. To buy oils from this company you need to have a subscriber number. Use mine — #1422496 — to register. To get the best prices, register as a wholesaler.

BIBLIOGRAPHY

Albers LL, Border N. (2007). Minimizing Genital Tract Trauma and Related Pain Following Spontaneous Vaginal Birth. *J Midwife and Women's Health*. 2007; 52(3):246-253.

Al-Khodairy AW, Bovay P, Gobelet C. (2006). Sciatica in the female patient: anatomical considerations, aetiology and review of the literature. *Eur Spine J*. 2007 Jun; 16(6):721-31. Epub Apr 19. PubMed PMID: 16622708; PubMed Central PMCID: PMC2200714.

American Pregnancy Association. Water Birth. Retrieved March 17, 2014 from http://americanpregnancy.org/labornbirth/waterbirth.html.

Aromaceuticals. Adverse Reactions to Peppermint Oil. Retrieved June 20, 2014 from http://www.aromaceuticals.com/blog/adverse-reactions-to-peppermint-oil.

Ayanniyi O, Sanya AO, Ogunlade SO, & Oni-Orisan MO. (2006). Prevalence and pattern of back pain among pregnant women attending ante-natal clinics in selected healthcare facilities. *African Journal of Biomedical Research*, 9, 149-156.

Baby Centre. TENS. Retrieved March 9, 2014 from http://www.babycentre.co.uk/a542581/tens.

Barakat R, Pelaez M, Lopez C, Montejo R, Coteron J. (2012). Exercise during pregnancy reduces the rate of cesarean and instrumental deliveries: results of a randomized controlled trial. *J Matern Fetal Neonatal Med*. 2012 Nov;25(11):2372-6. doi: 10.3109/14767058.2012.696165. Epub 2012 Jun 22.

Barakat R, Pelaez M, Lopez C, Lucia A, Ruiz JR. (2013). Exercise during pregnancy and gestational diabetes-related adverse effects: A randomised controlled trial. *Br J Sports Med* doi:10.1136/bjsports-2012-091788.

Birthing Naturally. Birth Plan Options for Pushing. Retrieved April 14, 2014 from http://www.birthingnaturally.net/birthplan/options/push.html.

The Birth Teacher. Ways to Push During Labor. Retrieved April 14, 2014 from http://thebirthteacher.blogspot.com/2009/12/ways-to-push-during-labor.html.

Buckle, J. (2003). *Clinical Aromatherapy.* Philadelphia: Elsevier Science.

Carr, CA. (2003). Use of a maternity support binder for relief of pregnancy-related back pain. *J Obstet Gynecol Neonatal Nurs*, 32(4), 495-502. Retrieved from http://www.ncbi.nlm.nih.gov/m/pubmed/12903699/?i=4&from=/19490291/related.

Carroll D, & Tramer M. (1997). Transcutaneous electrical nerve stimulation in labour pain: a systematic review. *Br J Obstet Gynaecol*, 104, 69-75.

Cohen SP, Chen Y, Neufeld NJ. (2013). Sacroiliac joint pain: a comprehensive review of epidemiology, diagnosis and treatment. *Expert Rev Neurother.* Jan; 13(1):99-116. doi: 10.1586/ern.12.148. Review. PubMed PMID: 23253394.

Conrad KP. (2011). Maternal vasodilation in pregnancy: the emerging role of relaxin. *Am. J. Physiol. Regul. Integr. Comp. Physiol.* (August 2011). 301 (2): R267–75. doi:10.1152/ajpregu.00156.2011. PMC 3154715. PMID: 21613576.

da Silva FM, de Oliveira, SM, Bick D, Osava R, Tuesta E, & Riesco ML. (2012). Risk factors for birth-related perineal trauma: a cross sectional study in a birth centre. *J Clin Nurs,* 21(15-16), 2209-18.

Depledge J, McNair P, Keal-Smith, C, & Williams M. (2005). Management of symphysis pubis dysfunction during pregnancy using exercise and pelvic support belts. *Phys Ther, 85*: 1290-1300. Retrieved from http://m.ptjournal.apta.org/content/85/12/1290.full.pdf.

England, Allison. (2000). *Aromatherapy and Massage for Mother and Child.* Vermont: Healing Arts Press.

Exercise during pregnancy and the postpartum period. (2002). ACOG Committee Opinion No. 267. American College of Obstetricians and Gynecologists. *Obstet Gynecol* 2002; 99:171–173.

Fast A, Shapiro D, Ducommun EJ, Friedmann LW, Bouklas T, Floman Y. (1987). Low back pain in pregnancy. *Spine;* 12:368–371.

Greenman PE. (2003). *Principles of Manual Medicine.* 3rd ed. Baltimore, MD: Williams & Wilkins.

Gutke A, Lundberg M, Östgaard HC, Öberg B. (2011). Impact of postpartum lumbopelvic pain on disability, pain intensity, health-related quality of life, activity level, kinesiophobia, and depressive symptoms. *Eur Spine J.* Mar; 20(3):440-8. doi: 10.1007/s00586-010-1487-6. Epub 2010 Jul 1. PubMed PMID: 20593205; PubMed Central PMCID: PMC3048223.

Gutke A, Ostgaard HC, Oberg B. (2006). Pelvic girdle pain and lumbar pain in pregnancy: a cohort study of the consequences in terms of health and functioning. *Spine* 31(5), 149-155.

Hastings-Tolsma M, Vincent D, Emeis C, & Francisco T. (2007). Getting through birth in one piece: protecting the perineum. *MCN Am J Matern Child Nurs, 32(3),* 158-164.

Herrera, Isa. (2014). *Ending Female Pain, Expanded 2nd Edition. A Woman's Manual.* New York, NY: Duplex Publishing, Inc.

Herrera, Isa. (2003). *The Pregnant Couple's Guide to Working Out Together.* Hoboken, NJ: John Wiley & Sons, Inc.

Ho SS, Yu WW, Lao TT, Chow, DH, Chung JW, & Li Y. (2009). Effectiveness of maternity support belts in reducing low back pain during pregnancy: a review. *J Clin Nurs,* 18 (11), 1523-32. doi: 10.1111/j.1365-2702.2008.02749.x.

Howell ER. (2012). Pregnancy-related symphysis pubis dysfunction management and postpartum rehabilitation: two case reports. *J Can Chiropr Assoc,* 56(2), 102-111. Retrieved from http://www.ncbi.nlm.nih.gov/pmc/articles/PMC3364059/.

Kaplan B, Rabinerson D, Lurie S, Bar J, Kreiser U, & Neri A. (1998). A transcutaneous electrical nerve stimulation (TENS) for adjuvant pain-relief during labor and delivery. *Int J Gynaecol Obstet,* 60, 251-255.

Keenan D, Simonsen L, & McCrain D. (1985). Transcutaneous electrical nerve stimulation for pain control during labor and delivery: a case report. *Phys Ther,* 65(9), 1363-1364.

Keskin EA, Onur O, Keskin HL, Gumus II, Kafali H, & Turhan N. (2012). Transcutaneuous electrical nerve stimulation improves low back pain during pregnancy. *Gynecol Obstet Intest,* 74 (1), 76-83.

Kordi R, Abolhasani M, Rostami M, Hantoushzdeh S, Mansournia MA, & Vasheghani-Farahani F. (2013). Comparison between the effect of lumbopelvic belt and home based pelvic stabilizing exercise on pregnant women with pelvic girdle pain; a randomized control trial. *J Back Musculoskelet Rehabil,* 26(2), 133-9. doi: 10.3233/BMR-2012-00357.

Lieberman, Adrienne B. (1992). *Easing Labor Pain: The Complete Guide to a More Comfortable and Rewarding Birth.* Boston, MA: The Harvard Common Press.

Lockstadt H. Back pain during pregnancy. Retrieved Nov 13, 2012 from http://www.spineuniverse.com/conditions/back-pain/back-pain-during-pregnancy.

Lowe, N. (2003). The nature of labor pain. *Am J Obstet Gynecol*, 86, 16-24.

Lyon, Erica. (2007). *The Big Book of Birth*. New York, NY: The Penguin Group.

Maigne JY, Rusakiewicz F, & Diouf M. (2012). Postpartum coccydynia: a case series study of 57 women. *European Journal of Physical and Rehabilitation Medicine*, 48(3), 387-92.

Mogren IM, Pohjanen AI. (2005). Low back pain and pelvic pain during pregnancy: prevalence and risk factors. *Spine*. 2005 Apr 15;30(8):983-91. PMID: 15834344.

Mojay, Gabriel. (1997). *Aromatherapy for Healing the Spirit: Restoring Emotional and Mental Balance with Essential Oils*. Rochester, Vermont: Healing Arts Press.

National Association for Holistic Aromatherapy. Exploring Aromatherapy: Safety Information. http://www.naha.org/explore-aromatherapy/safety.

Neumann DA. (2002). *Kinesiology of the Musculoskelatal System: Foundations for Physical Rehabilitation*. St. Louis, MO: Mosby.

NHS Choices. Pain Relief in Labor. Retrieved March 9, 2014 from http://www.nhs.uk/conditions/pregnancy-and-baby/pages/pain-relief-labour.aspx#close.

Nilsson-Wikmar L, Holm K, Oijerstedt R, & Harms-Ringdahl K. (2005). Effect of three different physical therapy treatments on pain and activity in pregnant women with pelvic girdle pain: a randomized clinical trial with 3, 6, and 12 months follow-up postpartum. *Spine, 30(8)*, 850-6. Retrieved from http://www.ncbi.nlm.nih.gov/m/pubmed/15834325/.

NYU Langone Medical Center. Aromatherapy. Retrieved June 20, 2014 from http://www.med.nyu.edu/content?ChunkIID=37427.

Okanishi N, Kito N, Akiyama M, Yamamoto M. (2012). Spinal curvature and characteristics of postural change in pregnant women. *Acta Obstet Gynecol Scand*.

2012 Jul;91(7):856-61. doi: 10.1111/j.1600-0412.2012.01400.x. PubMed PMID: 22429046.

Ostgaard HC, Andersson GB, Karlsson K. (1991). Prevalence of back pain in pregnancy. *Spine* 16(5), 549-552.

Pennick VE, Young G. (2007). Interventions for preventing and treating pelvic and back pain in pregnancy. *Cochrane Database Syst Rev.* 2007; (2):CD001139.

Pistolese, Richard A. (2002). The Webster Technique: a chiropractic technique with obstetric implications. *Journal of manipulative and physiological therapeutics* 25.6: E1-E9.

Preece SJ, Willan P, Nester CJ, et al. (2008). Variation in pelvic morphology may prevent the identification of anterior pelvic tilt. *J Man Manip Ther.* 16(2):113-117. PMCID: PMC2565125.

Prins M, Boxem J, Lucas C, Hutton E. (2011). Effect of spontaneous pushing versus Valsalva pushing in the second stage of labour on mother and fetus: a systematic review of randomised trials. *BJOG.* 2011 May;118(6):662-70. doi: 10.1111/j.1471-0528.2011.02910.x. Epub 2011 Mar 10. Review. PubMed PMID: 21392242.

Roberts J, Hanson L. (2007). Best practices in second stage labor care: maternal bearing down and positioning. *J Midwifery Women's Health.* 2007 May-Jun;52(3):238-45. Review. PubMed PMID: 17467590.

Saint Louis, Catherine. Surge in Narcotic Prescriptions for Pregnant Women. *New York Times.* Retrieved April 13, 2014 from http://www.nytimes.com/2014/04/15/science/surge-in-prescriptions-for-opioid-painkillers-for-pregnant-women.html?module=Search&mabReward=relbias%3Ar&_r=0.-.

Shorten A, Donsante, J, & Shorten B. (2002). Birth position, accoucheur, and perineal outcomes: informing women about choices for vaginal birth. *Birth*, 29(1), 18-27.

Simkin, Penny. (2013). *The Birth Partner: A Complete Guide to Childbirth for Dads, Doulas and All Other Labor Companions.* Boston, MA: The Harvard Common Press.

Simkin P, Bolding A. (2004). Update on nonpharmacologic approaches to relieve labor pain and prevent suffering. *J Midwifery Women's Health,* 49(6), 489-504.

Skaggs CD, Prather H, Gross G, George JW, Thompson P.A., Nelson D.M. (2007). Back and pelvic pain in an underserved United States pregnant population: a preliminary descriptive survey. *J Manipulative Physiol Ther.* 30(2):130–134.

Stær-Jensen J, Siafarikas F, Hilde G, Bø K, Engh ME. (2013). Ultrasonographic evaluation of pelvic organ support during pregnancy. *Obstet Gynecol.* 2013 Aug;122 (2 Pt1):329-36. doi: 10.1097/AOG.0b013e318299f62c. PubMed PMID: 23969802.

Tisserand, R, and Balacs, T. (1995). *Essential Oil Safety.* New York: Churchill Livingstone.

Van der Spank JT, Cambier DC, De Paepe HM, Danneels LA, Witvrouw EE, & Beerens L. (2000). Pain relief in labour by transcutaneous electrical nerve stimulation (TENS). *Arch Gynecol Obstet,* 264(3), 131-136.

Vladutiu CJ, Evenson KR, Marshall SW. (2010). Physical activity and injuries during pregnancy. *J Phys Act Health.* 2010 Nov;7(6):761-9. PMID: 21088307.

Wang S, Dezinno P, Maranets I, Berman MR, Caldwell-Andrews AA, & Kain ZN. (2004). Low back pain during pregnancy: Prevalence, risk factors, and outcomes. *Obstetrics & Gynecology,* 104(1), 65-70. doi: 10.1097/01. AOG.0000129403.54061.0e.

Wu WH, Meijer OG, Uegaki K, Mens JM, van Dieën JH, Wuisman PI, Ostgaard HC. (2004). Pregnancy-related pelvic girdle pain (PPP), I: Terminology, clinical presentation, and prevalence. *Eur Spine J.* Nov; 13(7):575-89. Epub 2004 Aug 27. Review. PubMed PMID: 15338362; PubMed Central PMCID: PMC3476662.

Yildirim G, Beji NK. (2008). Effects of pushing techniques in birth on mother and fetus: a randomized study. *Birth*. 2008 Mar;35(1):25-30. doi: 10.1111/j.1523-536X.2007.00208.x. PubMed PMID: 18307484.

Young, Gary. (2003). *Essential Oils Integrative Medical Guide;* 2nd Edition. Orem, UT: Life Science Publishing.

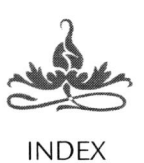

INDEX